HOMEOPATHIC SELF-CARE

THE QUICK & EASY GUIDE FOR THE WHOLE FAMILY

Robert Ullman, N.D.
Judyth Reichenberg-Ullman, N.D.

PUSTAK MAHAL®
Delhi • Bangalore • Mumbai • Patna • Hyderabad

Publishers
Pustak Mahal®, Delhi

J-3/16 , Daryaganj, New Delhi-110002
☎ 23276539, 23272783, 23272784 • *Fax:* 011-23260518
E-mail: info@pustakmahal.com • *Website:* www.pustakmahal.com

Sales Centre

- 10-B, Netaji Subhash Marg, Daryaganj, New Delhi-110002
☎ 23268292, 23268293, 23279900 • *Fax:* 011-23280567
E-mail: rapidexdelhi@indiatimes.com

- **Hind Pustak Bhawan**
6686, Khari Baoli, Delhi-110006
☎ 23944314, 23911979

Branches

Bengaluru: ☎ 080-22234025 • *Telefax:* 080-22240209
E-mail: pustak@airtelmail.in • pustak@sancharnet.in

Mumbai: ☎ 022-22010941, 022-22053387
E-mail: rapidex@bom5.vsnl.net.in

Patna: ☎ 0612-3294193 • *Telefax:* 0612-2302719
E-mail: rapidexptn@rediffmail.com

Hyderabad: *Telefax:* 040-24737290
E-mail: pustakmahalhyd@yahoo.co.in

Reprinted from: **'Homeopathic Self-Care'**

Published by: **Prima Publishing**

P.O. Box 1260BK, Rocklin, CA 95677

ISBN 978-81-223-0112-0

We dedicate this book to Dr. John Bastyr who, during his eighty-three years of compassionate, selfless service as a naturopathic physician, served as a model healer for us and for so many others, past, present, and future. He taught us the importance of combining never-ending study with tireless dedication to serving humanity.

May many follow in Dr. Bastyr's footsteps.

Contents

PART **2**

Medical Conditions You Can Treat Yourself

PART 3
Materia Medica

Foreword

There is a powerful popular movement abroad in the land, a movement for a new, more effective, less toxic, more humane, more people-centered kind of health care. One of its rallying cries is "homeopathy."

Homeopaths tell us that tiny doses of substances that in larger doses can produce symptoms, can be used to alleviate those symptoms, that *like* cures *like*. Though this concept pervades the thinking and practice of most of the world's great healing traditions, including our own Greek Hippocratic medicine, it is foreign to most of us. It is qualitative rather than quantitative. It seems "soft" to many, mystical, or, in the words of its critics, even bizarre.

Yet homeopathy works. There are now close to 150 controlled scientific studies on homeopathy, many of which document what Robert Ullman and Judyth Reichenberg-Ullman tell us in this book: homeopathic remedies *are* effective for common conditions such as asthma, arthritis, and allergies.

We in the United States once believed that homeopathy worked. At the turn of the century between fifteen and twenty percent of all M.D.s were homeopaths. Then, intimidated by orthodox medical pressure, homeopathy faded from the American healthcare scene. Now, it is making a powerful comeback. And the reasons are simple. It often works. It's inexpensive. Its principles are clear and its practice pleasing. And, it has very few side effects.

In recent years, there have been a number of books about homeopathy. Some are scholarly and technical. Fortunately, many are popular in the best sense of the word. Homeopathy is a system of medicine that lends itself to self care. One can observe one's own or a family member's symptoms without technology and ask simple questions. Are there blisters on the skin, or red bumps? Is the nose running, or just the eyes? Does it hurt more on the right or the left? Is it worse when you get up or go to sleep? One can, based on the answers, prescribe and see the results.

In this book Robert Ullman and Judyth Reichenberg-Ullman, naturopathic physicians, who previously focused on emotional problems, in particular, hyperactivity and attention deficit disorder, give us the guidance we need to successfully treat ourselves with homeopathic remedies. They give us succinct, easily remembered descriptions of commonly used remedies and list "key symptoms" that distinguish one condition from another. They give specific instructions for prescribing homeopathic remedies and how to decide when a remedy is working and what to do if it isn't.

Homeopathic Self-Care is clear, kindly (as I read, I felt as though the authors were at my side, gently helping me to see and think and prescribe), well organized and wonderfully useful. It is a powerful tool for those of us who want to enhance our own health and take back control of our health care and an enormous contribution to the field. I will recommend this book to my patients.

James S. Gordon, M.D., Clinical Professor of Psychiatry and Family Medicine, Georgetown Medical School and author of *Manifesto for a New Medicine: Your Guide to Healing Partnerships and the Wise Use of Alternative Therapies*

Why We Wrote This Book

JUDYTH

I had just moved to Seattle. That damp, bone-chilling first autumn knocked me for a loop. I was hacking and hawking and felt miserable. I tried herbs, vitamins, saunas, and all of the other natural methods that I knew, to no avail. In desperation, I sought the help of a naturopathic doctor who had the reputation of being an effective and compassionate healer. He was Dr. John Bastyr. I felt a warmth and trust the minute I met the kind, elderly gentleman. He reminded me of my father.

As I sat down with Dr. Bastyr, I knew that I had his full attention. He asked me a few questions about my symptoms. "You have bronchitis? A nagging cough that comes from a tickle in your throat? It's much worse when you lie down to go to bed? That's a *Rumex* cough." Short and sweet. Just a few questions, and Dr. Bastyr confidently handed me homeopathic *Rumex* (Yellow dock) to take until I felt better. I took a couple of doses. The tickle in my throat disappeared almost immediately. The cough improved significantly, and my normal energy and enthusiasm returned. I was impressed!

My life took a dramatic turn thanks to Dr. Bastyr. I enjoyed being a psychiatric social worker, but natural healing intrigued me. On the locked psychiatric ward and emergency room where I worked, we used powerful antipsychotic medications that had disturbing side effects. At home I used only natural medicine; I didn't even take aspirin. I began to feel like a hypocrite.

At this time, a naturopathic medical school opened in Seattle, named after Dr. Bastyr. I decided to attend. During my first year at the naturopathic college, I began to read about homeopathy. The philosophy made more sense to me than any other type of healing I had known. I had found my niche and my life's work.

BOB

My introduction to homeopathy was through a local study group of the National Center for Homeopathy. I first encountered the National Center at a health fair in 1975 when I was a graduate student in psychology at Bucknell University. I was fascinated by the "little white pills" and by how quickly and dramatically they were able to help people heal. Being an avid reader, I discovered that the books on homeopathy were fascinating, although in 1975 the reading list was quite short compared with the selection today.

I was introduced to naturopathic medicine that same year and, to my delight, learned that homeopathy was part of the curriculum at the National College of Naturopathic Medicine. I enrolled the following year, and, throughout the four years of naturopathic medical school, I developed a growing interest in homeopathy. Dr. Bastyr greeted our entering class, and I, too, was very impressed by this wise, gentle, humble healer.

I saw homeopathy perform seeming miracles at the school clinic, curing both acute and chronic illnesses—even in the hands of novices. Homeopathy was experiencing its first resurgence in the United States since the 1920s, and I was thrilled to be part of this exciting time. Reading *The Science of Homeopathy* by the Greek homeopath George Vithoulkas and attending conferences where he spoke was a great inspiration. Little did I know at the time that I would some day be teaching for, and be the vice president of, the International Foundation for Homeopathy (IFH), the organization that he founded to promote homeopathy. Taking the IFH Professional Course was a tremendous help to me when I first began my homeopathic practice.

Through fifteen years of practice—a word that aptly describes the learning curve—I have finally become a homeopath. I feel blessed to be able to carry on the two-hundred-year-old tradition of helping people, using the very best that nature has to offer.

JUDYTH AND BOB

Over the past twenty years, we have used homeopathy with ourselves and many thousands of patients, for a wide range of acute and chronic illnesses. We cannot begin to count the number of times we have seen immediate or overnight results from using *Arnica* for bruises, sprains, and strains—nor the times we have relied on *Cantharis* after accidentally touching a hot electric burner, only to find that the pain disappeared instantaneously. We have found the same to be true with our patients. Even people who have a hard time accepting the philosophy of homeopathy are often convinced of its effectiveness after their first experience with using *Arnica* for a smashed finger or a sprained ankle.

A number of books have already been written on the subject of homeopathic self-treatment. Why did we decide to write our own guide? Although some of these books contain accurate and useful information, we believed that we could write a simple, practical, highly informative yet user-friendly guide to self-treatment.

Having treated patients for fifteen years, we have had many opportunities to learn exactly which questions to ask. A busy practice has taught us to make the process of acute prescribing as quick and efficient as possible. We have also learned a great deal from fifteen years of teaching students how to treat themselves and their families. It is extremely important to differentiate between which conditions are appropriate for self-treatment and which are not. Many books on homeopathic self-care do not make this distinction clear. Some are written by authors who have no clinical experience.

But most importantly, we wanted to write a book on self-treatment that would lead to treatment success: a book that a bleary-eyed, half-awake parent could pick up in the middle of the night to help a screaming baby; a book that contains enough information to provide effective self-care for many conditions, but not so many unnecessary details that the self-prescriber would become lost and discouraged; a book that is laid out clearly enough that the best medicine will jump out at the reader.

We hope that we have accomplished all of these goals with this book. We use icons extensively for visual appeal and quick learning. We include those medicines that you are likely to use frequently and a few more uncommon medicines that you may need when nothing else will do. We teach you to ask the questions and make the observations that we have consistently found invaluable in our own prescribing. For those of you who do not yet have a homeopathic medicine kit, we make one available by mail-order that you can use along with our book.

Homeopathic self-care for first-aid conditions is extremely simple to learn and is often quickly and dramatically effective. Learning to self-prescribe for acute illnesses is sometimes easy, and sometimes more complex, depending on the situation. With this book, we simplify the process as much as possible. Homeopathy is a subtle yet powerful medical science and healing art. We hope this book inspires you to help yourself and your family and that the wisdom and benefits of homeopathy will flourish.

We thank all of our teachers of homeopathy for sharing their wisdom and all of our patients for their trust. Most of all, our gratitude goes to Dr. Samuel Hahnemann for developing the brilliant science and art of homeopathy, which has helped so many in their healing. We also give special thanks to Jeff and Gaby Hansen, parents of two beautiful little girls, who worked closely with us to design this book so that a desperate parent can find the one right homeopathic medicine for a screaming toddler in the middle of the night. We are also grateful to Dr. James Gordon for his kind and insightful foreword.

PART 1

WHAT YOU NEED TO KNOW TO SELF-PRESCRIBE

CHAPTER 1

As Easy as One, Two, Three: How to Make the Most of This Book

JENNY NEEDS YOUR HELP

Jenny, your normally cheerful two-year-old, is not herself. It is the first snowfall of the year, and Jenny bounds out of bed as fast as her legs will carry her to build a snowman. She remembers her down jacket and mittens but forgets her wool hat. The air is quite nippy. Jenny is so enthralled with making huge snowballs for her snowman that she doesn't even think about her cold head.

Two hours later, she comes running inside screaming that she has a terrible earache. One of her cheeks is beet red. You take Jenny's temperature and are surprised to find that she has a fever of 102°F. You are astonished at how quickly your daughter went from being perfectly fine to having a high fever and severe ear pain. Your spouse wants to take her to the pediatrician immediately. Is there anything you can do to relieve Jenny's pain naturally?

Homeopathy can help Jenny feel better rapidly and safely. To anyone who knows homeopathy, this is a very clear-cut case. Jenny needs homeopathic *Aconite*. By reading this book and learning how to prescribe for uncomplicated acute ear infections and other minor and acute illnesses, you can help Jenny and others to find an effective, natural, drug-free alternative treatment for their everyday health problems.

QUICK AND EASY HOMEOPATHY

Homeopathy is extremely effective for most first-aid situations and many acute illnesses. The methods you will learn here are designed to help you readily find an effective homeopathic medicine for yourself and others. The methods are easy to learn and quick to apply; they work very well if you carefully follow the principles outlined in this book.

Prescribing homeopathic medicines for yourself and your family can be easy when you follow a step-by-step process. Take time to study the process and learn the steps of *first aid* and *acute prescribing*. Practice on yourself and your willing family members until you know that you can apply the principles in the book to actual situations and help someone get better rapidly and easily. The more you practice prescribing for yourself and those close to you, the better your results will be. With even a little study and practice, you will find that helping Jenny and others like her is often simple and very rewarding. As you go through this book, be sure to use the examples and practice cases to enhance your understanding of the process so that you can use it when you or your loved ones are ill.

An overview of the process follows. The actual steps and procedures will be covered in detail in later chapters.

Look, Listen, and Ask

In order to select homeopathic medicines, you must first understand in exactly what way the person you are treating is sick. Homeopaths call this process *casetaking*. It involves observing and interviewing the sick person, even if it is yourself, until you know all the ways in which the illness is affecting the person and how that condition is different from his normal state. In other words, you are looking for everything about that person that has changed since the acute illness symptoms began to develop. These changes are what make up the *symptom picture* of the illness. You will match this symptom picture to descriptions of various homeopathic medicines so that you can decide which one medicine is appropriate for the person and the illness. Three steps are involved:

1. *Look* carefully at the person who is ill in her environment.
2. *Listen* to what she says to you about her illness.
3. *Ask* the right questions to get the information you need to discover the correct medicine to help her heal.

These steps of "look, listen, and ask" are the "one, two, three" of homeopathic casetaking. For each illness we cover in this book, you will be guided through these steps so that you can collect all the information you need quickly and easily. Once you know what kind of medical condition you are treating, use the Look, Listen, and Ask sections (indicated by the eye, ear, and question mark icons) under each medical condition to guide you in taking the case history.

Analyze the Case and Choose the Medicine

After you have taken the sick person's case, you will need to organize, understand, and analyze the information you have collected. You need to make a list of the symptoms, noting anything about the symptoms that is intense, striking, or unusual. This makes up the symptom picture that you will match with possible homeopathic medicines until you determine which is the best one for the person who is ill.

This three-step process will help you find the correct medicine:

1. *Analyze* the illness and the symptoms you have collected. Understand the specific kind of problem the person you are treating has and what he is experiencing as a result of the illness.
2. *Find* the type of illness that is closest to the person's problem in the list of conditions. Use the casetaking steps and the descriptions of each homeopathic medicine listed under that condition to select the medicine that best matches the individual's symptoms.
3. *Read,* in the *Materia Medica* section of this book (Part 3), about the homeopathic medicine you have chosen to see if it fits the person and the illness as well as you thought. If it doesn't really match well after all, continue to look for another medicine that matches better, and give the person that one.

These are the three steps of homeopathic case analysis that you will use to select the correct medicine. You will be guided through each step of this process in Chapters 6 and 9.

Give the Medicine

Once you have selected the best medicine, give it, then observe whether the person gets better. The proof of a homeopathic medicine's effectiveness is in its catalyzing an observable healing process that definitely improves the person's condition.

The steps in this stage are:

1. Give the medicine.
2. Observe the medicine's effects on the person.
3. Repeat the medicine when needed, or change it if it is not working.

These three steps constitute administering the homeopathic medicine and evaluating the results. We will more fully describe each step in Chapters 7 and 9.

WHAT YOU WILL FIND IN THIS BOOK

It is possible to use this book on several different levels of interest and involvement, depending on your needs. First, we'll introduce you to homeopathy itself—what it is, how it works, and what it can do. We will describe the medicines, show you how to get a homeopathic medicine kit, and tell you how to use the medicines properly. Then we will lead you in depth through a simplified form of the process homeopaths use in prescribing for minor illnesses, including all the steps listed above: taking the case, analyzing the case, and giving the homeopathic medicine.

Some of you, we know, will not take the time to learn the whole process that gives the best results, hoping for a quick-and-easy solution to your problem. You can also find that here if you turn to Part 2: Medical Conditions. There we provide basic information on each medical condition and its symptoms and complications. Charts for each condition list the most useful medicines for treating that problem, their key indicating symptoms, and other symptoms that can help you decide which medicine to give. Complete information on dosage and what to expect from the medicine is also provided for you.

In Part 2 there are also simple pointers for finding the correct homeopathic medicine, drawn from our own experience in treating thousands of patients. If you cannot decide which homeopathic medicine to give someone or to take yourself, or if you want additional healing help, we also provide other naturally oriented self-care suggestions that can help resolve the illness.

For a more in-depth description of each homeopathic medicine, turn to the *Materia Medica* section in Part 3; it can help you decide if the medicine you are considering matches other features of the person who is sick. You can use this section to become familiar with the medicines in your kit so that you will readily recognize them when you need them.

The Appendix, How to Find Out More About Homeopathy, will guide you to books on homeopathy and sources of homeopathic medicines. The Glossary will help you understand the language of homeopathy, which may not yet be familiar to you.

Whether you are a serious student of homeopathy or you just want to feel better, you will find something useful in this book. If you can, take some time to read the introductory material and learn as much as you can about how to prescribe. Otherwise, cut to the chase and quickly find the right medicine for the symptoms at hand. Do what works for you. The rest of the information is here for you when you need it. We want you to get the best results possible and use homeopathy in a way that truly helps you attain the health and healing you desire.

CHAPTER **2**

Homeopathy: Safe, Effective Family Medicine

THE FASCINATING EVOLUTION OF HOMEOPATHY

What exactly is homeopathy? Homeopathy is not a new form of medicine. In fact, it celebrated its two-hundredth birthday in 1996. Homeopathy provides an *alternative* to conventional medicine in that it can be effective in situations where conventional medicine fails. It is also considered *complementary* because it works well with, and adds to the existing benefits of, standard medical treatment. It is one of the most popular forms of alternative or complementary medicine in use today. Homeopathic medicines are derived from natural substances and are given in very small, specially prepared doses to stimulate the body's ability to heal itself mentally, emotionally, and physically.

The concept of *like cures like,* which is the basic principle of homeopathic medicine, means that the same substance that can *cause* a particular set of symptoms in a healthy person can *cure* the same or similar symptoms in a person who is ill. This idea, also called the *law of similars,* dates back over five thousand years to the ancient medical texts of China and India. Hippocrates, in 400 B.C., and Paracelsus, the renowned medieval physician, also referred to this same idea.

Samuel Hahnemann (1755–1843) is the founder of homeopathy. A German physician, chemist, and medical translator, he was discouraged with the harsh, often dangerous, medical methods commonly used in his time. He sought to discover a more gentle and effective type of medicine. Hahnemann expanded the ancient idea of "like cures like" into a complete medical system for the first time. He coined the term *homeopathy*, from the Greek roots for *similar* and *suffering*, to describe the new system that he evolved from the law of similars.[1]

Although many of Hahnemann's contemporaries attempted to discredit his ideas as being radical and contrary to accepted medical theory, homeopathy was such a successful medical innovation that it spread throughout much of Europe and to the United States as well. The growing popularity of homeopathic medicine has continued in Europe to this day. The national healthcare systems of a number of European countries, including the United Kingdom, France, and Norway, utilize homeopathic medicine.

Homeopathy took a more roundabout route, however, in the United States. Initially, homeopathy received considerable recognition for its effectiveness in treating epidemics of life-threatening illness, including cholera, scarlet fever, and yellow fever. By 1900, approximately one in every five medical doctors was a homeopath. More than one hundred homeopathic hospitals, over twenty homeopathic medical schools, and at least one thousand homeopathic pharmacies flourished in the United States at that time.[2]

Political opposition from conventional physicians in the early 1900s, however, led to eventual closing of all of the homeopathic medical schools and nearly led to the demise of homeopathy in the United States. People who managed to discover homeopathy and wanted to learn more had to study on their own or find others to establish homeopathic study groups.

Fortunately, the homeopathic scene has advanced dramatically over the past twenty years. More books and articles have been published about homeopathy worldwide in the last five years than in the preceding fifty. There are more than one thousand medically trained homeopaths now practicing in the United States, including medical doctors, naturopathic physicians, chiropractors, physician's assistants, acupuncturists, dentists, nurses, nurse practitioners, and veterinarians, as well as a growing number of trained but unlicensed homeopathic practitioners who are currently seeking certification.

The tremendous resurgence of interest in homeopathy is being fueled to a large degree by public demand for safer, effective, and natural health care. In 1992, the National Institutes of Health appointed a group of respected health professionals to evaluate the effectiveness of alternative therapies, including homeopathy. This process is beginning to stimulate research on alternative medicine in this country for the first time. These studies have not been published yet, but this was a break-

[1]Robert Ullman and Judyth Reichenberg-Ullman, *The Patient's Guide to Homeopathic Medicine* (Edmonds: Picnic Point Press, 1995), 2.

[2]Dana Ullman, *Discovering Homeopathy: Medicine for the 21st Century* (Berkeley: North Atlantic Books, 1988), 48.

through toward eventual mainstream acceptance of homeopathy and other effective alternative therapies. A survey published in the January 28, 1993, issue of the *New England Journal of Medicine* revealed that more than one-third of Americans were using some form of alternative medicine, including homeopathy. The total number of visits to all categories of alternative practitioners was greater than those to primary care physicians.[3]

WHAT YOU NEED TO KNOW

THE HEALING POWER OF THE VITAL FORCE

The correctly chosen homeopathic medicine sets into motion a process of healing that can continue for days, weeks, or months. How is this possible?

Homeopaths use the term *vital force* to describe the intelligence that animates each and every person. This is a concept that has been recognized universally for thousands of years and called by many different names, including *life force, breath, chi, ki, prana,* and *mana,* depending upon the particular culture or tradition. This vital force is an energy force or a kind of innate wisdom, which is why homeopathy, along with acupuncture, is considered a form of "energy medicine." The *defense mechanism* is that aspect of the vital force which keeps each person in balance. *Symptoms* are the language of the defense mechanism.

Homeopaths spend a great deal of time learning to communicate with the defense mechanism by discovering how to interpret symptoms. Each individual is unique, and each defense mechanism communicates through its own particular set of symptoms. The homeopath's job is to carefully listen to each person to discover what is unique about that individual and his symptoms. While conventional medical doctors try to fit people into diagnostic categories based on the commonality of their symptoms, and select among a limited number of medicines that apply to the category, homeopathic doctors are continually trying to figure out the uniqueness of the individual's symptoms and how they may be matched to a single homeopathic medicine. The individual's particular way of being sick is the disease to be treated, not the common symptoms that are similar to everyone else who would be given the same diagnosis by a conventional doctor.

Take a sore throat, for example. One person will say that her sore throat is worse on the left side, made much worse by swallowing, and made better by drinking cold drinks and will complain of a lump in her throat. A homeopath would call this a *Lachesis* sore throat. Another person will complain that the sore throat hurts more on the right side and feels much better after he swallows warm drinks. This person will feel much better if he takes *Lycopodium.*

[3]David M. Eisenberg, Ronald C. Kessler, Cindy Foster, et al., "Unconventional Medicine in the United States," *New England Journal of Medicine* 328, no. 4 (January 28, 1993):246–52.

Which side the sore throat is on, whether it is worse or better when swallowing, and particular sensations such as a lump in the throat make up the uniqueness of a particular symptom picture, composed of a pattern of specific individual symptoms. One factor that makes a specific symptom unique is what makes that particular symptom feel better or worse. In homeopathy, this is called a *modality*. As in the example above, one sore throat may be relieved by cold drinks and another by warm drinks. This fact, when put together with other factors such as sensation and sidedness, makes up the symptom picture. Different symptom pictures require different homeopathic medicines.

These fine distinctions are essential to the homeopath in order to help heal the person, but would mean nothing to a medical doctor in terms of differentiating between one type of medicine and another. The medical doctor is more interested in which organism is apparently causing the sore throat in order to select an antibiotic to kill it. The homeopath is looking for the substance in nature which can stimulate the person to heal himself, restoring an internal ecological balance which also relieves the sore throat.

HOMEOPATHY TREATS THE WHOLE PERSON AS A UNIQUE INDIVIDUAL

Many forms of healing claim to treat the whole person yet still focus on prescribing different pills or therapies for each part of the body or for each symptom. A homeopath always tries to take into account the person as a whole. Even in the case of an injury or other first-aid situation, the homeopath tries to understand how each individual has her own unique response. One person who is involved in a minor collision will refuse help and say she is just fine. This is an *Arnica* state. Another person, having experienced the identical circumstances, will develop an intense panic reaction. She will experience a racing heart, sweaty palms, and trembling, and will not be able to let go of the fear that she could have died. This is an *Aconite* state. Each person is an individual and reacts to the events and challenges of life in a unique way. For this reason, even those who experience similar life circumstances are likely to need different homeopathic medicines.

HOMEOPATHY TREATS THE PERSON, NOT THE DISEASE

This is one of the most essential and special features of homeopathic medicine. A homeopathic medicine restores balance to the health of each person. Symptoms are the clues to what is out of balance. Homeopathy places the emphasis on what is needed to trigger a renewed state of health for each individual. When the rebalancing occurs, symptoms will automatically improve. However, the converse is not necessarily true. Just because particular symptoms are eliminated, such as with conventional drugs, it does not necessarily mean that the person will experience an overall state of well-being.

Homeopaths seek the medicine that will result in a *fundamental* shift in the person from disease to health. To that end, it is essential to use the principle of "like cures like" to match the state of the disturbance to precisely the substance from nature that would cause such an imbalance in a healthy person. Homeopaths seek to bring about genuine healing. The conventional approach, though well intentioned, often temporarily rids the individual of an annoying symptom only to have it return, perhaps even stronger, once the conventional medicine is discontinued.

A UNIQUE MATCH: ONE MEDICINE AT A TIME

Once the homeopath is able to perceive the uniqueness of the person and his symptoms, the next step is to select a single homeopathic medicine, made from the natural substance that is known to cause those same symptoms. This medicine, paradoxically, can treat what its parent substance causes. A very highly diluted, specially prepared medicine is made from the original substance, which stimulates the body to heal itself.

There are over two thousand homeopathic medicines made from substances in the plant, animal, and mineral kingdoms. Any substance that you can possibly think of has either been made into a homeopathic medicine or could potentially become a medicine. Each substance in nature possesses its own unique traits. Think for a moment about a honeybee, from which the medicine *Apis mellifica* is made. Everyone knows that bees are busy and protective of their hives and that they don't like to be crossed. So, even if you know nothing about homeopathy, it will not be too surprising that people who need the medicine *Apis* can demonstrate all of these same traits.

Now think of iron, which comes from the mineral kingdom and is prepared homeopathically as the medicine *Ferrum metallicum*. Just as iron has the property of being strong and unbending, of becoming molten, and of being used to make prisons and armor, people needing the medicine *Ferrum* tend to be red-faced, irritable, and strong-willed and tend to engage in battles with other people. Another example is poison ivy, commonly known in homeopathy as *Rhus toxicodendron*. Just as poison ivy can cause a stinging, blistering rash with great itching that is very distressing, a person who needs *Rhus toxicodendron* will feel terribly restless, with itching or discomfort, and will go to great lengths to stretch and squirm to try to find a comfortable position.

In this same way, any substance in nature can be made into a homeopathic medicine and, depending on which symptoms it causes in a healthy person, can be of great benefit in relieving similar symptoms in a person who is ill. Understanding which medicine to give when is actually quite logical. Once you are familiar with symptoms and with the medicines that treat them, finding the needed medicine is like recognizing a friend you have met before. As long as you remember the principle that the symptoms a substance can cause are the same symptoms it will cure when it is made into a medicine, you will be able to understand how homeopathic medicines are discovered and used.

CLINICAL SUCCESS STORIES

The philosophy of homeopathy may be fascinating to some and bewildering to others. What speaks most loudly are the clinical success stories that every practitioner of homeopathy sees again and again. Here are a few typical case studies of people with acute illnesses who were helped dramatically by homeopathy.

Peter: Eye Injury

Peter, eight years old, was a patient of ours. His mother called, frantic, late on a Friday afternoon to tell us that a branch had flipped into Peter's right eye and scratched his cornea. He immediately felt great pain in his eye, and his mother rushed him to the local emergency room. The emergency room physician examined Peter's eye, gave him pain medication, and warned that if the pain continued into the next day, he would need surgery. Peter's mother picked up *Arnica* from us, and we asked her to hold on to *Symphytum* in case the *Arnica* didn't help. She called the next morning to say that Peter was feeling much less pain. The doctor again examined Peter's eye, felt that it was healing nicely, and said surgery was unnecessary. Peter's eye improved quickly, and he had no further problems with it. He never needed to take the *Symphytum*.

Claire: Bladder Infection

Claire, age thirty-two, came to see us complaining of an excruciating bladder infection. The burning in her bladder and urethra had come on very suddenly. She noticed an increasing amount of blood in her urine. She felt an intolerable need to urinate all the time. We gave Claire *Cantharis*. Within ten minutes, the pain began to subside. The pain continued to lessen, and within four hours it was gone entirely.

Lila: Sore Throat

Lila, sixteen, could barely swallow because her throat was so sore. The first thing we noticed when she opened her mouth was that her breath smelled bad. When we looked at her throat, we noticed several white, pus-filled ulcers on her tonsils. Lila remarked that she had much more saliva since her throat became sore. We gave her *Mercurius*. By the next morning, Lila had only a slight sore throat. By the next evening she felt fine.

Herman: Flu

Herman, forty-five years old, felt fine when he went to work one morning, but by mid-afternoon he felt awful. A number of his co-workers seemed to be coming down with the same symptoms. Herman's head pounded, his eyelids felt like lead, he experienced chills up and down his spine, and all he wanted to do was go to bed. He felt like every muscle of his body ached. He called us before leaving work and picked up a dose of *Gelsemium* (Yellow jasmine). This is a commonly prescribed homeopathic medicine for people who feel dizzy, drowsy, droopy, and dull with the flu. Herman called us the next morning to say he woke up feeling seventy-five percent better. He was able to go back to work and did not develop any other flu symptoms.

These are typical cases from our homeopathic practice. The best thing about homeopathic treatment is how well it works and how rapidly. You can relieve many short-term or acute illnesses in twenty-four to forty-eight hours if you give the correct homeopathic medicine. First-aid situations such as injuries and shock may respond immediately. Sore throats, the flu, and earaches are speedily relieved by the appropriate homeopathic medicines. If you read this book carefully and follow our recommendations, you will see the same kinds of results when you treat yourself and your family.

A GROWING BODY OF HOMEOPATHIC RESEARCH

Due to limitations in funding, there has not been as much opportunity to conduct homeopathic clinical research as many of us would like. Some sound studies have been published nonetheless, and there is a committed group of people dedicated to conducting more research. Here is a brief summary of some of the best work done to date.

In a 1991 review article in the *British Medical Journal,* a group of Dutch researchers reported their evaluation of 107 controlled clinical research studies on homeopathy published in medical journals between 1966 and 1990. Eighty-one of these studies showed positive results in such conditions as respiratory and other infections, digestive disorders, influenza, hay fever, recovery after surgery, rheumatoid arthritis, fibromyalgia, and psychological problems.[4]

An excellent study by Jennifer Jacobs, M.D., M.P.H., on the effectiveness of homeopathy in treating childhood diarrhea was published in 1994 in *Pediatrics.*[5] Dr.

[4]J. Kleijnan, P. Knipschild, and G. ter Riet, "Clinical Trials of Homeopathy," *British Medical Journal* 302 (February 9, 1991):316–23.

[5]Jennifer Jacobs, Dean Crothers, L. Margerita Himenez, and Stephen S. Gloyd, "Treatment of Acute Childhood Diarrhea with Homeopathic Medicine: A Randomized Clinical Trial in Nicaragua," *Pediatrics* 93, no. 5 (1994):719–25.

Jacobs and her associates conducted a double-blind, placebo-controlled study that demonstrated a statistically significant difference between children treated with a homeopathic medicine and those given a placebo.

The most recent major study was published in the prestigious British medical journal *The Lancet*. Dr. David Taylor Reilly and his associates found that eighty-two percent of asthma sufferers who were treated with homeopathic dilutions of their principal allergens improved significantly, as compared to the thirty-eight-percent improvement in the placebo control group.[6]

We are currently participating in a preliminary study of the results of our best cases using homeopathic treatment for attention deficit hyperactivity disorder (ADHD). Hopefully many other studies on the efficacy of homeopathic treatment will follow once more funding is available.

WHY CHOOSE HOMEOPATHY OVER CONVENTIONAL MEDICINE?

A growing number of people are dissatisfied with the overspecialized and compartmentalized approach of conventional medicine. Many people feel skeptical about taking prescription medications which have long lists of potential side effects. We have also heard many complaints that conventional medicine does not address the root of a problem.

Homeopathy provides a safe, effective, natural, nontoxic treatment for many acute and chronic illnesses. Homeopathy is safe even for newborns, pregnant women, the elderly, and animals. It uses only natural substances that are gentle yet extremely effective when used properly. Homeopathic medicines are highly individualized. Ten different people with coughs are likely to need ten different homeopathic medicines. Homeopathy individualizes rather than stereotypes. The medicines are inexpensive and often work rapidly. They address mental and emotional as well as physical complaints, and they treat the whole person. It is easy to see why homeopathy is becoming so popular.

WHICH CONDITIONS YOU CAN TREAT YOURSELF AND WHICH YOU SHOULD NOT

In order to prescribe a homeopathic medicine, you must find out specifically how the person is ill, which symptoms and changes in the body and mind characterize the dis-

[6]David Reilly, Morag Taylor, Neil Beattie, et al., "Is Evidence for Homeopathy Reproducible?" *Lancet* 344 (1994):1601–6.

ease, and which substance in nature matches those symptoms. This process may be simple or complicated, depending on the disease. A minor illness with a few well-defined symptoms is easy to prescribe for. A complicated, chronic illness with many factors involved is much more difficult. It is helpful to divide medical conditions into three different groups: *first-aid, acute,* and *chronic.*

First-Aid Conditions

Examples of first-aid conditions are emergency situations such as injuries, burns, insect bites, and sunstroke. Homeopathy is extraordinarily helpful in these situations, and it is generally very easy to select a homeopathic medicine for first-aid situations.

Acute Illnesses

Acute illnesses are, by definition, self-limiting, meaning that the person who is ill will either recover on her own or will die from the illness in a relatively short time. Severe acute illnesses which would normally require medical or surgical intervention in a doctor's office, emergency room, or hospital are not appropriate for home treatment, except for giving first aid (including homeopathic medicine) until professional homeopathic or conventional medical assistance can be obtained. More minor problems such as colds, influenza, hay fever, bladder infections, earaches, headaches, indigestion, bruises, cuts, minor bleeding, strains, and sprains can often be treated effectively using homeopathy. Acute emotional states such as anger, sadness, grief, and anxiety can also respond to homeopathic treatment.

Learning to treat acute problems at home can be a very gratifying experience. You will see yourself and your family respond well to homeopathy, and you will feel great satisfaction at being able to relieve suffering and bring healing to those who need it. It can also save a lot of unnecessary and costly visits to the doctor or emergency room for simple problems you can treat yourself.

Chronic Illnesses

These are long-standing conditions such as allergies, asthma, headaches, eczema, menstrual problems, and mental and emotional conditions such as depression, anxiety, and attention deficit hyperactivity disorder (ADHD).

This book is dedicated to teaching you how to treat first-aid and acute conditions. The homeopathic method, when applied correctly, leads to predictably good results. We will teach you the method and the tools that we use to make quick and accurate decisions about which medicine to give to a sick person to promote rapid relief.

The first-aid and acute conditions described in this book may be treated safely and effectively with a small amount of training. We need to emphasize, though, that it is important to get competent homeopathic assistance if a person's symptoms have not been relieved after a few attempts with the methods and medicines described in this book. Sometimes what appears to be a simple acute illness is only a sign of a deeper and more complicated condition—like a headache that is, in fact, the early sign of a brain tumor, or a "stomach ache" that is actually appendicitis. If you are not getting results, get help. It is necessary to give the right medicine in order for homeopathy to be effective, and sometimes more experience is needed to find that medicine.

This book is not for the treatment of chronic illness, which must be treated by a professional homeopath who has received hundreds or thousands of hours of training. It is like the difference between treating a cold and treating colitis. A cold is treated simply and easily and tends to go away by itself over time, even if you do nothing but suffer through it. Colitis (an inflammation of the large intestine or colon with ulceration, bleeding, and mucous discharge) is a serious, long-term illness that can be fatal in some people.

Finding the homeopathic medicine for a person with a cold that has clear, definite symptoms is a relatively easy task. Discovering the prescription for a person with colitis is much more complicated, involving an extensive interview, physical examination, and laboratory testing; it deals not only with physical symptoms, but with complex mental and emotional factors as well.

Clearly, treating a serious chronic illness like colitis is no job for a beginner. Chronic illnesses are complex, and their treatment requires years of homeopathic training in addition to medical knowledge. You can become very skilled in treating first-aid and acute conditions by following the directions in our book. Do not even think about treating someone with chronic illness. You will not be doing him a favor, and could harm him. Refer that person to an experienced homeopathic physician or other qualified medical practitioner.

We also advise against treating anyone for an acute condition who is already receiving constitutional treatment for chronic disease under the care of a professional homeopath. In such a case, instruct the person to first call his homeopathic practitioner for suggestions. Many homeopaths prefer to treat all acute illnesses themselves, or at least to consult with their patient before he takes any medicine for an acute condition. If a person under *constitutional* treatment (a more extensive process in which a professional homeopath treats the whole person, generally for chronic illness) self-treats or is treated for an acute illness by someone else, it is possible that the self-treatment will interfere with the constitutional treatment causing the chronic symptoms to return or worsen.

THE SUCCESS OF HOMEOPATHY IN TREATING CHRONIC DISEASE

This book is about self-prescribing for minor illnesses. However, we want you to also be aware that homeopathic medicine, in the hands of an experienced and highly trained practitioner with adequate medical knowledge, can be extremely effective in treating chronic disease. Homeopaths commonly treat patients who have a wide variety of physical complaints, including allergies, eczema, arthritis, chronic fatigue, headaches, asthma, ear infections, menstrual problems, and digestive complaints. Homeopathy can be very beneficial in treating mental and emotional problems, including anxiety, depression, fears, attention deficit hyperactivity disorder (ADHD), and other behavioral and learning problems. Homeopathy can often be helpful even if the person has suffered from the problem for many years.

The process of homeopathic treatment for chronic illness involves an extensive interview and careful follow-up care. The homeopath must understand the patient in depth, as a whole, in order to choose the best homeopathic medicine. The medicine is given either once or repeatedly, depending on the situation. The patient should notice an improvement within hours to weeks. There should be a minimum of a sixty- to seventy-percent improvement in most conditions if the correct medicine is chosen. In the case of most chronic illnesses, treatment needs to continue for at least one to two years, although appointments are scheduled less frequently once the patient begins to improve.

Here are a few case studies from our two books on homeopathic treatment of patients with chronic illness, *The Patient's Guide to Homeopathic Medicine* and *Ritalin-Free Kids*. These cases will hopefully give you an idea of what is possible with homeopathy:

Cliff: Allergies

"It wasn't until I got better that I saw how sick I was. My typical day for most of my thirty-six years consisted of slowly waking from a not-so-restful sleep, feeling haunted by past events for most of the day, crashing, dog-tired, by 4:00 in the afternoon, and then going home to be alone. From time to time, I sneezed. At the time, I thought my life was just like everyone else's, except that I had allergies. I battled allergies since I was fourteen. A series of skin tests indicated that I was allergic to tomatoes, dusts, trees, grass, and molds, all of which seemed unavoidable. I began taking injections of a dark syrupy substance that relieved the congestion and sneezing. After taking the injections for a few years, I concluded that I was cured. Unfortunately, a few years later my allergies not only returned, but were worse.

"My medical doctors suggested surgical desensitization by scraping the nerve endings out of my nose. It seemed so barbaric. After considerable study on my part, I found that if I ate only rice and frozen vegetables and took seventy-five assorted pills each day I was fine. I was spending a fortune on pills each month and wanted someone to help me determine which ones I didn't really need. I found my homeopathic doctor. He listened to me a lot during that first appointment. Then, without saying much about my medicine cabinet full of pills, he gave me a little envelope filled with a small amount of white granules. He said it was a preparation of salt. I took it in the evening before bed.

"I awoke the next morning from the most restful sleep I had had in years. To my disbelief, both of my nostrils were open and clear. I felt fifteen years younger, could breathe easily, and had high energy throughout the day. My body worked better, and I felt that something deep inside had changed. Over the next few months, I noticed that my attitude toward myself gradually improved.

"During the five years that I have been under homeopathic care, my life has improved steadily and dramatically. I am no longer held captive by the old negative feelings that guided my life. Allergies are no longer a problem. I can eat any food. I have more energy. Homeopathy helped me release my fears about intimate relationships, which enabled me to get married and have a child. My wife and daughter have also enjoyed the benefits of homeopathy."[7]

Sonya: Menopause

Sonya, a forty-four-year-old artist, had received homeopathic treatment periodically for years. During that time, she was treated successfully for depression, headaches, and digestive problems. She consulted us because of anxiety that seemed to come on with menopause.

Sonya told us, "My brain has been used up. I feel pressure in my head. My mind does not want to function. I have burning hot flashes from the slightest excitement; they spread from my head and face to my whole body. My whole body sweats. I constantly think about business. I wake frequently at night. I am always figuring things out during my sleep. I organize things in my mind for work.

"My fingers and arms get numb easily on waking. It is worse when I sleep on my left side. I have an aching sensation in my forearms and wrist, especially on the right side. It is almost a burning, but it kind of feels icy cold and tingles. My lower eyelids, back, and legs are twitching lately. I have a hurried feeling. It's overwhelming. There's not enough time. I have to tell myself to slow down. I can't think. It's an effort. Nothing connects. I lose my train of thought. I forget words. I get so speedy that I forget half of what I'm thinking about. I'm bloated and I have gas. My bowels are sluggish. I have an inner gnawing feeling. If I get hungry, watch out and don't get near me! I have a tightness in my larynx. It feels tense."

[7]Robert Ullman and Judyth Reichenberg-Ullman, op. cit., 73–75.

Sonya had had no menstrual period for the previous five months. She was much warmer since the hot flashes began. She couldn't find a comfortable sleeping position because her mind was "chewing" all the time. The sun and light were bothering her again lately, and she noticed recently that she was more afraid of heights. Sonya was very anxious to feel better.

We treated Sonya with *Iodum* (Iodine). She called us several weeks after she took the remedy to say how well it had worked. The rushed feeling in her mind and the restlessness were gone within twenty-four hours. Within two weeks, she was "back on track." The hot flashes disappeared completely and have not returned. The numbness in her fingers and arms was gone, as well as the aching in her wrist. These symptoms were still not bothering her two years later.[8]

Sumi: Attention Deficit Hyperactivity Disorder

Six-year-old Sumi was a very cute little girl who could not sit still for more than five minutes at a time. It was impossible for her to stay in one place. Sumi kissed, poked, prodded, and pulled. She blurted things out loudly. School was a struggle because of her difficulty concentrating, following directions, and staying at her desk. She wandered around and was always busy. Her verbal skills lagged far behind the other children's at her grade level. It was particularly hard for her to remember words. This sweet child seemed to lack any awareness of how her behavior affected others. She often came on too strong but did not realize it. She also bit her nails down to the quick and even nibbled on her toenails.

We began treating Sumi with *Veratrum album* (White hellebore) three years ago. She is a different child now. Just weeks after starting homeopathic treatment, she began making excellent progress with her speech. She spent less time searching for words, and her focus was greatly improved. She did not stumble or rush so much. Before, she could only color one page at a time in her coloring book. Within three weeks of beginning homeopathic treatment, she was completing eight pages at a time.

Over time, Sumi's progress continued. Her nail-biting diminished. She no longer kissed inappropriately. Her actions became more purposeful, and she became more aware of her impact on others. Her teachers no longer complained that her behavior was disruptive. She could connect phrases, and her vocabulary grew. She has continued to blossom into a delightful, bright, engaging, well-behaved child.[9]

These are all typical of chronic cases that you should refer to an experienced homeopathic practitioner.

[8]Ibid., 77–78.

[9]Judyth Reichenberg-Ullman and Robert Ullman, *Ritalin-Free Kids: Safe and Effective Homeopathic Medicine for ADD and Other Behavioral and Learning Problems* (Rocklin: Prima Publishing, 1996), 158–59.

CHAPTER **3**

The Homeopathic Medicine Chest

WHAT ARE THE SOURCES OF HOMEOPATHIC MEDICINES?

Homeopathic medicines can be made from literally any substance in nature. The majority of medicines are derived from the mineral and plant kingdoms, and a minority from the animal kingdom. Hahnemann, during his lifetime, tested out many substances through a process that is called a *proving*. In a proving, a number of healthy people repeatedly take a particular substance, then keep meticulous notes about any symptoms or experiences that result. In this way, it is possible to discover which symptoms that same substance can cure in a person who is ill. The thirty or so most commonly used homeopathic medicines, called the *polychrests*, appear often in this book. They include such diverse substances as sodium chloride (table salt), charcoal, flowers, sea creatures, and snake venom. Each of these substances can cause, and therefore treat, a variety of physical, mental, and emotional symptoms. There are over two thousand homeopathic medicines available, and more provings are being conducted worldwide.

WHAT MAKES A MEDICINE HOMEOPATHIC?

There are two things that make a medicine homeopathic: the way it is prepared, and the way it is used. We have already explained the way a homeopathic medicine is used: how a homeopath bases each prescription on the symptoms of the whole person—called the *totality of symptoms*—and uses the law of similars to select the one medicine that best fits the person's situation. Another aspect that makes homeopathic medicines radically different from conventional medications is their preparation.

Hahnemann found that, in order to avoid the harmful side effects of the medicines of his day, he could dilute natural substances into microdoses. He discovered further, through extensive experimentation, that the more he diluted the substances the longer their healing effects lasted. Homeopathic medicines are still prepared in the same way they were during Hahnemann's time.

The medicines are prepared on one of two scales: a *decimal* scale or, more frequently, a *centesimal* scale. In a decimal preparation, one part of the original *mother tincture* of the substance, which is prepared in a specific and standardized way, is mixed with nine parts of water or alcohol. This is called a "1X" preparation or *potency*. In a 6X potency, which is widely available in pharmacies or health food stores, one part of the 1X has been mixed again with nine parts of water or alcohol, and this process has been repeated a total of six times. Each time a dilution is made, the substance is vigorously shaken in order to distribute the material thoroughly. This shaking, called *succussion,* also seems to alter the energy of the substance. Because homeopathic medicines are diluted many times, even poisonous substances such as strychnine, arsenic, and various snake venoms are rendered completely safe, even for a newborn.

Homeopaths commonly used the potencies from the centesimal scale, and that is what we recommend in this book. In a centesimal preparation, one part of the original substance is mixed with ninety-nine parts of water or alcohol to form a "1C" medicine. This process is repeated a number of times. Each time the medicine is diluted and shaken, it actually becomes stronger, rather than weaker. Dilutions of various strengths are inoculated onto sugar pellets.

We prefer 30C medicines for acute prescribing because they are strong enough medicines to last at least several hours or more, and they do not need frequent repetition. Some people use 6X preparations for acute prescribing, but we find these impractical since they may need to be repeated every fifteen to thirty minutes. What is most important, however, is to select the best homeopathic medicine for the person, because the right medicine will generally work in any potency.

Potencies of 200C and above are usually called *high potency* homeopathic medicines. Potencies below 200C are called *low potency* medicines. Professional homeopaths generally use 200C (diluted two hundred times), 1M (one thousand dilutions), or 10M (ten thousand dilutions). The effects of these high-potency medicines can last for months or years in chronic cases; they should only be used by experienced prescribers, except in emergency situations where a rapid, dramatic effect is needed. Although homeopathic medicines are quite safe when used properly, people can experience reactions to the higher potencies.

HOW DOES ONE TAKE A HOMEOPATHIC MEDICINE?

Homeopathic medicines are prepared in the form of tiny pills or pellets which are to be placed on or under the tongue. In some parts of the world, homeopathic medicines are administered in water, but that is not generally the case in the United States.

The administration of homeopathic medicines is different from conventional drugs in that you only need to take the medicine until you notice a change for the better. As soon as your symptoms have improved, under most circumstances, you can stop taking the medicine. The correct homeopathic substance sets into motion a healing process. Once this process has begun, it will continue unless something interrupts it. There are specific guidelines as to when or how often to take homeopathic medicines, depending partly on the person's situation and partly on the potency of the medicine. Exactly when to give, change, or stop giving a medicine will be discussed in detail later in the book.

WHERE CAN ONE FIND HOMEOPATHIC MEDICINES?

Manufacturing pharmacies all over the world prepare the thousands of medicines which homeopaths use in daily practice and which people use at home to heal themselves. In most countries, the standards for homeopathic medicines are regulated by government agencies like the Food and Drug Administration in the United States, where most homeopathic medicines are considered over-the-counter rather than prescription medications. In many countries in Europe, homeopathic medicines are widely available. Each of the 23,000 pharmacies in France not only carries homeopathic medicines, but displays them prominently on its signs.

Until recently, homeopathic medicines were only available by mail order from a handful of pharmacies in this country. Now many health food stores and some pharmacies carry homeopathic medicines, and they can be ordered from a growing number of homeopathic pharmacies. Many retail outlets carry only the standard medicines, sometimes in limited potency selections. If you are looking for a more obscure medicine, you generally need to order it from a homeopathic pharmacy. In some cases, particular homeopathic medicines or particular potencies are available only to physicians. There are also a limited number of homeopathic medicines made from controlled substances that are not available in the United States.

We recommend that you have a home kit so that you can have the medicines you need readily available. For information on our specific Homeopathic Self-Care Medicine Kit suggestions, turn to Chapter 4.

TOPICAL PREPARATIONS

There are a couple of extremely useful homeopathic medicines that are available in the form of creams, lotions, ointments, tinctures, or sprays and which should be added to your kit.

The first of these is *Calendula* (Marigold), which is invaluable for cuts, scrapes, burns, sores, and non-fungal eruptions. Since you will apply it often in the case of an open wound, some preparations are water-based and tend to burn less, which is especially nice for children. We cannot begin to tell you how many thousands of times we have recommended *Calendula* to our patients for skin conditions and later heard them rave about the results. If you only buy one topical product to include in your kit, make it *Calendula*.

The other topical preparation that is very useful is *Arnica* (Leopard's bane). A common and attractive mountain flower, *Arnica* is said to have been munched on by mountain sheep when they injured themselves and is extremely useful for sprains, strains, or bruises. *Arnica* should *not* be used on open wounds because it can cause an angry rash in some people. It is fine to just use *Arnica* internally according to the instructions for the other homeopathic medicines in this book, but many people also like to use it topically for muscle soreness and bruising.

STORING AND HANDLING HOMEOPATHIC MEDICINES

Homeopathic medicines can last indefinitely as long as you take a few simple precautions:

- Store your kit away from direct sunlight, extremely high temperatures, and the aromatic substances named on the *antidote* list (an antidote interferes with the medicine's action; see Chapter 7).
- Avoid touching the pellets with your hands.
- Open only one bottle at a time to avoid contamination and confusion.
- If a medicine spills or falls on the floor, discard it.
- When traveling, pass the kit around the airport X-ray machine.

CHAPTER **4**

Your Homeopathic Self-Care Medicine Kit

DON'T LEAVE HOME WITHOUT IT!

Knowing which homeopathic medicine to use for a particular first-aid or acute situation can be of great benefit as long as you have the medicine. You never know when you or a family member will be in need of homeopathic care. The best time to administer a homeopathic medicine is immediately following an injury or at the beginning of an acute illness, when the symptoms are clear but before they have a chance to progress. The more available your self-care kit, the more useful it will be.

Kits come in a variety of sizes, shapes, and potencies, suited to different needs. Some are made for use at home or when traveling; others are smaller for hiking or bicycle trips. We recommend a kit of at least thirty medicines. If space is not an issue, a kit containing fifty medicines is even better. We used to put together a traveling kit with only a dozen homeopathic medicines, but there is nothing more frustrating than knowing what a person needs and not having the medicine.

Several years ago, we attended a homeopathic seminar on Maui which included a special snorkeling trip to the island of Molokini. The water was very choppy and a number of us became terribly seasick, including Judyth. She knew exactly what she needed: *Tabacum* (see Motion Sickness in Chapter 9). But not one of the thirty or more homeopaths on that boat had brought any remedies. Don't let yourself get into such an unfortunate predicament. The best advice we can give you regarding your self-care kit is: Don't leave home without it.

We have put together the Homeopathic Self-Care Medicine Kit in conjunction with this book in order to save you the time and money of compiling or locating your own kit. Our kit contains the fifty medicines we use most commonly. We do not include every medicine mentioned in this book in our kit, but we do include the medicines you are most likely to need for first aid and for common acute illnesses. An order form is available at the back of the book. A variety of other kits are also available (see Appendix) and sold by retailers or homeopathic practitioners.

Regardless of which kit you choose, the most important thing is to have the medicine you need when you need it. Homeopathic prescribing is extremely effective when the right medicine is available, and fairly useless when it is not. If you intend to use homeopathy, it is much more cost-effective and convenient to buy a kit than to buy individual medicines. A homeopathic self-care kit does not, however, replace the need for other essential items, including bandages, scissors, tape, and an elastic bandage, as well as any other specific travel-kit items you might need, such as water-purification tablets and other preventive aids.

WHAT TO INCLUDE IN YOUR KIT

We recommend using a kit that contains 30C potency medicines. Many kits contain 6X, 12X, 12C, or 30X potencies. The correct homeopathic medicine will work in any potency, but these lower potencies need to be repeated more often, some up to six times a day. We find it much easier to recommend a 30C potency, which needs to be used every four hours at the most, and often only one or two times.

The following are the medicines we include in our Homeopathic Self-Care Medicine Kit:

Aconite
Allium cepa
Antimonium tartaricum
Apis
Arnica
Arsenicum album
Belladonna
Bryonia
Cantharis
Carbo vegetabilis
Chamomilla
China
Cocculus
Coffea
Colocynthis
Drosera
Euphrasia
Ferrum phosphoricum
Gelsemium
Glonoine
Hepar sulphuris
Hypericum
Ignatia
Ipecac
Kali bichromicum
Lachesis
Ledum
Lycopodium
Magnesia phosphorica
Mercurius
Natrum muriaticum
Nux vomica
Petroleum
Phosphorus
Phytolacca
Podophyllum
Pulsatilla
Rhus toxicodendron
Rumex
Ruta
Sarsaparilla
Sepia
Silica
Spongia
Staphysagria
Sulphur
Symphytum
Tabacum
Urtica urens
Veratrum album

CHAPTER 5

Taking the Homeopathic Case

PRACTICE MAKES PERFECT

Homeopathic casetaking is an art and a skill that is learned through practice and experience. As soon as you have an opportunity to treat yourself or someone in your family, look, listen, and ask to learn everything you can about that person and her illness. You will become increasingly familiar with how to elicit the information you need quickly and easily. After years of experience, we can solve most acute cases in under fifteen minutes. You may take a little longer at first, but the amount of suffering you can save yourself or relative is well worth whatever time it takes to find the medicine needed.

USING THE MEDICAL CONDITIONS CHAPTER AND THE LOOK, LISTEN, AND ASK SECTIONS

The person you are treating will usually tell you in general terms the kind of illness she is having, such as a headache, a sprained ankle, a sore throat, a cold, or an earache. With a child, you may have to make that assessment from a description like "Mommy, my stomach hurts." This book is set up to help you self-treat a variety of medical conditions (listed in the Table of Contents) once you have identified the main problem.

Select a medical condition that most resembles the symptoms of the person you are treating, such as eye infection, cold, ear infection, flu, bladder infection, sore throat, or headache. Choose the condition that seems to match best by reading the description of the common symptoms that occur in that kind of problem. If most of the symptoms are similar, you are in the right place. If you don't know which medical condition to choose, pick the one you think most closely applies and read the description of the condition. If it seems right, use it. If not, read other related conditions until you find the one that fits best. Keep looking until you find the right one. If the situation is too complicated to match any of the conditions listed, it is probably too difficult for you to treat at home and you should find a professional homeopath who can treat the person or seek other medical assistance.

Use the Look, Listen, and Ask sections under each condition to guide you in your casetaking so that you can acquire the specific information that will allow you to choose the correct medicine. The Look section (indicated by the eye icon) gives you instructions on what to observe about the patient. The Listen section (indicated by the ear icon) helps you be attentive to what you may hear about the problem. The Ask section (indicated by the question mark icon) gives you specific questions to ask to find out more about the symptoms of the case.

Look Carefully

Read the Look section (eye icon) under the appropriate medical condition for tips on what to observe.

A person who is acutely ill will develop definite symptoms that can lead you to find the right homeopathic medicine. You need to be able to paint the entire picture of the illness from the person's point of view. The signs of illness are readily apparent if you know what to look for and how to observe. Observation is essential for good casetaking.

When a person is ill, he often looks different than when he feels well. The color and expression of the face, general skin color and tone, body posture, brightness of the eyes, and color of the ears, tongue, and throat are all things you can observe to find out what kind of illness is present, and to get an impression of the individual's level of energy, emotional state, and extent of physical illness. You can notice injuries, bleeding, skin rashes, discoloration, bruising, and the color, odor, and consistency of mucus, stool, and urine.

Use all of your five senses when you observe, as well as your sixth sense, intuition. If you know the person you are treating, observe how she looks, sounds, or smells as compared to her usual condition: if she usually has a red face, but now is pale; if she usually smells sweet, but now smells sour; if she usually walks normally, but now has a limp; if she usually smiles, but now has a distressed or pained expression. All these changes are part of her homeopathic symptom picture. Write down your observations so that you don't forget them when it comes time to analyze the case.

When observing, it is useful to survey your patient from top to bottom in order to note any changes. Look at her facial expression for signs of weariness, sadness, pain, or other feelings. Watch for postures, movements, and gestures that are out of the ordinary or that signal injuries. Observe the skin for discoloration, rashes, and other skin eruptions, perspiration or bleeding, lumps, bumps, and swollen lymph nodes.

Notice any discharges from the eyes, mouth, ears, nose, anus, or genitals. Note their color, odor, and consistency. Observing carefully bodily secretions, urine, stool, vomit, and blood may be important in understanding the illness and selecting the appropriate medicine. Whether the nasal discharge is thick, thin, green, yellow, bloody, or clear, for example, can be very important in differentiating which homeopathic medicine is the most appropriate one for a sinus infection.

If you have a flashlight and a tongue depressor (a spoon will do), look in the mouth and throat. Take the pulse at the wrist. Count the number of breaths per minute (fifteen is average). If you have no medical experience, go to the beach or the gym and become familiar with looking at different types of bodies so that you can learn what general appearance is normal in a healthy person and what is abnormal.

Also be aware of the sick person's environment and how it has changed since he became ill. Does he want it dark or bright, clean or messy, cold or warm? Is the bed rumpled or freshly made? Is the window open or closed? Does he have any beverages by his bed? If so, is the glass or bottle empty or full? Is he desiring cold drinks or warm ones? Does she prefer company or would she rather be left alone? Is food present, and what and how much has she eaten? The patient's environment will give you clues as to her likes and dislikes and what makes her feel better or worse—crucial information in selecting a homeopathic medicine. If you are taking the case by telephone and cannot observe her environment, ask her about it to learn if there is anything unusual or unique.

Signs and symptoms of extreme distress and danger should be noted first and treated as emergency situations. Difficulty breathing, severe pain, shock, extreme paleness, unconsciousness, bleeding, profuse vomiting or diarrhea, involuntary urination or defecation, and convulsions are signs of possibly life-threatening illness, and medical attention should be sought immediately. If you are certain of the appropriate homeopathic medicine, give it immediately, depending on the situation, and use CPR (cardio-pulmonary resuscitation), call an ambulance, or take the person to the emergency room or an appropriate physician.

Listen, Listen, Listen

Listen to everything the person has to say about her problem. A thorough interview, even for an acute problem, is a very important part of homeopathic casetaking. If you are able to crawl into that person's skin, so to speak, and understand what she is experiencing, you will be more likely to choose a medicine that can help her.

Rather than asking a long list of questions, begin by allowing the person to tell you what is bothering him. Ask an open-ended question like "Can you tell me how you're feeling?" to initiate the interviewing process. Simply allow the person to talk while you listen. Pay careful attention not only to what he is saying but to how he expresses himself. Listen for clues to his emotional state that would indicate pain, anger, sadness, anxiety, or fear. Let the person talk until he has said all that immediately comes to his mind. Allow some time for him to collect more thoughts. If he runs out of information, you can prompt him with a simple "What else?" or "Tell me more" or "What else has changed since you became ill?"

The Listen section under each medical condition gives sample quotes of what the person might say if he needed a particular homeopathic medicine.

WHAT YOU NEED TO KNOW

Ask the Right Questions

After the individual has told you all about his problem, ask any relevant questions necessary to select a homeopathic medicine for him. At first you may not know what kind of questions to ask, but with practice the questions will become more obvious. The Ask section under each condition in this book includes a list of potential questions. The descriptions of medicines found in the Medical Condition section (Chapter 9) can also be a guide to gathering the information you need. The more specific information you can gather to help you understand what is unique about that person's condition, the more accurate your choice of medicine will be, and hence the better your results will be.

There are two kinds of symptoms in homeopathic casetaking: *general* symptoms and *particular* symptoms. General symptoms describe how the person feels as a whole, including mental and emotional symptoms as well as physical experiences that are felt in the entire body. Examples of general symptoms are "I feel sad since my father died," "I am sleepy," "I am hungry at 2:00 P.M.," and "I have a fever." When she says: "My throat is sore" or "I have a sharp pain across my forehead" or "My eye is irritated," she is describing a particular physical symptom. It is useful to know if the symptom is confined to one part of the body, or if it actually affects the whole person. General symptoms, such as mental and emotional states, sensitivity to temperature and weather, food desires and aversions, sleep patterns, hunger, and thirst, are considered to be indicators of the overall condition of the person and are often given considerable weight in choosing the homeopathic medicine. You will find both general and particular symptoms listed under each medicine in the Medical Conditions and *Materia Medica* sections of the book.

It is important to collect enough information to understand the person's condition and select a medicine, but not so much that you get lost in irrelevant details. Do ask specific questions about the location of the pain or sensation, the time when and circumstances under which the symptoms first began, and what makes the symptoms better or worse (*modalities*). Here are some sample questions for each area to get you started:

Suggested Questions

Onset:	When did the symptom first start? At what time? Did it occur suddenly or gradually?
Duration:	How long has it been present? Does it come and go or just stay?
Time of day:	When do the symptoms occur?
Causation:	What brings on the symptoms? Are the symptoms affected by changes in body position such as standing, sitting, or lying? Are the symptoms affected by activities such as eating, sleeping, or walking? Are the symptoms affected by environmental factors such as cold, noise, and light? Are the symptoms affected by emotional states such as anger, sadness, or grief?
Observation:	If the symptom can be perceived, what does it look, sound, smell or taste like?
Sensation:	What does it feel like? Is there any pain? What kind of specific sensation does the person experience?
Location:	What part of the body is affected? Is the symptom located on one side or the other?
Extension:	Does the sensation travel to any other part of the body?
Intensity:	How strong is the symptom? How much does it affect the patient—for example, on a scale from one to ten?
Character:	What makes the symptom(s) unique, striking, or unusual?
Along with:	What other symptom(s) commonly occur at the same time as or along with the symptom you are investigating?
Modalities:	What makes the symptom better or worse?

THE STATE OF THE PERSON

Just as important as the specific physical symptoms is the *state* of the individual. Professional homeopaths use this state, which includes the attitude, temperament, and nature of the person, as a major factor in treating people with chronic diseases. The state can also be important in acute prescribing, and is reflected by the mental and emotional symptoms and by any psychological factors which brought on the acute illness.

It is rarely an accident when a person becomes acutely ill immediately following a certain stressful circumstance or event. This *etiology*, or causation, will generally provide an insight into that person's state. This is obvious in the case of a person who develops a sore throat with a sensation of a lump and difficulty swallowing just after a close friend dies in a collision. The state of the person is grief. The medicine needed is *Ignatia.* Take another example of a man who tells you that he developed a stomach flu immediately after filing his income tax return. Exploring further, you discover that he is extremely worried about his finances and security, to the point that he wonders whether he will survive. The state is one of tremendous insecurity, fear of poverty, and fear of dying. The medicine called for is *Arsenicum album,* which fits the state.

Of course the physical symptoms are extremely important in acute prescribing, but so is the state. We include the basic characteristics of some of the major mental symptoms that would be treated by each medicine listed in this book. Make sure that you take these mental characteristics into consideration in choosing the most appropriate medicine.

WHAT YOU NEED TO KNOW

A MODEL CASETAKING

Homeopath	Tell me what's going on.
Patient	I have a really bad sore throat.
Homeopath	Tell me more.
Patient	It started yesterday afternoon at about 4:00 P.M.
Homeopath	Tell me what was happening just before your throat became sore.
Patient	I had a big oral exam at school yesterday morning. I was really scared that I would fail. I think it went okay, but a couple of hours later I started feeling awful.
Homeopath	Describe your throat pain.
Patient	It first started on the right side. Now it's on the left. It hurts most when I swallow liquids. For some reason, all I feel like drinking is warm tea.

Homeopath	Anything else?
Patient	I'm feeling chilly—like I want to take a hot bath.
Homeopath	Do you usually tend to feel cold?
Patient	No, it's odd. I'm usually quite warm.
Homeopath	Any other symptoms?
Patient	No, that's it. I tried gargling with salt water, but it didn't help much. Neither did Vitamin C. I sure hope you can help me.
Homeopath	I hope so, too. Tell me a little more about how you felt before your oral exam.
Patient	I'd been preparing for it for weeks. I was very nervous that I would make a mistake. I was afraid that I'd look like a fool in front of all my professors.
Homeopath	I think I have a medicine that will help you.

Starting with the simple statement, "I have a really bad sore throat," a homeopath is able to bring out a complete picture that clearly matches the homeopathic *Lycopodium* (Club moss). (See Sore Throat in the Medical Conditions section or *Lycopodium* in the *Materia Medica* section for a description of the medicine.) In more complicated situations, such as a flu with a sore throat, headache, and cough, you will need to explore several symptoms in depth in order to put together the complete symptom picture that will lead you to the correct homeopathic medicine.

PUTTING IT DOWN ON PAPER

It is important to write down whatever you discover about the person you are helping. This becomes the record of the homeopathic case that you can analyze to find the correct medicine. In the case of a professional homeopathic practitioner, this is an essential component of the patient's chart. For your purposes, you need a written case for several reasons:

- to provide the information source that will help you analyze the case and select a medicine
- to use one or several days later in case the person has not improved and you need to restudy and select another medicine
- if you are serious about becoming a good prescriber, to keep all of your written cases in a notebook for the purpose of future study.

Homeopaths emphasize certain symptoms in a case by *underlining* them in the case history or chart to indicate how much weight should be given to a particular symptom in the analysis:

Underlined once	Symptoms are somewhat clear, mildly intense, and elicited after questioning.
Underlined twice	Symptoms are more clear, more intense, or spontaneously expressed by the patient.
Underlined three times	Symptoms are very clear and quite intense and offered spontaneously.

You can either actually underline the symptom the appropriate number of times or put the number in parentheses as we do in this book. Even if you are just prescribing for yourself and your family, underlining is extremely useful to remind you, when you look over the case history, how strong and clear each symptom was.

WHAT YOU NEED TO KNOW

KEEPING A PERMANENT HOMEOPATHIC SELF-TREATMENT RECORD

We recommend that you keep a written record of your own and your family's self-treatment for a number of reasons. First, it is common that a person needs the same acute medicine at various times in his life. If you keep a record of which medicine you gave for what symptoms, when it was administered, and in which potency, it can be very helpful for future self-treatment. Imagine for example, that you find the correct medicine for your husband's hay fever. He has a dramatic recovery and is grateful to be cured of his fits of sneezing and nose-blowing. The following spring his symptoms return. If you have kept a record of exactly what worked, you can quickly relieve him of his misery again. If you have forgotten what you gave him, you need to begin again at square one.

Another benefit of a complete health record is that, if you consult a homeopathic practitioner about a chronic condition or a difficult acute condition at a later date, it will be useful for the homeopath to know which medicines have and have not been helpful in the past.

> A Sample Written Case History
> (Remember that the numbers in parentheses indicate underlines.)
> Two-year-old girl.
> Chief complaint: Eye infection
> Symptoms: Redness (3) and burning pain (2) of both eyes. Swelling of the eyelids (3). It started yesterday evening after dinner around 7:00 P.M. Discharge

of green pus from the lower lids (2). Child is weepy (3) and desires to be carried (2). Desire for pastries (2) and pizza (3). (These are not new food desires.) Not thirsty (3), which is unusual for her. Changeable mood, one minute crying, the next laughing (2). Wakes at night and cries for her mother (3). Child feels worse in a warm, stuffy room (1). Wants to be outside or to be near an open window (2).

Medicine and Potency Given: *Pulsatilla 30C*

Results: The eye symptoms and moodiness rapidly resolved, allowing the little girl to happily resume her play.

CHAPTER 6

Analyzing the Case and Selecting the Medicine

ANALYZING THE CASE

Once you have the information you need, the choice of a homeopathic medicine for a first-aid or acute condition often becomes relatively easy. Follow these steps:

1. Read the Description of the Medical Condition

For each condition, there is a description given in Chapter 9 of the kind of problem it is, the usual diagnostic characteristics, and the normal course of the illness, including any complications of which you should be aware. As you read about the condition, match the symptoms in your case history to the description of the medical condition to make sure you have selected the right condition. Pay attention to any immediate instructions about caring for the person prior to or after giving a homeopathic medicine.

2. Read the Pointers and the Listen Sections If You Have Not Already Done So

The Pointers for Finding the Homeopathic Medicine give capsule summaries of the main homeopathic medicines for each condition, with distinguishing characteristics. The Listen section has quotes similar to what you might hear a person say who needs a particular medicine.

3. Read the Description of Each Homeopathic Medicine in the Chart

- First read the Key Symptoms.
- If there are mental and emotional symptoms, read the Mind symptoms. If there are no mental symptoms, or *if none of the symptoms listed match your patient, disregard them.*
- Read the Body section.
- Read the Worse and Better symptoms.
- Read the Food and Drink section if there is one. This section indicates a patient's *desire for* or an *aversion to* certain food and drink.

Each medicine is described according to the typical pattern of symptoms for which it is likely to be effective in that particular illness. As you read about each one, evaluate how closely it matches the symptoms of the case you have taken. The person may not have all the symptoms that are described for a particular homeopathic medicine, but the symptoms which she does have should mostly fall within the group of symptoms listed. The descriptions are short, yet they contain the most typical symptoms covered by that medicine. You can see all the symptoms for each medicine by reading across the chart. You can compare the symptoms in each section for different medicines by reading down the chart.

CHOOSING THE BEST MEDICINE

The match should be the best possible one out of the medicines listed. We have chosen to list the most commonly prescribed medicines and, for some conditions, a few less commonly used medicines. If you cannot decide between two or three of the medicines, read each one in the *Materia Medica* section to see how well it matches your case.

There are two ways to use this book to select the one best homeopathic medicine for a person:

- Read the list of symptoms for each medicine described under the appropriate medical condition in Chapter 9. This will give you a picture of how a person with that condition needing that medicine will be.
- Consult the *Materia Medica* in Chapter 10. This section describes each homeopathic medicine in greater depth so that you can understand the typical symptoms that it matches in many kinds of illness, not just the particular illness you are treating. The more you learn about the characteristics of each medicine, the better you will be able to know if it matches your case.

In both the Medical Conditions (Chapter 9) and *Materia Medica* (Chapter 10) sections, read about all of the medicines that correspond to the case you are studying.

Discard the ones that do not fit at all. Choose the one that fits best, even if it is not a perfect match. A person will never have all of the characteristics of the medicine, and a medicine may not cover all of the symptoms of the person. You are simply looking for the best match.

It can be helpful to separate the symptoms in your case into Key Symptoms, Mind, Body, and Worse/Better symptoms so that you can see a pattern in the symptoms more easily and match it to the description given for a particular medicine. The bold-faced symptoms listed under each medicine are the ones that are most typical for that medicine. If your case has symptoms that you underline two or three times, it is likely that the symptom will be in boldface under the description of the medicine.

Choose the medicine that matches best. If no medicine matches well, make sure you have all the information you need. If necessary, ask a few more questions. You may not have been specific enough when first taking the case, but now you know what you need to ask to differentiate among the different medicines you are considering.

If you still can't find a good match, suggest that the person use the other self-care recommendations in this book, or refer the patient to a qualified homeopath.

CHAPTER 7

Administering the Homeopathic Medicine

WHAT TO EXPECT FROM A HOMEOPATHIC MEDICINE

Once you have selected the appropriate homeopathic medicine, the next step is to give it. It is essential to know what you can expect in terms of the person's response, whether and how often to repeat the medicine, and when to change to a different medicine. After you have given the medicine, you need to allow it time to act. One of the following situations will occur:

Nothing Changes

What is happening The person is neither better nor worse. The symptoms are unchanged.

What to do In most cases, three doses of the medicine have been given over twelve hours without change, you have not chosen the correct medicine. With some conditions such as tendinitis, it is best to wait several days before you decide that the chosen medicine has not acted. Find another medicine and give it. If no medicine seems to fit, the person may need a constitutional medicine or may need a more unusual acute medicine that is not in this book. In either case, seek professional homeopathic or other medical care.

> Example:
> A two-year-old child has an ear infection with severe pain, restlessness, whining, crying, and a desire to be carried. Twelve hours and three doses of

Pulsatilla later, the same symptoms remain with the same intensity. A new medicine *Chamomilla* is found and given, yielding rapid improvement.

WHAT YOU NEED TO KNOW

There Is Some Definite Change for the Better

What is happening Symptoms are less intense. Some symptoms go away. The person's energy and feeling of well-being increase. The medicine has acted.

What to do Wait for more improvement. Do not give another dose unless the patient begins to become worse again in the same way as before (*relapse*).

> Example:
> A man has a flushed face, a high fever, and a severe headache over his right eye, which is pounding and made worse by light, noise, and jarring. A dose of *Belladonna 30C* causes an immediate improvement, but twelve hours later he still has some head pain. His fever is gone and his face is still red, but less so. His energy is better and he doesn't feel so sensitive. He continues to improve, but later that day, his headache begins to get worse again and his temperature begins to climb. A second dose of *Belladonna 30C* causes a complete cure of his symptoms.

There Is Complete, Rapid Relief

What is happening All the symptoms resolve quickly. The person feels healthy again.

What to do The medicine has acted very well. Only repeat if there is a definite relapse.

> Example:
> A woman with a bladder infection complains of burning pain at the end of urination and a feeling of pain in the urethra extending inward. She feels a frequent urge to urinate and feels like she needs to stand up while urinating. After one dose of *Sarsaparilla 30C*, she is completely relieved of all of her symptoms in one hour. She does not need any more doses and remains well.

Symptoms Are Aggravated; No Improvement

What is happening The person feels worse twelve hours after taking the homeopathic medicine. Some symptoms are more intense, but the pattern is mostly the same.

What to do Either the medicine was not correct or it was *antidoted* (see the last section of this chapter), resulting in no improvement. If the condition is an acute flare-up of a chronic condition, however, the medicine may take a day or two to act. Assuming this is not the case, look for another medicine that may match the case. If you find a better one, give it. If you find an antidoting factor, remove it and give the first medicine again. Otherwise, wait another twelve hours (in a non-emergency situation). If there is no improvement, seek professional homeopathic or other medical care.

> Example:
> A young man who has been camping in the summer complains of gushing, watery diarrhea with lots of rumbling in his abdomen. The diarrhea comes every few hours and it smells very offensive. A dose of *Arsenicum 30C* makes him feel worse. The diarrhea becomes much more frequent, with more gurgling and rumbling. Twelve hours later, he is given *Podophyllum 30C*, followed by rapid improvement.

Symptoms Are Aggravated, but Definite Improvement Follows

What is happening The person feels worse briefly, followed by feeling considerably better.

What to do The medicine is correct. Repeat the medicine only if the same symptoms begin to return.

> Example:
> A ten-year-old child has a fever, a croupy cough, and a sore throat that feels like a fish bone is stuck in his throat. He is extremely sensitive to cold and does not want to be uncovered. He is very irritable. One dose of *Hepar sulphuris 30C* causes a worse sore throat and cough. He feels so chilly that he has to be under ten blankets. But six hours later he breaks out in a sweat, his fever goes away, and his throat stops hurting. The cough becomes considerably lessened. The medicine is repeated twice over the next twenty-four hours, leading to complete cure.

The Original Symptoms Go Away Partially or Completely, and a New Symptom Picture Emerges

What is happening The picture is changing.

What to do Restudy the case and give the medicine which most nearly matches the new set of symptoms.

> Example:
> A woman has severe indigestion after eating a pizza. She suffers from severe abdominal bloating and gas pains which only feel better when she burps. She

feels weak and exhausted and needs to lie down. She feels better when she is fanned. A dose of *Carbo vegetabilis 30C* completely relieves her gas and bloating, but she continues to be exhausted, feels very apathetic, and develops a painless, profuse diarrhea with a craving for fruit and refreshing drinks. Two doses of *Phosphoric acid 30C* four hours apart completely relieve her symptoms.

REPETITION OF THE DOSE

It is sometimes difficult to tell at first whether the medicine has acted or exactly how long to wait before repeating it. A homeopathic medicine only needs to be repeated when its effects have worn off. You may choose between the following options:

- You may give the medicine only once and, when you see that the person is improving, repeat the medicine only if and when the person starts to get worse again.
- You may begin by giving the medicine on a schedule, such as every two to four hours until you see an effect, then repeat it if there is a relapse. Stop when you see improvement.

What is happening and what to do:

- If the illness is severe, with rapid onset, doses may need to be given more frequently.
- In case of an emergency or very severe illness, you may need to repeat the dose as often as every fifteen to thirty minutes, in addition to seeking immediate medical care, because the effect of the medicine may last only for a brief time in those situations.
- If the symptoms develop slowly and are not severe, the medicine will generally not need to be repeated as often.
- If you see an aggravation or worsening of symptoms after giving a dose of medicine, do not give more until the aggravation has gone away. The best time to give another dose is after some improvement has been noted, but the improvement has slowed or stopped and signs of relapse are beginning.
- If you have given three doses of medicine without any difference in how the person feels or looks, give the next best medicine, unless there is a possibility that something is antidoting the action of the first medicine.

The proof that you have given the correct medicine is improvement in your patient's condition. There is no use repeating a medicine more than three times if neither of you notices any change. If there has been a change for the better, though, stay with the same medicine and give doses whenever they are needed.

The best rule of thumb is to repeat the medicine only after the first dose has shown a positive effect, or when the symptoms have begun to reappear after being relieved for a time. If the improvement is brief—perhaps only for an hour or two—the medicine will have to be repeated frequently, at least at first. If the improvement lasts for a long time—hours or days—it is only necessary to repeat the medicine if the symptoms that have been relieved eventually return. If you are still confused about what to do, wait and do nothing. Observe for a while, then reassess the situation.

Repeat the Medicine

1. Up to three times, every two to four hours, depending on the potency, until you observe an effect.
2. When symptoms return after initial improvement, even if the improvement has been brief.
3. Whenever the original symptom picture recurs.
4. If the medicine has been antidoted.

CHANGING THE MEDICINE

You should expect a significant improvement, often at least fifty to ninety percent, after giving the correct homeopathic medicine. If the first medicine does not help the person in a definite way, find a new one. A medicine that is close to the correct one may have a partial effect, helping some of the symptoms but not all of them.

There Is Slow Improvement

What is happening The person is continuing to improve.

What to do Do not change the medicine, even if improvement seems slow. The pace of improvement depends on the type of illness and the strength of the person's vital force. The correct medicine will produce a reduction in the intensity of the symptoms and heal the problem over time.

The Symptom Picture Changes

What is happening The first medicine has worked, but the pattern of symptoms has changed significantly since.

What to do The original medicine may no longer work, and a new medicine will have to be selected. Find out exactly how the symptoms have changed and, once again, go through the process of choosing a medicine that best matches the person's new symptom picture.

> Example:
> Your sister is suffering from a severe left-sided sore throat. You have recommended the medicine *Lachesis.* If the pain switches to the right side, the person may still need *Lachesis* or may progress to need *Belladonna, Lycopodium, Apis,* or *Phytolacca,* depending on the specific symptoms. Or the throat pain may go away entirely and be replaced by a dry, raspy cough that sounds like a seal barking, in which case *Spongia* would be indicated. If the symptom picture has changed to match *Spongia,* only that medicine will work. *Lachesis* will be ineffective, no matter how many doses you give. For that reason, it is necessary to communicate with the person to find out how the symptoms are changing, especially if the last dose of medicine had no effect.

WHAT YOU NEED TO KNOW

Change the Medicine

1. If the first medicine does not work at all.
2. If the symptoms change markedly.
3. If the original medicine no longer works after initial improvement.

As long as the first medicine is producing benefit, even if improvement is slow, do not change it. Simply repeat it when needed.

ANTIDOTING FACTORS

If a medicine is not working, it is important to check for factors that may interfere with the medicine's action. The following substances and exposures should be avoided during homeopathic treatment in order to get the best results possible:

Coffee This is the one substance that most often interferes with homeopathic treatment. Even one sip of coffee or a small amount of coffee ice cream, Kahlua, or coffee candy may be sufficient to disturb the treatment, especially in sensitive individuals. Other forms of caffeine, such as black tea and cola drinks, do not interfere.

Electric blankets These affect the action of medicines by altering your body's electromagnetic field.

Aromatic substances Avoid camphor, eucalyptus, and menthol and any products that contain them, including Vick's VapoRub, Noxema, Tiger Balm, BenGay, calamine lotion, and cough drops and lozenges containing these substances. This includes some aromatherapy oils as well as mouthwashes that contain menthol and other aromatic compounds. Other substances that may interfere due to their aromaticity include citronella oil, pennyroyal, and other aromatic herbal mosquito repellents; all tea-tree products; peppermint oil; lavender oil; Olbas spray; and Ricola lozenges. Chapstick, Blistex, Carmex, and other aromatic lip balms should also be avoided, although fruit-flavored balms are fine. Strong fumes from oil-based paint, turpentine, paint thinner, and certain household cleaning agents, such as Pine-Sol, Lysol, and strong-smelling industrial chemicals, may also interfere, depending on individual sensitivity.

Medications Homeopathic medicines will not prevent prescription drugs from working, but some prescription drugs may interfere with homeopathic remedies. When treating yourself homeopathically, it is usually best to avoid topical or internal over-the-counter medications except to relieve pain. *Do not discontinue any prescription medications without conferring with your physician.*

Dental work Dental drilling and the use of Novocain may disturb the effects of homeopathic medicines.

Drugs Avoid all recreational drugs including marijuana, cocaine, LSD, barbiturates, and amphetamines. Alcohol in moderation is not a problem.

Beauty treatments Permanent waves, electrolysis, and aromatic facial and skin products may interfere with homeopathic treatment.

Other therapies Acupuncture and therapeutic ultrasound have been known to disturb homeopathic treatment in some cases.

Avoid During Homeopathic Treatment

- coffee
- products containing camphor, eucalyptus, tea-tree oil, menthol (such as Tiger Balm, Carmex, Vick's VapoRub, Ben-Gay, Olbas, Ricola)
- aromatic herbs and aromatherapy
- acupuncture
- ultrasound
- dental work
- permanents
- electric blankets
- strong solvents
- Lysol
- Pine-Sol
- some prescription medications, particularly antibiotics and steroids (consult your physician)
- other homeopathic medicines (unless prescribed by the person's homeopath)

CHAPTER **8**

Practice Cases for Homeopathic Self-Care

It is time to put into practice what you have learned. Here are some examples of what you or your family members might experience. The numbers in parentheses indicate the underlining from one to three that shows the intensity of each symptom. Follow all of the instructions that we have given you and select the medicine that best fits each case. Answers are in the back of the book.

The Steps for Homeopathic Self-Care

Take the case:

1. Find out the person's main complaint and any symptoms of the acute illness.
2. Find the closest medical condition in the Table of Contents.
3. Use the Look, Listen, and Ask sections to gather all the information you need.

Analyze the case:

1. Read the descriptions of medicines for that medical condition.
2. Choose the medicine that seems to fit the best.
3. Read the description of the medicine in the *Materia Medica* section to confirm your choice.

Give the medicine:

1. Choose the potency and give a dose of medicine
2. Observe the effects of the medicine.
3. Repeat the medicine when needed, or change it if it is not working.

---

1. PUNCTURE WOUND

John, a twenty-five-year-old carpenter, accidentally stepped on a board with a rusty nail sticking out of it. It penetrated the sole of his foot at the heel. He doesn't remember when he had his last tetanus shot. John's heel is unusually cold to the touch (3). He is experiencing a sharp pain in his heel (3). There is no numbness, tingling, or radiating pain.

You recommend that John get a tetanus shot and give him ______________.

2. BURN

Your cousin Melody, age five, goes to a wedding. Her brother, Brian, chases her around the room and she bumps into her aunt, whose hot coffee spills on Melody's leg. She starts screaming. You happen to be nearby with your homeopathic kit and offer to help. There is a two-inch area on Melody's right thigh that is very red (3). There is no swelling. She says that it burns (3) and stings (3), almost like someone pricked her with something.

You give Melody ________________.

3. FLU

Your uncle Jack, a forty-year-old stockbroker, tells you that he feels awful with the flu. It started two days ago. His joints ache all the time (2), especially when he tries to walk around (3). He tried to jog this morning, but he only made it halfway around the track because he was in so much pain. The only thing he feels capable of doing is lying around quietly and reading. Jack tells you that he is extremely thirsty for very cold water (3) and that his mouth and lips feel very parched. The symptoms began two days after the stock market dropped one hundred points. Jack hadn't slept the first night afterward because he kept worrying about his clients.

You give Jack ____________________.

4. COUGH

Your granddaughter, Tracy, is three. Your daughter, Shannon, calls to ask if you can help with Tracy's croupy cough, which began two nights ago. The cough has become violent (3). Once Tracy starts coughing, she goes on and on for up to twenty minutes and can't stop (3). The cough began after Tracy played outside. The air was quite brisk and she became chilled. Now she is so cold that she shivers, even under a down comforter (3). Tracy has a sore throat (2) with pus on her tonsils (2). It feels like she has splinters in her throat (2). She is much fussier than usual (3). The only thing she feels like eating is a salad with vinegar and oil, which she normally doesn't like.

Tracy needs ______________________.

WHAT YOU NEED TO KNOW

5. BLADDER INFECTION

Jan, age thirty-two, just returned from her honeymoon in Hawaii. She had a great time but started having bladder pain on the flight home. She knows that you are interested in homeopathy and asks for your help so that she can avoid taking antibiotics. She and her husband were very sexually active during the honeymoon. She has burning pain in her urethra during urination (2). She feels like urinating often, but nothing comes out most of the time (3). She mentions that she got into a big argument with her mother just before the wedding.

Your choice for Jan is ______________.

6. EAR INFECTION

Seven-month-old River, your cousin's son, has been pulling on his ears and crying for the past two nights (2). The pain seems to be bothering him in both ears. He screams at the top of his lungs with the pain (3), and his parents are very concerned. They would like to try homeopathy before resorting to antibiotics, but if he's not better by tomorrow they will take him to the pediatrician. He has just begun to teethe and is unusually fussy (3). He'll point to his favorite toy, then when his mother hands it to him, he throws it on the floor (2). Nothing seems to please him except when his mother carries him around (3). His mother has also noticed that he has had greenish diarrhea the past few days (2).

You tell her that you think homeopathy can help and give River ____________.

7. FEVER

Nellie, your four-year-old niece, has a high fever. Her mother knows that you are learning about homeopathy and asks for your help. Nellie's fever started last night; it is 103°F (3). Nellie's little cheeks are bright red (3). Her eyes are glassy (2) and her face is hot (3) and dry (3). She's not tugging on her ear and doesn't complain of any ear pain, but she does say that the right side of her throat burns (2). Her mother looked at her throat and sees that it, too, is bright red. The only thing that Nellie feels like eating or drinking is lemonade.

Nellie needs ________________.

8. ABDOMINAL PAIN

Jay, your brother-in-law, has an acute gastrointestinal flu. He went to an Italian restaurant with friends last night for his birthday. He ate a lot of heavy food and drank a little too much. He woke up at 4:30 this morning (2) with severe abdominal cramping (3) and had to run to the bathroom immediately (3). He is having explosive diarrhea (3) and can hear his abdomen rumbling and gurgling (2). He has had three episodes of diarrhea already today. He is feeling exhausted (3). He knows that it will pass with time, but some friends want to take him out for a belated birthday dinner again tonight, and he hopes you can fix him quickly.

Jay should feel a lot better after he takes ____________________.

9. SORE THROAT

Catherine has had a sore throat for the past few days. Her throat feels raw (2) on the right side. Her cervical glands on the right side are swollen (2). Her throat seems to hurt more in the late afternoon around 4:00 or 5:00 P.M. (2). The throat pain started the day after she had to give a big presentation at work. She was very nervous about it and was afraid that she'd look like she didn't know anything. The only thing that relieves Catherine's sore throat is tea that's cooled to room temperature.

You suggest that Catherine take ____________________.

10. BRONCHITIS

Carl, fifty years old, just got bronchitis. He sings in a choir and has been going to a lot of practices because a big performance is coming up. He feels soreness in his chest (2) and is beginning to lose his voice (2). Now his voice sounds hoarse (2). He has a dry cough that is much worse from drafts (3). Carl works as an animal rights advocate.

Carl needs ____________________.

11. COMMON COLD

Your mother, Sally, calls you for help with an awful cold. Her sinuses feel incredibly stuffed (3), and it is hard to breathe through her nose. The worst symptom is severe pressure in her cheekbones (3) and at the top of her nose, where her glasses sit (3). She has tried hot packs, but they only provide relief for ten minutes or so. She has lots of very thick (3), yellowish-green (3), stringy mucus (3) coming out of both nostrils.

You give your mother ______________________.

WHAT YOU NEED TO KNOW

12. MINOR COLLISION

Your partner comes home at the end of the day and tells you that she was rear-ended at a traffic light a couple of hours earlier. Her neck feels a bit sore (2), and her body feels sore and bruised all over (2). She didn't bother calling her doctor or going to the emergency room because she didn't feel that she needed any help.

You tell her to take _______________ and suggest that she see her doctor the next morning to get checked out and have any injuries documented.

13. HEATSTROKE

You and Phil go to the beach the first sunny day of the year. He is red-headed and fair-skinned and doesn't do well in the sun. It's such a nice day that you lie on the beach reading for several hours. You notice that Phil has a very red face (3). His skin is hot (3) and he has a bursting headache (3). Phil seems rather disoriented and spacey.

You give Phil ______________. If it doesn't help within half an hour, your second choice is _________________.

14. SHOCK AFTER A BLOOD DRAW

Sarah has a tendency to be anemic and goes to her doctor to have her blood tested to see whether her iron levels have gone up to normal. Right after the tube of blood is drawn, Sarah starts to feel weak (3) and dizzy (3). She has to put her head between her legs to avoid fainting. The person who drew her blood suggests that she lie down for ten minutes or so. When she gets up, she still feels somewhat weak.

Sarah needs ____________.

15. HAY FEVER

You father, Tom, is fifty. He gets a bad case of hay fever every March. This year, he calls you before trying antihistamines to see if homeopathy can help. His nose is running like a faucet (3). He is sneezing incessantly (3). He is blowing his nose all the time, and the area right under his nose is starting to get red and raw (2). His eyes are also watering a lot (2).

You give your dad __________, and he thinks you're the greatest.

PART 2

MEDICAL CONDITIONS YOU CAN TREAT YOURSELF

CHAPTER 9

The Medical Conditions

USING THIS SECTION EFFECTIVELY

Choose the Correct Medical Condition

1. Select the name of a medical condition that most resembles the symptoms of the person you are treating (the Table of Contents may be helpful here).
2. Read the description of the common symptoms that occur in that kind of problem to see if they match the patient's symptoms; if more than one condition might apply, choose the best match.

Read About the Condition

When the description matches the symptoms of the person who is ill, read carefully the information provided about that condition.

Description
Defines the condition and what causes it.

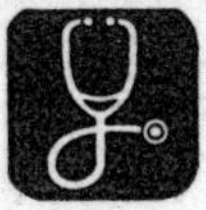

Symptoms
Tells you the common symptoms of the condition.

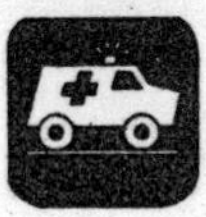

Complications
Indicates problems that may develop in this kind of condition, possible medical emergencies, when to seek medical help, and what kind of help you need.

Use the Look, Listen, and Ask Sections to Guide You in Your Casetaking

Look
Gives you instructions on what to observe about the person who is ill.

Listen
Helps you be attentive to what you may hear about the problem that correlates with the characteristic symptoms of particular homeopathic medicines.

Ask
Gives you specific questions to ask to find out more about the symptoms of the case.

Read the Pointers Section for Finding the Homeopathic Medicine

Pointers for Finding the Homeopathic Medicine
Provides capsule summaries of symptoms you may encounter, and indicates which medicines should be considered or definitely given for those types of symptoms.

Use the Chart of the Homeopathic Medicines

You can read the chart either vertically or horizontally:

- Reading vertically allows you to compare the medicines in relation to a particular criterion. For example, you can read down the column of Key Symptoms for all the listed medicines and compare them.
- Reading horizontally gives you a list of all the symptoms for a particular medicine:

1. First read Key Symptoms for particularly strong or striking symptoms that are characteristic for this homeopathic medicine.

2. Read the Mind entry next for relevant mental and emotional symptoms characteristic for this medicine.

3. Read Body entry next for other physical symptoms covered by the medicine.

4. Read Worse and Better entries next for the factors that affect the person negatively or positively if they need this medicine.

5. Read Food and Drink section next for the characteristic food and beverage desires and aversions, and relative hunger and thirst, of those who need this medicine.

Compare Symptoms

Compare the symptoms you have collected from the sick person with the symptoms that are listed for each medicine.

- Focus on the Key Symptoms.
- If the case has no mental symptoms, disregard the Mind section, but if mental symptoms are prominent make sure to take them into account.
- Pay attention to the other Body symptoms listed and compare them to the symptoms of the person who is ill.
- Match the factors that make the person feel worse or better with the items listed in the Worse and Better categories.
- If there are any strong desires for food or drinks, or anything particularly striking about hunger or thirst, compare the person's desires with those listed under Food and Drink.

Read About the Medicines

Turn to the *Materia Medica* section (Chapter 10) and read about the medicines you find that seem to fit best, based on your casetaking and your reading in this chapter.

- See if any of the other symptoms the person has are listed here under the name of the medicine.
- See if there is a good match between the person's symptoms and the overall impression given by the symptoms listed under the name of the medicine.

Choose the Best Medicine

Most of the sick person's symptoms should be included in the symptoms listed. However, the sick person will probably not have *all* of the symptoms listed for each medicine. The sick person may also have other symptoms which are not listed. That is okay. The medicine that seems to match most closely is probably the correct one; the match does not have to be perfect for the medicine to work.

After Selecting a Medicine

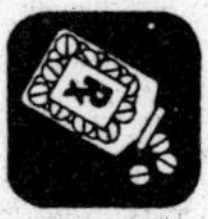

Dosage

Read Dosage to find out how to give the medicine.

What to Expect from Homeopathic Self-Care

Read the What to Expect from Homeopathic Self-Care section to establish a time frame for treatment.

Other Self-Care Suggestions

Read Other Self-Care Suggestions to learn other valuable, effective, and natural therapies to help the person regain health.

Abscesses

(See also Skin Infections.)

Description

An abscess is an enclosed pocket in the tissue filled with pus, usually caused by the body's reaction to bacterial infection.

Symptoms

Abscesses are accompanied by heat, pain, swelling, redness, and tenderness over the site of the abscess. Fever may be present, but not always. Abscesses are difficult to heal without treatment.

Complications

Sometimes abscesses must be surgically drained in order to release the pus. If the abscess is severely painful, or if you observe any red streaks radiating from the area, get immediate medical attention.

Look

What do you observe about the abscess?
Is the abscess draining? If so, what color is the pus? Is it bloody?
Is there redness of the skin around the site of the abscess? Discoloration?
Is the abscess red? If so, bright or dark red? Is it blue?
Is there swelling? Tenderness?
Are there swollen lymph nodes nearby?

Listen

"Ow! Don't touch it! Quick, cover it up again!" *Hepar sulphuris*
"It feels like it's going to explode from the pressure." *Lachesis*
"I have a bad taste in my mouth and I've been drooling." *Mercurius*
"I've been sweating a lot more than usual and it smells bad." *Mercurius*
"It feels like there is something inside the abscess." *Silica*

Ask

How much does it hurt?
What does the pain feel like?
What makes it feel better or worse?

Do you feel warm or chilly?
Have you been craving anything to eat or drink?

Pointers for Finding the Homeopathic Medicine

Hepar sulphuris and *Silica* are the most common medicines for abscesses. ▮ For an abscess that is exquisitely sensitive to pain, cold, and touch, in a very irritable chilly person, give *Hepar sulphuris.* ▮ For an abscess from a foreign body give *Silica* unless the symptoms are particularly like *Hepar sulphuris.* ▮ For abscesses that are purplish or mottled, left-sided, and much better from discharging, in a talkative, intense person, give *Lachesis.* ▮ For abscesses that are very foul-smelling in a chilly, sweaty person with bad breath and a bad or metallic taste in the mouth, give *Mercurius.*

Dosage

- Give three pellets of 30C every four hours until you see improvement.
- If there is no improvement after three doses, give a different medicine.
- After you first notice improvement, give another dose only if symptoms begin to return.
- Lower potencies (6X, 6C, 30X) may need to be given more frequently (every two to four hours).
- Higher potencies (200X, 200C, 1M) usually only need to be given once, but can be given again if there is a definite relapse.

What to Expect from Homeopathic Self-Care

Homeopathic medicines reduce fever and inflammation and may stimulate the body to promote spontaneous drainage of the abscess. If you are not getting results within two to three days, seek medical attention, especially if high fever or red streaks are present.

Other Self-Care Suggestions

If the abscess is draining, cover it with a gauze dressing and keep the area clean. ▮ Alternating hot (five minutes) and cold (one minute) wet compresses stimulates circulation and healing. ▮ Use massage techniques that specifically promote drainage of the lymph system. ▮ A combination of echinacea and goldenseal (two dropperfuls of tincture in water three times a day or two capsules four times a day) can be useful to stimulate the immune system to fight infection. ▮ Apply *Calendula* tincture (diluted one part to three parts water) to the area once it has drained. ▮ Give beta-carotene: 50,000 IU once a day. ▮ Give zinc: 30 mg once a day. ▮ Give vitamin C: 1000 mg three times a day.

	Key Symptoms	Mind	Body	Worse	Better	Food & Drink
Hepar sulphuris *(Calcium sulfide)*	**Extreme sensitivity to pain, cold, and touch** **Extreme sensitivity to cold air, a cold cloth, or an ice pack** **Splinter-like pains**	**Very irritable** **Quarrelsome** **Complaining**	**Abscess is very painful, especially to touch** **Thick pus and bad-smelling discharges, smelling sour or like rotten cheese** Helps expel foreign bodies	**Cold** Drafts Uncovering any part of the body	Warmth	Desire for vinegar Desire for fat and sour flavors
Lachesis *(Bushmaster snake)*	**Abscess has bluish-purple or black appearance** **More likely to be on the left side of the body or to go from left to right**	**Talkative** Intense Jealous	**Abscesses feel better as soon as they drain** Abscesses form at the roots of the teeth, in muscles, tonsils, lymph glands, or organs Abscesses filled with pus	**Constriction** Heat During and after sleep	Open air	Desire for oysters
Mercurius *(Mercury)*	**Abscesses form ulcers and discharge bad-smelling pus** **Made worse by both heat and cold; sensitive like the mercury in a thermometer**	Suspicious Hurried Hesitant Reserved	**Bad breath** **Increased saliva** Abscesses have inflammation with burning and stinging pain Rapid formation of pus Metallic taste in the mouth Chilly and sweaty Trembling of the extremities	**Night** Sweating	Moderate temperature	Desire for bread and butter
Silica *(Flint)*	**Abscesses may originate from a foreign body like a splinter** **Abscesses have not yet drained** **Low stamina and energy** **Refined, delicate features**	Refined Delicate Timid Precise	**Lymph nodes are swollen and hard** **Abscess is filled with bad-smelling pus** Slow to heal, with an irritating, thin, offensive discharge Sour, offensive foot sweat, and perspiration on head and neck Chilly and exhausted	**Suppression of sweat by antiperspirants** Cold, drafts New or full moon	Warmth	Desire for sweets and eggs Aversion to fat and milk

Allergic Reactions

(See also Hay Fever, Insect Bites and Stings, Hives, Poison Ivy.)

Description

Allergic reactions can be mild or severe. They occur when the body is exposed to an allergen—a substance in the environment that causes an immune-system response. The response is triggered by the release of histamine from the mast cells, which are part of the immune system. Allergic reactions are caused by an immune-system response that is greater than is needed to respond to the presence of a foreign substance in the body.

Symptoms

Allergic symptoms include swelling, itching, redness, inflammation, sneezing, mucous discharges, hives or other skin rashes, asthma, and systemic shock, as seen in an anaphylactic response.

Complications

Anaphylactic shock and respiratory arrest: If the person has a severe reaction to an allergen, including significant itching and swelling of lymph nodes, swelling of the mucous membranes of the nose and ears, and difficulty breathing due to constriction of the air passages, this is likely to be an anaphylactic response and requires emergency care. If untreated, anaphylaxis can be rapidly fatal.

Look

Is there respiratory distress, collapse, unconsciousness, rapid pulse, sweating, or paleness, indicating an anaphylactic reaction or asthmatic attack? If so, get emergency medical attention immediately.
Do you see hives, skin rashes, inflammation, or swelling?
Is there mucous discharge, especially from nose? What color and consistency?
Is the person sneezing, with watery eyes?

Listen

"My nose is running like a faucet." *Allium cepa*
"I can't breathe," or "I feel like I'm going to pass out" (get emergency medical attention immediately). *Apis* (see Insect Bites and Stings)
"My eyelids are so swollen that I can barely open them." *Apis*

"These allergies are so bad that I'm afraid I'm going to die!" *Arsenicum*
"The blisters are so itchy that I can't stop scratching." *Rhus toxicodendron*
"Whenever I eat clams, I get hives." *Urtica urens*

Ask

What did the exposure occur and the symptoms start?
What is the nature of the reaction?
How intense is it?
What are you experiencing now?
Are you in any pain or acute distress?
Are you having any particular sensations anywhere in your body?
What do you need to feel better now?
Does anything make your symptoms feel better or worse?
Have you had any mental or emotional changes just before or since the reaction?
Are you desiring anything to eat or drink?
Do you feel warm or chilly?

Pointers for Finding the Homeopathic Medicine

If the person's nose runs like a faucet with streaming eyes, think of *Allium cepa.* ▮ If swelling and stinging pains are the most prominent symptoms, consider *Apis.* ▮ If anxiety and restlessness are the most significant symptoms, think of *Arsenicum.* ▮ If symptoms occur after getting wet or overwork, and stiffness and itching eruptions are present, give *Rhus toxicodendron.* ▮ If the allergic reaction is to shellfish, or feels like stinging nettles or a burn, give *Urtica urens.*

Dosage

- Give three pellets of 30C every two hours until you see improvement.
- In severe allergic reactions, you can give a dose up to once an hour.
- If there is no improvement after three doses, give a different medicine.
- After you first notice improvement, give another dose only if symptoms begin to return.
- Lower potencies (6X, 6C, 30X) may need to be given more often (every one to four hours, depending on the severity of the allergic reaction).
- Higher potencies (200X, 200C, 1M) generally need to be given only once except in a very severe allergic reaction. In the case of anaphylaxis,

you can give a dose up to every fifteen minutes while the person is transported to emergency care.

What to Expect from Homeopathic Self-Care

Homeopathic medicines relieve the symptoms of an acute allergic attack rapidly. Constitutional treatment helps remove the underlying predisposition to allergy, helping the immune system have a more appropriate response to allergenic exposures.

Other Self-Care Suggestions

For shock: lie down, keep warm, drink fluids. ▮ For itching: soak in a bathtub of warm water with one cup of baking soda or one cup of raw oatmeal. ▮ For swelling: ice pack or cold wet compresses. ▮ Give a glass of one to two Alka-Seltzer Gold tablets dissolved in water. ▮ Give one teaspoon baking soda in a glass of water. ▮ Give 500 mg buffered Vitamin C every two hours until symptoms pass, up to 3000 mg per day.

	Key Symptoms	Mind	Body	Worse	Better	Food & Drink
Allium cepa *(Red onion)*	**Thin, watery, irritating nasal discharge, pouring like a faucet** **Eyes and nose run as if person were peeling an onion**	Fear that the pain will become unbearable	**Burning nasal discharge, especially from the left nostril** **Red, very watery eyes with a non-irritating discharge** **Sneezing** Hacking, tickling cough; worse from breathing cold air	Warm room	Cool, open air	Desire for onions Aversion to cucumbers
Apis *(Honeybee)*	**Swelling** **Stinging pain that feels better from a cold cloth or ice pack** **Anaphylactic shock (see Insect Bites and Stings)**	**Busy** Active Irritable if crossed	**Heat, redness, and stinging pain, with lots of swelling** **Affected area is hot, worse from heat, and better from a cold cloth or ice pack** **Hives with burning, stinging, and itching after a bite or sting** Itching is intolerable at night	Heat, hot drinks, or bath	**Cool air, cold baths** Uncovering	Not usually thirsty
Arsenicum album *(Arsenic)*	**Thin, watery, burning nasal discharge** **Burning in the eyes** **Asthmatic attacks with great anxiety**	**Restless and anxious** **Needy and demanding** Fear of being alone Fear of dying	**Burning pains anywhere in the body** **Hives (can be from shellfish)** Heart palpitations Sneezing	**Cold; cold cloth or ice pack** **Cold food and drink**	**Warmth** **Hot cloth or hot water bottle** Warm food	**Thirsty for small sips frequently** Desire for fat and sour foods and drinks

		get well Insomnia from midnight to 2:00 A.M.		**midnight** Bad food or meat Vegetables		
Rhus toxicodendron *(Poison ivy)*	**Skin eruptions like poison ivy** **Water-filled blisters** **Terrible itching** **Hives**	Restless Jovial	**Extremely restless; can't get comfortable** **Allergic skin eruptions along with joint stiffness**	**Cold baths or showers** **Scratching** Night Rest	Hot baths or showers	Desire for cold milk
Urtica urens *(Stinging nettle)*	**Allergy to shellfish** **Hives** **Stinging, burning pains**	Restless	**Itching, raised red welts or hives** **Burning, itching skin (see Burns)** Insect bites and stings	Cold baths or showers Cool, moist air	Rubbing Lying down	

Amebic Dysentery (Amebiasis)
(See also Diarrhea and Food Poisoning.)

Description

Amebiasis is a parasitic infection caused by a microorganism called *Entamoeba histolytica,* more commonly known as amebas. It is usually contracted by ingesting cysts in drinking water or food contaminated with stool. It is more frequent in parts of the world where sanitation is poor, and is a problem often encountered by travelers to developing countries.

Symptoms

The main symptoms of amebic dysentery are painful abdominal cramps, loose watery stools, and gas. The stools may contain mucus and blood, and are infectious. Amebas frequently cause liver swelling and tenderness and, less commonly, abscesses in the liver. The diagnosis is confirmed primarily by a laboratory examination of the stool called an "ova and parasite" test. Sometimes several stool samples are needed to find the amebas.

Complications

Since amebiasis may be confused with ulcerative colitis, irritable bowel syndrome, and other parasitic infections, diagnosis by a qualified medical professional is recommended. Dehydration, blood loss, and death are possible complications.

Look

Observe the stool, if possible. Note the color, consistency, and odor of the stool.
Are the eyes sunken?
Are the lips dry and chapped?
Get the stool tested for parasites.

Listen

"My stools are like jello." *Aloe*
"I'm afraid that I'm really sick and will die." *Arsenicum album*
"I feel so nauseated that I just want to vomit." *Ipecac*
"My bowel movements shoot out all over the toilet." *Podophyllum, Croton tiglium, Gambogia*

Ask

When did the diarrhea start?
How long has it been going on?
What is the stool like?
Is there pain or cramping?
Is there gas?
What makes the diarrhea better or worse?
What time of day does it occur?
Did any other physical symptoms start along with the diarrhea?
Are there any mental or emotional symptoms with the diarrhea?
How is your sleep?

Pointers for Finding the Homeopathic Medicine

If the person is extremely anxious and restless with diarrhea, give *Arsenicum album.* ▮ If the person has exhausting diarrhea with lots of cramping, think of *Arsenicum album* and *Podophyllum.* ▮ If the stool is explosive, consider *Croton tiglium, Gambogia,* or *Podophyllum.* ▮ If there is significant nausea and vomiting, first consider *Ipecac,* then *Arsenicum album.* ▮ If there is lots of rumbling and gurgling in the abdomen, give *Podophyllum, Croton tiglium,* or *Gambogia.* ▮ If there is profuse diarrhea and cramping with sweating and shivering, first think of *Veratrum album* then *Arsenicum album.*

Dosage

- Give three pellets of 30C every two hours until you see improvement.
- If the diarrhea is severe, give a dose every hour.
- If there is no improvement after three doses, give a different medicine.
- After you first notice improvement, give another dose only if symptoms begin to return.
- Lower potencies (6X, 6C, 30X) may need to be given more often (every one to four hours depending on the severity of the symptoms).
- Higher potencies (200X, 200C, 1M) generally need to be given only once, but may be repeated if the diarrhea is profuse and very frequent or if there is severe pain.

What to Expect from Homeopathic Self-Care

Diarrhea, cramps, and gas should disappear over several hours to several days.

Other Self-Care Suggestions

Drink plenty of fluids and replenish electrolytes, including sodium and potassium. Recharge, Gatorade, Emergen-C, and electrolyte solutions available from pharmacies are useful. Clear liquids such as water, vegetable broth, and diluted fruit juice help replace fluids. ▮ The diet should be light and bland; include vegetable soup, whole-grain toast, brown rice, bananas, and applesauce. ▮ A warm pack over the abdomen is soothing and may reduce cramping. Calcium (1000 mg) and Magnesium (500 mg) per day may also help to reduce cramping. ▮ One tablespoon of psyllium seed husks per day often helps to firm up stools.

	Key Symptoms	Mind	Body	Worse	Better	Food & Drink
Aloe *(Aloe socotrina)*	**Feeling of insecurity in the rectum as though stool would come out** **Hemorrhoids bleed and protrude like a bunch of grapes**	Irritable, discontented, or angry, with abdominal pain or constipation Does not want to be around people	**Stools are lumpy, gelatinous, slimy, bloody, and watery** **Feels like stool will come out while passing gas, and it does** Stool may be bright yellow Mucus and burning pain in the rectum after stool Rumbling and gurgling in the bowels; sudden urging to pass a watery, gushing stool Beer and oysters cause diarrhea	Heat, summer, hot damp weather After eating or drinking	Cool open air, cold bathing, cold cloth or ice pack Passing gas	
Arsenicum album *(Arsenic)*	**Severe abdominal cramping** **Burning pains in the abdomen and rectum** **Diarrhea is worse after eating and drinking, especially fruit and cold food or drinks**	**Restless and anxious** Needy and demanding Afraid of being alone Afraid of death Complains that she won't get well Insomnia 1:00 to 2:00 A.M.	**Very weak and wiped out** **Extremely chilly** Stools are frequent, dark, watery, and foul-smelling, with blood and mucus	**After midnight, 1:00 to 2:00 A.M.** Cold	Heat Warm food and drinks	**Thirst for frequent sips of cold water** Desire for milk, fat on meat, sour foods
Croton tiglium *(Croton oil seed)*	**Diarrhea gushing like a fire hydrant combined with skin rash like poison ivy** **Diarrhea immediately after eating or drinking**	Anxious, as though something bad will happen, during the diarrhea	**Diarrhea shoots out explosively in one big gush** **Strong urge to have a bowel movement with lots of watery diarrhea**	**Drinking or eating the least amount** Washing	After sleep Gentle rubbing	

continued on next page

	Key Symptoms	Mind	Body	Worse	Better	Food & Drink
Croton tiglium *(Croton oil seed)* *continued*			**Gurgling in the intestines from drinking even a little liquid or from eating a small amount of food** Sensation of sloshing in the intestines as if there is only water in them Emptiness in the stomach Nausea with retching and vomiting Skin eruption feels thick and stiff			
Gambogia *(Gummi gutti tree)*	**Severe diarrhea** **Stools come out suddenly and in gushes**	Cheerful and talkative Depression alternating with diarrhea	**Stools come out in thin, prolonged gushes** **Rumbling and rolling in abdomen** **Gurgling before stool** Diarrhea with vomiting Burning of anus	Toward evening and at night After stool Motion Open air	After stool	
Ipecac *(Ipecac root)*	**Vomiting and nausea with nearly all complaints**	Hard to please Does not know what he wants Disgusted with everything	**Extreme vomiting** **Constant nausea, not relieved by vomiting** **Sinking sensation in the stomach and nausea at the smell of food** Tongue is usually clean despite vomiting Cutting, clawing, cramping pains in the abdomen, especially around the navel Very painful straining with bowel move-	Warmth Eating or drinking Overeating, especially rich food Vomiting	Cold Fresh air	

Podophyllum *(May apple)*	**Traveler's diarrhea** **Rumbling and gurgling before the stool** **Abdominal cramping with diarrhea, leading to exhaustion**	Fidgety, restless, and whining Imagines she will become very ill or die	**Stools are frequent, profuse, and liquid** **Stools shoot out forcibly with gas into the toilet** **Stools smell bad** Diarrhea is often painless Yellowish-green stools Liver pain	**Early morning around 4:00 or 5:00 A.M.** **Hot weather** Sour fruit Eating or drinking Motion	Rubbing the liver Lying on the abdomen Bending forward	
Veratrum album *(White hellebore)*	**Violent vomiting and diarrhea** **Icy cold with cold sweat**	**Very active and busy** Restless	**Diarrhea profuse, painful, watery** **Forceful diarrhea followed by exhaustion and cold sweat** **Collapse with bluish color of the face** Stools like rice water (as in cholera)	**Cold** **Cold drinks** **Menstrual period** **Fruit**	Warmth Hot drinks Covering up	**Desire for sour juicy fruits, lemons, salt, cold drinks, and ice**

Back Pain, Acute

(See also Sciatica.)

Description

Pain in the back may be caused by a strain or sprain, by misalignment of the spinal vertebrae, or by pelvic bones causing pressure on nerves. Back tension and spasms may also be caused by emotional states such as anger or fear.

Symptoms

Pain is present in the affected part of the back. The low back and neck are the most common sites of acute back pain. It is sometimes difficult and painful for the person to move or straighten up. Pain may be either dull or quite sharp, particularly when moving about. Muscles around the site of the pain are often in spasm.

Complications

Some acute back pain may be caused by a herniated vertebral disk. This type of pain usually extends into a limb and may be quite severe and accompanied by numbness. It is usually worse when sneezing, coughing or holding the breath, and bearing down. (See Sciatica.) Acute pain in the mid-back may be caused by kidney stones or a kidney infection. Medical attention should be sought immediately for proper diagnosis, especially if fever is present or the pain is excruciating.

Look

Does the person need a particular position or posture to be comfortable?
Are there any visible signs of injury?

Listen

"There is nothing wrong with me. Go away!" *Arnica*
"I'm stressed out and I want to go home." *Bryonia*
"My tailbone hurts!" *Hypericum*
"I feel stiff all over." *Rhus toxicodendron*

Ask

Was there any injury?
Where is the pain?

What does the pain feel like?
What makes it better or worse?
Does the pain extend to anywhere else?
Are there any mental or emotional symptoms with the back pain?

Pointers for Finding the Homeopathic Medicine

Give *Arnica* for sore, bruised back pain after an injury or trauma. ▮ *Arnica* is used before and after back surgery to promote healing. ▮ *Bryonia* is the best medicine when the main symptom is pain that is made worse by moving. ▮ *Hypericum* is good for direct injuries to the spine or nerves, with shooting pain. ▮ Give *Rhus toxicodendron* when the pain is made worse by overexertion and getting wet, and better by limbering up and moving around.

Dosage

- Give three pellets of 30C three times a day until you see improvement.
- If there is no improvement after three doses or two days, give a different medicine.
- After you first notice improvement, give another dose only if symptoms begin to return.
- Lower potencies (6X, 6C, 30X) may need to be given more often (every four hours).
- Higher potencies (200X, 200C, 1M) usually only need to be given once. Repeat only if the symptoms definitely return after being relieved.

What to Expect from Homeopathic Self-Care

Homeopathic medicines can produce quick results in acute back pain, often helping a person get over it in a day or two.

Other Self-Care Suggestions

When the injury first occurs, apply an ice pack if there is swelling or inflammation. ▮ After twelve to twenty-four hours, apply moist heat to the area. ▮ Take a hot bath with one cup of Epsom salts added. Whirlpool baths or hot tubs are also good. ▮ Rest in bed in a comfortable position. ▮ Acupuncture, chiropractic, osteopathy, physical therapy, Bowen therapy (an Australian bodywork technique), massage, or other bodywork techniques are often helpful if homeopathy is not producing immediate results. Do not use acupuncture, however, if the homeopathy is effective for the back pain, because it may interfere. ▮ Take Calcium (1500 mg) and Magnesium (750 mg) daily to reduce muscle spasms. ▮ *Arnica* gel or oil or *Traumeel* ointment is very helpful when applied locally to the area. (If you are under constitutional treatment, consult your homeopath before using *Traumeel,* since it is a combination homeopathic medicine.) ▮ Back strengthening exercises and proper lifting techniques are essential to preventing future back injuries. ▮ Being overweight contributes to chronic or recurrent back pain. Consider losing some weight. ▮ Yoga or other stretching techniques are excellent to strengthen back muscles once the acute pain or injury has passed.

	Key Symptoms	Mind	Body	Worse	Better	Food & Drink
Arnica *(Leopard's bane)*	**Back pain after an injury or trauma** **Bruised, sore feeling in the back**	**Wants to be left alone** **Says there is nothing wrong with him**	Wants to lie down, but the bed feels too hard and he looks for a softer spot	Touch Lying on hard surfaces Motion	Lying down, especially with the head low	
Bryonia *(Wild hops)*	**Back pain worse from any movement** **Neck very stiff and painful**	Very irritable Stressed out from business; talks only of business matters Wants to go home	Sharp pain and stiffness in the small of back is made worse by walking or turning Low back pain, made worse by bending over	Motion Coughing Sneezing	Lying on the painful side Pressure	
Hypericum *(St. John's wort)*	**Injuries to the spine, nerves, or tailbone with sharp, shooting pains** **Pain in the coccyx (tailbone) from a fall or blow** **Numbness and tingling** **Shooting pain radiating upward from the injured area**	Sad	**Herniated disk (also consult a physician)**	Touch Jarring the injured area	Rubbing Lying face-down Bending backward	
Rhus toxicodendron *(Poison ivy)*	**Back pain from overexertion** **Back pain worse from cold, damp, or getting wet** **Stiffness of the joints on first getting up**	**Restless and hurried** Jovial	**Pain when getting up from sitting or lying** **Must stretch or walk around** **Extreme restlessness in the body** Chilly	**Cold, damp** **Sitting for long periods of time**	**Continued motion** **Stretching** **Hot baths**	

Bladder Infections (Cystitis)

Description

Bladder infections are caused by microorganisms that colonize the bladder in susceptible patients. Bladder infections may have no apparent symptoms even though bacteria can be cultured from the urine. Symptoms may also occur with no apparent infection.

Symptoms

The most common symptoms are urgent desire to urinate, frequent urination, bladder pain, low back pain, and burning pain before, during, or after urination. Bladder infections occur most commonly in women following sexual intercourse, especially with a new partner. Bladder infections can also occur after waiting too long without urinating or going too long without drinking liquids. Catheterization is a common source of bladder infections in hospitals and nursing homes. Bladder infections often come on with sudden severity, but can progress gradually.

Complications

There is risk of bladder infections ascending up the ureter to cause acute pyelonephritis, a serious infection of the kidneys. Pain along the sides of the mid-back along with urinary frequency, urgency, and pain is indicative of a kidney infection and requires immediate treatment.

Look

Does the person need to urinate frequently?
Do they urinate in an unusual posture or position?
What color is the urine?
Is there sediment in the urine?

Listen

"My bladder and urethra feel very swollen and stinging." *Apis*
"I have a terrible burning pain in my bladder and blood in my urine, and both came on very suddenly." *Cantharis*
"I've got to go, I can't hold it back, but it hurts so badly to urinate." *Mercurius corrosivus*

"I feel burning where the urine comes out at the end of urination."
Sarsaparilla
"I get a bladder infection whenever I have sex with a new partner."
Staphysagria

Ask

When did the symptoms begin? Was there a causative factor?
How quick was the onset of symptoms?
How severe are the symptoms?
Do you experience pain? Where? What type of pain?
What makes the pain better or worse?
Do you have frequent urination?
Do you have urgency (have to run to the bathroom)?
Do you feel any pain in your back?

Pointers for Finding the Homeopathic Medicine

The most common medicines for bladder infections are *Cantharis* and *Staphysagria.* ▮ Think of *Apis* if the pain is mostly stinging and burning, there is any swelling, the last drops feel scalding, and the urine will not come out easily. ▮ Give *Cantharis* if blood in the urine is prominent or the pain is excruciating. *Cantharis* has the most extreme bladder symptoms. ▮ If the major symptom is frequent, intense urging with very severe pain, give *Mercurius corrosivus.* ▮ *Sarsaparilla* is a very common medicine for women's bladder infections. ▮ If the major symptom is burning in the urethra at the close of urination, give *Sarsaparilla.* If it doesn't work, look at *Staphysagria* or *Cantharis.* ▮ If the bladder infection comes on after sex, consider *Staphysagria* first.

Dosage

- Give three pellets of 30C every one to two hours until you see improvement.
- If there is no improvement after three doses, give a different medicine.
- After you first notice improvement, give another dose only if symptoms begin to return.
- Lower potencies (6X, 6C, 30X) may need to be given more often (every one to four hours depending on the severity of the pain and urgency).

- Higher potencies (200X, 200C, 1M) usually need to be given only once but may need to be repeated if the symptoms of the bladder infection are severe or return after initial improvement.

What to Expect from Homeopathic Self-Care

Bladder infections respond best if homeopathic treatment is begun as soon as the symptoms first appear, since they can progress very rapidly in some cases. Homeopathic medicines can relieve the pain of the bladder infection and stimulate the immune system to eliminate the infectious microorganisms. Where inflammation is present without infection, homeopathic medicines are also effective. Acute homeopathic treatment will only address the immediate infection. Constitutional homeopathy is highly effective in reducing underlying susceptibility to prevent future bladder infections.

Other Self-Care Suggestions

Drink as much water as possible. ▮ Take cranberry concentrate or capsules to acidify the urine. Cranberry juice is adequate if that is all that is available, but it has a high sugar content. ▮ Urinate whenever you have the urge. ▮ Avoid horseback riding or other activities that put pressure on the urethra and bladder. ▮ Take bladder herbs such as Oregon grape, *Bucchu, Pipsissewa,* and *Uva ursi* every two hours until symptoms improve. The dosage will depend on whether it is a tea, capsule, or tincture. ▮ Some people get bladder infections from being chilled; if so, bundle up. ▮ If citrus fruits aggravate your bladder, avoid them. ▮ Prevention suggestions include drinking liquids frequently and urinating as soon as possible after you feel the urge and after sex.

	Key Symptoms	Mind	Body	Worse	Better	Food & Drink
Apis *(Honeybee)*	**Scalding urine, especially the last drops** **Stinging, burning pains** **Swelling of parts of the body**	**Busy** Active Irritable if crossed	**Urination is frequent and can be involuntary** **Feels as though the urine will not come out** Urine tends to be suppressed or difficult to pass Sediment in the urine looks like coffee grounds Infant goes a long time without urinating then cries out with pain	**Heat, hot rooms, hot drinks, a hot bath, or lying under covers in bed** Pressure After sleep Lying down Exercise	**Cool air or cold bath or shower** Uncovering Motion Sitting erect	
Cantharis *(Spanish fly)*	**Extreme symptoms** **Very rapid onset of bladder symptoms** **Intolerable pain** **Bloody urine** **Tremendous urgency and frequency**	In a frenzy	**Intense stinging, cutting, and burning pain on urination** **Urine is scalding and comes out drop by drop with intolerable pain** **Constant desire to urinate** **Strains tremendously to urinate** Fever and chills Strong sexual desire	**Urinating** Cold drinks Hearing the sound of water	Rubbing Rest Warmth Lying quietly on her back	
Mercurius corrosivus *(Mercuric chloride)*	**Tremendous urge to urinate** **The urge to urinate is not relieved by urination** **Urine is only passed drop by drop with great pain** **Intense burning in the urethra** **Urine is hot and burning**	Anxious and restless Difficulty thinking and speaking clearly	Bleeding of urethra after urination Spasm of bladder and rectum	Urination	Rest	

continued on next page

	Key Symptoms	Mind	Body	Worse	Better	Food & Drink
Sarsaparilla *(Wild licorice)*	**Severe pain in the urethra at the end of urination**	Anxious and depressed from the pain	**Urine may be difficult to pass while sitting, only dribbling out** Can only urinate while standing Urine is scanty, slimy, flaky, sandy, or bloody Pain from the right kidney extending downward Gas released from the bladder during urination Bladder is tender and swollen Child screams before and during urination	At night Yawning Motion	Standing Uncovering the neck and chest	
Staphysagria *(Stavesacre)*	**"Honeymoon cystitis" (occurs following sexual intercourse)**	**Symptoms come on after suppressed anger, indignation, embarrassment, or insult** Mild personality Wants to please	**Desires to urinate but can't after sex with a new partner or during pregnancy** **Sensation of a drop of urine continuously rolling along the urethra** Burning in the urethra while urinating Urging and pain after urination Frequent urge to urinate results in a scanty or profuse discharge of watery urine	**Too much sex** Masturbation	Warmth Rest Expressing emotions	

Bleeding
(See also Nosebleeds.)

Description
Bleeding, or hemorrhage, is a flow of blood from the arteries, veins, or capillaries, occurring internally or through any of the natural openings of the body or from damage to the tissues or blood vessels. There are many causes of abnormal bleeding, ranging from wounds, trauma, and acute conditions, such as a nosebleed, to chronic conditions such as hemorrhoids, hemorrhagic disorders, or cancer.

Symptoms
Bleeding is characterized by a flow of blood, ranging in color from bright red to black, from anywhere in the body. The blood may spurt if it comes from an artery, or flow more passively if it originates in a vein. The most common symptoms of blood loss are weakness, fatigue, dizziness, a fai feeling, thirst, perspiration, and, later, changes in pulse and breathing. Anemia is confirmed through a complete blood count.

Complications
Extreme blood loss due to injury, postpartum hemorrhage (after childbirth), uncontrolled uterine bleeding due to other causes, or undetected internal bleeding can result in anemia, dehydration, shock, or death. Get medical attention immediately if blood loss is severe.

Look
What is the source of the bleeding?
What is the color of the blood?
How much blood is being lost?
Is the blood flowing passively or is it spurting?
Has there been an injury?
What is the person's position and attitude?
Is immediate care required?

Listen
"I'm just fine. I don't need your help" *Arnica*
"I feel like I'm going to faint." *China*

"My blood is black and comes out slowly. I don't know if I can trust you." *Crotalus horridus*
"I always get anemia after I bleed. Could you please talk more softly?" *Ferrum metallicum*
"I feel like my veins are going to burst." *Hamamelis*
"I started bleeding after I ran around the block. The blood is bright red." *Millefolium*
"I always bleed easily. Could you please get me some ice water?" *Phosphorus*

Ask

What happened?
How are you feeling?
What are your symptoms?
Has this happened before?
Do we need to get help?
What makes the bleeding better or worse?
Are you in pain? If so, where? Describe the pain.
What makes the pain better or worse?
Are there any mental or emotional symptoms since the bleeding began?

Pointers for Finding the Homeopathic Medicine

The first medicine to give for bleeding resulting from injury or trauma is *Arnica.* ▮ For bleeding in which the person has bright red cheeks, consider *Belladonna* or *Ferrum metallicum.* ▮ For blood loss in a weak, pale, collapsed person, give *China.* ▮ If there is dark blood oozing from various parts of the body, give *Crotalus horridus.* ▮ For bleeding from the veins with a full feeling in the veins, the medicine is *Hamamelis.* ▮ If the bleeding is caused by a fall or overexertion and the blood is bright red, look at *Millefolium.* ▮ For a person who bleeds easily and the blood is fluid, bright red, and without clots, give *Phosphorus.*

Dosage

- Give three pellets of 30C every ten to thirty minutes until you see improvement.
- In an emergency situation, give a high potency if you have it. Higher potencies (200X, 200C, 1M) usually only need to be given once, but can be given again if there is a definite relapse, especially in an emergency.

- If there is no improvement after three doses, give a different medicine.
- After you first notice improvement, give another dose only if symptoms begin to return.
- Lower potencies (6X, 6C, 30X) may need to be given more often (every five minutes to an hour).
- Higher potencies (200X, 200C, 1M) usually need to be given only once, but may need to be repeated if the symptoms of the bladder infection are severe or return after initial improvement.

What to Expect from Homeopathic Self-Care

Homeopathic medicines can stop or slow down bleeding within fifteen minutes to several hours. If bleeding is profuse, or if bleeding continues, seek immediate medical attention. Chronic bleeding should be diagnosed by a qualified medical professional, and often responds to constitutional homeopathic treatment depending on the cause. Iron supplementation is often required, depending on the type of anemia.

Other Self-Care Suggestions

Take whatever first-aid measures are necessary to stop the bleeding, including applying pressure directly to the injury with a clean cloth or by applying pressure to the pressure points above the injured area or by wrapping the injury with gauze or cloth. ▮ Bach Rescue Remedy, taken five drops under the tongue every ten to thirty minutes, is helpful for shock if *Arnica* is not available. ▮ Apply *Calendula* tincture or a combination of *Calendula* and *Hypericum* tinctures directly to the bleeding area. ▮ Never apply topical *Arnica* preparations to open wounds because they can cause a rash. ▮ Dried cinnamon applied directly to the area can sometimes stop bleeding. ▮ *Geranium, Trillium,* and Shepherd's purse can all be taken internally for bleeding. Take one-half teaspoon of tincture every one to two hours up to four times a day. ▮ If weakness occurs from bleeding, take iron supplementation. The dosage depends on the form of iron, the degree of anemia, and the cause and degree of bleeding. ▮ Consult a book on Chinese medicine to learn about specific acupressure points to stop bleeding.

	Key Symptoms	Mind	Body	Worse	Better	Food & Drink
Arnica *(Leopard's bane)*	**Bleeding from any area of the body due to trauma** **Bleeding followed by bruising** **Body feels sore and bruised after bleeding**	**Refuses help** **Says she is just fine**	Internal and external bleeding	**Injuries** **Touch**	Lying down with the head low	
Belladonna *(Deadly nightshade)*	**Bright red bleeding** **Sudden bleeding or other symptoms** **Right-sided symptoms** **Flushed face**	Hallucinations during shock or fever Angry rages	**Active bleeding from blood vessels or capillaries causing congestion of blood, throbbing, and dilation of the arteries**	Letting the affected part hang down	Bending backward Bed rest	**Desire for lemons or lemonade** Either very thirsty or not thirsty at all
Cinchona officinalis *(China)*	**Weak, pale, collapsed** **Profuse, exhausting bleeding**	**Irritable, sensitive, and moody** **Fantasies about great things he'd like to do** **Feeling of persecution**	Bleeding with coldness of the body Perspiration with weakness	Touch Drafts	Hard pressure Loose clothing Warmth	Desire for cherries, sweets, salty and spicy foods
Crotalus horridus *(Rattlesnake)*	**Bleeding from all openings of the body** **Dark, unclotted blood** **Slow, oozing hemorrhages**	Feels someone is behind her	**Profound weakness and shock**	Lying on the right side	Motion	

Ferrum metallicum *(Iron)*	**Bright red hemorrhages with small clots** **Bright red cheeks or pale face** **Anemia after bleeding**	**Very sensitive to noise, even the rustling of paper** Irritable	Throbbing in the blood vessels Paleness alternating with flushing	Loss of blood Sudden motion	Walking around slowly	
Hamamelis *(Witch hazel)*	**Bleeding from veins** **Full feeling in the veins** **Dark bleeding causing weakness** **Injuries with bruising and bleeding**	Feels peaceful while bleeding Irritable	**Sore, bruised feeling** **Varicose veins, hemorrhoids**	Injuries Pressure		
Millefolium *(Yarrow)*	**Wounds bleed profusely, especially after a fall** **Profuse, bright red, painless bleeding** **Bleeding after overexertion**	Doesn't know what she's doing or wants to do Sad	**Bruised, sore feeling** **Oozing of blood from edges of closed wounds**	Injury Violent exertion Stooping	Bleeding	
Phosphorus	**Small wounds bleed a lot** **Fluid, non-clotted blood** **Tendency to bleed easily**	**Outgoing** **Sympathetic** **Friendly** **Desires company** Afraid of the dark, thunderstorms, and ghosts	**Nosebleeds** Blood-streaked discharges	Lying down Lying on the left side	**Lying on the right side** **Washing the face in cold water**	**Very thirsty for cold and carbonated drinks** Desire for chocolate, ice cream, salty and spicy food

Bruises

Description
Bruises are caused by trauma that doesn't break the skin, resulting in blood leakage into the tissues.

Symptoms
Black and blue or purplish-green discoloration under the skin with sore, aching, pain.

Complications
Discoloration may take a long time to go away. The area can remain tender.

Look
Where is the bruised area?
How extensive is it?
What color is it?

Listen
"I'm fine. I don't need any help." *Arnica*
"I got a huge hematoma after a blood draw." *Bellis perennis*
"I hit my finger with a hammer and got a bad bruise. The only thing that makes it feel better is to ice my finger." *Ledum*
"I was going really fast and I fell off my bike and got a terrible bruise. *Arnica* didn't help." *Sulphuric acid*

Ask
How did the injury occur?
How long has the bruise been there?
How much does it hurt?
Does anything make the bruise feel better or worse?
Are there any mental or emotional symptoms since the injury?

Pointers for Finding the Homeopathic Medicine
Arnica is the first medicine to think of for any bruise. ▮ Give *Bellis perennis* for bruises to the veins or from leakage from the veins after blood

drawing or for ordinary bruises if *Arnica* fails. ▮ Give *Ledum* if the bruise is cold and feels better from cold. ▮ Give *Ruta* for bruises on the outer covering of bones (periosteum), such as on the shins. ▮ If the bruising tendency is chronic or recurrent, *Phosphorus* may work. ▮ Think of *Sulphuric acid* if *Arnica* doesn't work after injuries.

Dosage

- Give three pellets of 30C every four hours until you see improvement.
- If there is no improvement after three doses, give a different medicine.
- After you first notice improvement, give another dose only if symptoms begin to return.
- Lower potencies (6X, 6C, 30X) may need to be given more often (every hour).
- Higher potencies (200X, 200C, 1M) may need to be given only once unless symptoms definitely return after being relieved.

What to Expect from Homeopathic Self-Care

Homeopathic medicines can be very effective in relieving pain and healing bruises quickly, sometimes in less than a day, though the discoloration may take longer to disappear.

Other Self-Care Suggestions

Ice a bruise right away to keep more blood from leaking out into the tissues. ▮ Wrap an Ace bandage around the area, not too tightly, to support the area and control the extent of the bruise. ▮ After twelve hours, a hot bath can relieve soreness of the muscles. After twenty-four hours, alternating hot and cold moist packs can speed healing and remove discoloration. ▮ If a person is susceptible to bruising, bioflavonoids (1000 mg per day) strengthen the veins.

	Key Symptoms	Mind	Body	Worse	Better	Food & Drink
Arnica _(Leopard's bane)_	**Sore, bruised feeling in the injured part** **Bruising after injury or blunt trauma**	**Wants to be left alone and refuses help** **Says there is nothing wrong with him**	**Black eyes** Wants to lie down, but the bed feels too hard	Touch Lying on hard surfaces Motion	Lying down, especially with the head low	
Bellis perennis _(English daisy)_	**Bruises to veins or deeper tissues, especially after surgery or having blood drawn** **Ordinary bruises (if _Arnica_ fails)**	Restless	Swelling sensitive to touch	Touch	Cold applications Motion	
Ledum _(Marsh tea)_	**Bruises that feel cold and are better from a cold cloth or ice pack** **Black eyes**	Angry	**Bruises resulting from puncture wounds**	Warmth or a warm cloth Motion	Cold cloth or ice pack	
Phosphorus	**Chronic tendency to bruise and bleed easily**	**Outgoing** **Sympathetic** **Friendly** **Desires company** Afraid of the dark, thunderstorms, and ghosts	**Small wounds that break open and bleed easily**	Cold	Sleep Motion	**Great thirst for cold or carbonated drinks** Desire for chocolate, ice cream, salty food, and spicy food
Ruta _(Rue)_	**Bruises to the periosteum (the outer layer of bones), such as the shin**	Dissatisfied	Skin becomes chafed easily	Overexertion Lying down	Warmth Rubbing Motion	
Sulphuric acid	**Bruises that occur after blows or trauma (if _Arnica_ doesn't work)**	**Very hurried**	**Hemorrhage of black blood from any body opening**	Cold air, cold cloth, or ice	Warmth	**Desire for alcohol**

Burns

Description

Burns are caused by heat, electricity, radiation, hot water (scalds), or particular chemicals. The skin may be inflamed (first-degree), blistered (second-degree), or charred (third-degree). The most common burns are sunburn and burns from fire or touching something hot.

Symptoms

First-degree: redness, heat, swelling, and pain
Second-degree: all of the above plus blistering and oozing
Third-degree: significant charring of tissues

Complications

Burns can be serious, even fatal, depending on the extent of the body that is burned and the degree of the burn. Any extensive burn—even first-degree—should receive medical attention. First-degree burns will heal without extensive treatment in most cases. Palliative treatment will help relieve pain and inflammation. Second- and third-degree burns may cause scarring and infection. Third-degree burns can be life-threatening if extensive and may require treatment in a hospital setting. Get medical attention immediately for a third-degree burn.

Chemicals will continue to burn the skin as long as they are present; wash them off immediately with lots of water. Get medical attention for serious electrical burns.

Look

Is the burn inflamed, blistered, or charred?
What percentage of the body is burned?
Is the patient conscious and alert?
Is she in any apparent distress?

Listen

"I was scalded by boiling water." *Urtica urens* or *Cantharis*
"I just burned myself on the stove and it really hurts." *Cantharis*
"I was out in the sun all day and got terribly burned." *Cantharis*
"This burn never healed well." *Causticum*
"I got burned when I touched the live wire." *Phosphorus*

Ask

How did the burn occur?
When did it happen?
How bad is the pain?
What does the pain feel like?
Does anything make it better or worse?

Pointers for Finding the Homeopathic Medicine

The first medicine to consider in most burns is *Cantharis.* ▮ For scalds, either give *Cantharis* first, then *Urtica urens* if there is not improvement within thirty minutes, or, if the other symptoms fit *Urtica urens,* give it first. ▮ For chemical burns, the after-effects of old burns, or burns that are slow to heal give *Causticum.* ▮ For electrical burns, give *Phosphorus.*

Dosage

- Give three pellets of 30C every two hours until you see improvement. Give a dose hourly only in the case of severe burns.
- If there is no improvement after three doses, give a different medicine.
- After you first notice improvement, give another dose only if symptoms begin to return.
- Lower potencies (6X, 6C, 30X) may need to be given more often (every one to four hours, depending on the severity of the burn).
- Higher potencies (200X, 200C, 1M) generally need to be given only once. Repeat only if the burn is very severe and the person is not improving.

What to Expect from Homeopathic Self-Care

The pain of the burn should improve within minutes to an hour. Homeopathy will prevent or decrease scarring of mild burns and promote more rapid healing of more severe burns.

This is one condition in which, even if you have found the correct medicine, also apply *Calendula,* diluted (one part tincture to three parts water), to the burn.

Other Self-Care Suggestions

Soak the burned part in cold water or ice water, or apply cold wet compresses to relieve pain and inflammation. *Calendula* or *Hypericum* tincture may be added to the water as described next. ▮ Apply *Calendula* spray, gel or tincture, diluted one part tincture to three parts water. Dilute more if the tincture hurts to apply. *Hypericum* tincture may be used, diluted 1:3 as well. On first-degree burns, *Calendula* gel or salve may be applied. *Calendula* tincture, diluted one part *Calendula* to three parts water, can be very useful in first- and second-degree burns. ▮ Aloe vera juice, either directly from a leaf of the plant or commercially prepared, is very helpful for burns. ▮ Do not pop the blisters, because they protect the burns. ▮ Cover the burn with a non-adhesive dressing if there is a risk of rubbing or contamination of the burned area. Otherwise, leave open to the air. Change the dressing twice a day.

	Key Symptoms	Mind	Body	Worse	Better	Food & Drink
Cantharis *(Spanish fly)*	**Any burn, especially if severe or painful** **Intense burning pain**	In a frenzy	**Burns have blisters** After-effects of burns Chemical burns to the eyes		Cold water	
Causticum *(Potassium hydrate)*	**Deep burns and the after-effects of severe burns** **Burns that are slow to heal** **Chemical burns**	Fear that something bad will happen	Wounds that reopen	Extremes of temperature Drafts	Washing	
Phosphorus	**Electrical burns**	**Outgoing** **Sympathetic** **Friendly** **Desires company** Fear of the dark, thunderstorms, and ghosts				**Great thirst for very cold water**
Urtica urens *(Stinging nettle)*	**First- or second-degree burns with stinging, intense burning pains, and itching** **Scalds**	Restless		Cold water		

Canker Sores

Description

Canker sores or apthous ulcers are small oval ulcerations of the mucous membranes of the mouth and tongue. The cause is unknown, but deficiencies of some vitamins and minerals, including iron, Vitamin B-12, and folic acid, may predispose a person to canker sores. They often occur, in susceptible people, after eating too much acidic food. They usually resolve on their own in seven to fourteen days.

Symptoms

Small, painful ulcers with a raised border, surrounded by a red ring of inflammation. They can be extremely painful. The pain is often aggravated by acidic foods and drinks.

Complications

None.

Look

What is the color and size of the canker sores?
Is there just one sore or are there several?
Exactly where are the sores located?

Listen

"My canker sores really burn." *Arsenicum album*
"My mouth feels hot and dry and is really sensitive to sour things, salt, and spices." *Borax*
"I have a chubby baby with canker sores who sweats on his head." *Calcarea carbonica*
"I get canker sores and herpes in my mouth often." *Natrum muriaticum*
"I get bad canker sores with lots of saliva and a bad taste in my mouth." *Mercurius*

Ask

What brought on the canker sores?
How severe is the pain?
What makes the pain better or worse?

Pointers for Finding the Homeopathic Medicine

The most common medicines for canker sores are *Natrum muriaticum* and *Borax.* ■ *Arsenicum* is useful for burning canker sores in a chilly, anxious, needy person. ■ The most frequently used medicine for canker sores in infants is *Borax,* especially if there is also a tendency to have thrush. ■ Give *Calcarea carbonica* if the infant is flabby and sour-smelling with a large, sweaty head. ■ If there is also a tendency to get herpes, try *Natrum muriaticum* first. ■ If the canker sores seem to come on after excessive exposure to the sun, try *Natrum muriaticum.* ■ If the person has bad breath, is drooling, and has a metallic taste in the mouth, give *Mercurius.* ■ Give *Sulphur* if the person has a hot, dry, burning mouth and desires sweets and spicy food.

Dosage

- Give three pellets of 30C every four hours until you see improvement.
- If there is no improvement after three doses, give a different medicine.
- After you first notice improvement, give another dose only if symptoms begin to return.
- Lower potencies (6X, 6C, 30X) may need to be given more often (every one to four hours).
- Higher potencies (200X, 200C, 1M) usually only need to be given once. Repeat only if the symptoms return and are still severe.

What to Expect from Homeopathic Self-Care

Homeopathic medicines shorten the course of canker sores and help to relieve pain and inflammation. If canker sores are frequent, consult a qualified homeopath for constitutional care in order to prevent future recurrences.

Other Self-Care Suggestions

Reduce stress. ■ Take a high-potency multivitamin with B-complex. ■ Avoid citrus, tomato sauce, vinegar, and other acidic foods. ■ Apply pharmaceutical-grade alum powder to the canker sore with a cotton swab several times a day.

	Key Symptoms	Mind	Body	Worse	Better	Food & Drink
Arsenicum album *(Arsenic)*	**Canker sores with burning pain in the mouth and bad breath** **Chilly and thirsty for sips of warm water**	**Restless and anxious** Needy and demanding Afraid of being alone Complains that she won't get well	Bleeding gums Bites the glass when drinking	**Cold** After midnight, 1:00 to 2:00 A.M.	Heat	**Desire for frequent sips of cold water** Desire for fat
Borax	**Canker sores in children, especially if thrush is also present** **Hot, sensitive, canker sores that bleed if touched** **Dread of downward motion**	**Startled easily by noise** **Sensitive** Nervous	Mouth feels hot and dry Mouth is sensitive to acids, salty foods, and spicy foods	Nursing Fruit		
Calcarea carbonica *(Calcium carbonate)*	**Canker sores in infants who have large, sweaty heads and flabby bodies** **Sour taste in the mouth and sour perspiration**	**Independent** **Obstinate** Gets illnesses from taking on too much responsibility	Tip of tongue feels scalded Cold air makes the teeth hurt	**Teething** Cold, damp weather		**Desire for eggs, sweets, and salty food**
Mercurius *(Mercury)*	**Excess saliva, bad breath, and a metallic taste in the mouth** **Inflammation and ulceration of the mouth** **Symptoms are worse from heat and cold, sensitive like the mercury in a thermometer**	Hurried Hesitant Suspicious	**Gums are spongy and bleeding** **Tongue is moist and has the imprint of the teeth on the edges** **Chilly and sweaty, with trembling of the extremities**	Night Sweating		**Desire for bread and butter** Aversion to sweets

continued on next page

	Key Symptoms	Mind	Body	Worse	Better	Food & Drink
Natrum muriaticum *(Sodium chloride)*	**Canker sores inside the mouth and cold sores on the lips**	**Feelings hurt very easily** **Sensitive, depressed, weepy, and with-drawn** **Wants to be left alone when sick**	**Canker sores in the mouth, and on the gums and tongue** **Sores burn when food touches them** **Lips are dry with a crack in the middle of the lower lip** Cold sores on and near the lips Bitter, salty mucus from the throat	**10:00 A.M.** **Sunlight** Heat At the ocean	Outside in the fresh air Sweating Cold bath or shower	**Desire for salt, pasta, bread, and lemons**
Sulphur	**Canker sores with a hot, dry mouth, and a red face and lips** **Burning pains**	**Critical** **Impatient** Opinionated Messy	**Becomes overheated and perspires easily** The tongue is white, with a red tip and borders The mouth is sore in nursing children Saliva is profuse, with a bad taste in the mouth	Heat 11:00 A.M.		**Desire for sweets, alco-hol, fat, and spicy food** **Aversion to eggs, fish, and squash**

Carpal Tunnel Syndrome

Description

Carpal tunnel syndrome is a compression of the median nerve as it passes through the tendon sheath in the wrist. It may occur in either or both wrists as a result of too much work involving flexing the wrist, or from swelling of the wrists during pregnancy or due to hypothyroidism. It is common in people who spend a lot of time typing at a keyboard.

Symptoms

The symptoms are usually pain and numbness in the outer side of the hand in the three fingers nearest the thumb, the wrist, and the forearm. The symptoms are usully chronic with acute flare-ups.

Complications

If carpal tunnel syndrome is not treated, permanent injury to the nerves may result.

Look

Is there any limitation of movement in the wrist or hand?
Is any paralysis present?
Are the joints red or swollen, indicating arthritis?
Are both wrists affected?

Listen

"I have right wrist pain and the tendons feel very contracted." *Causticum*
"I have carpal tunnel pain in the same place where I fractured my wrist." *Calcarea phosphorica*
"The muscles in my forearm feel too short." *Guiacum*
"When I stretch my hand or wash it in hot water, my wrist feels better." *Rhus toxicodendron.*
"It feels like my wrist is bruised." *Ruta*
"I play the violin and have right-sided carpal tunnel syndrome." *Viola odorata*

Ask

What type of activity brought on the carpal tunnel syndrome?
How severe is it?
How long has it been present?
Is it an acute flare-up or a chronic condition?
What makes it better or worse?
Do you have any desire for particular foods or drinks?
Are there any mental or emotional symptoms that came along with the carpal tunnel syndrome?

Pointers for Finding the Homeopathic Medicine

The most common medicines for carpal tunnel syndrome are *Causticum* and *Ruta*. ▮ If there is a history of fractures or other bone problems, look at *Calcarea phosphorica*. ▮ If the pain is only on the left side and is better from cold water, give *Guiacum*. ▮ If there is considerable stiffness which is better from moving the hands, *Rhus toxicodendron* will probably help. ▮ If there are no clear symptoms for another medicine, give *Ruta*. ▮ *Viola odorata* is useful for the right wrist in sensitive, intellectual, and musical people—often violinists.

Dosage

- Give three pellets of 30C twice daily until you see improvement.
- If there is no improvement after three days, give a different medicine.
- After you first notice improvement, give another dose only if symptoms begin to return.
- Lower potencies (6X, 6C, 30X) may need to be given more often (every two to four hours).
- Higher potencies (200X, 200C, 1M) generally only need to be given once in the case of carpal tunnel syndrome. Repeat only if the symptoms return with intensity or severity.

What to Expect from Homeopathic Self-Care

Homeopathic medicines can often relieve carpal tunnel syndrome. The acute flare-up can be treated in twelve to twenty-four hours. The chronic condition should be treated by a qualified homeopath and may take several months to improve. If the medicines and self-care suggestions described in this section are not effective, consult a qualified homeopath. If all other options fail, see an orthopedic surgeon.

Other Self-Care Suggestions

Rest the wrist as much as possible, especially avoiding repetitive motions. ▮ A removable wrist splint or brace may be useful if the pain is severe from moving the wrist. ▮ Take Vitamin B-6, 100 mg per day. ▮ Soak the hands and wrists to stimulate circulation and relieve pain. Alternate hot and cold water: five minutes hot, one minute cold, then repeat twice for a total of three hot/cold soaks. Do soaks twice a day. ▮ Consult a physical therapist specializing in the upper extremities regarding specific exercises for carpal tunnel syndrome. ▮ Get a wrist support for your computer keyboard, and, if necessary an ergonomic keyboard.

	Key Symptoms	Mind	Body	Worse	Better	Food & Drink
Calcarea phosphorica *(Calcium phosphate)*	**Sore tendons in the wrist that are worse from cold and drafts** **Problems with bones or teeth in general** **Worse from cold damp weather, particularly when it is snowing**	**Dissatisfied** **Loves to travel** **Always looking for greener pastures**	**Cramping and pain in the wrist, when moving or using it** Pain in the right wrist, with weakness, as if it had been beaten	**Change of weather** **Lifting** Melting snow	Warm dry weather Lying down	**Desire for smoked meats, salty food, and ice cream**
Causticum *(Potassium hydrate)*	**Contractions of the finger tendons** **Writer's cramp** **Lack of tolerance for any injustice**	**Fear that something bad will happen**	**Right-sided paralysis of the hand** **Numbness of the hands** **Pain in right wrist, as if sprained, with weakness of the joint**	Wind Dry, cold air	Cold drinks Damp weather	**Desire for smoked meat, beer, salty food, and cheese. Aversion to sweets**
Guiacum *(Resin)*	**Left-sided carpal tunnel syndrome**	Critical	**Muscles seem too short** **Wants to stretch the hand** Arthritis of the wrist	**Heat** Touch Motion Exertion	**Cold cloth or ice pack** Yawning and stretching Apples	Desire for apples
Rhus toxicodendron *(Poison ivy)*	**Wrist stiff on first motion, then better when continuing to move it** **Carpal tunnel syndrome from overuse of wrist** **Desire to constantly stretch or move the wrist** **Wrist feels better after washing or soaking in hot water**	**Restless** Jovial	May have stiffness in other joints of the body also	At night With warmth At rest	**Continuing to move**	**Desire for cold milk**

Rutà *(Rue)*	**Injuries to tendons and ligaments** **Sore, bruised feeling with stiffness** **Sensation like a sprain and stiffness in the wrist**	Dissatisfied with himself and others	**Weakness and stiffness of the wrist** **Wrist hurts from lifting** **Pain as if bruised in the bones of the wrist and the back of the hand at rest and when moving the hand** Wrenching or shooting pain in wrists Fibrous growths on the tendons from overuse of the hands Numbness and tingling in hands after working	**Over-exertion** Cold, damp weather	Lying down Warmth Motion	
Viola odorata *(Sweet violet)*	**Carpal tunnel syndrome of the right wrist, especially in women** **Sensitivity or aversion to music, especially the violin**	People who think more than they feel	Pain in wrist along with pain in the right shoulder Pressing pain in the finger bones	Cold air Waking in the morning	After getting up	Desire for meat.

Chicken Pox

Description

Chicken pox is an acute viral disease, usually in young children, associated with the varicella-zoster virus, which also causes shingles. It is spread by infected droplets from the nose or throat.

Symptoms

A period of mild headache, fever, and general discomfort followed by numerous fluid-filled sores, which crust over. Once crusts form, the contagious period is over. Normally once a person has chicken pox she will never get it again.

Complications

Chicken pox is very contagious and may cause scarring. The sores may become infected. Do not give aspirin to a child with chicken pox, because they may get Reye's syndrome—a type of brain and liver illness characterized by nausea and vomiting and a sudden change in mental functioning with lethargy, loss of memory, and disorientation, leading to coma.

Look

What do the skin eruptions look like? Blisters? Pus-filled? Color?
Where on the body are the eruptions located?
How big are the eruptions? Are they oozing any liquid?
Has the color of the face changed from usual?
Are there any other visible symptoms?

Listen

"Don't leave me alone. I just want you to stay here with me." *Pulsatilla*
"Just leave me alone. Don't even look at me." (Turns head away). *Antimonium crudum*
"I can't stop scratching and moving around." *Rhus toxicodendron*

Ask

When did the symptoms begin?
Has your mood changed since you got chicken pox?

Have your habits, hunger, thirst, or anything else changed since you started to get sick?

Pointers for Finding the Homeopathic Medicine

The most common medicine for a very itchy chicken pox is *Rhus toxicodendron.* ▮ If the sores ooze a honey-like discharge and scab over, and the tongue is coated white, think of *Antimonium crudum.* ▮ If the main symptom is a loose, rattling cough, take a look at *Antimonium tartaricum.* ▮ For out-of-the-ordinary fussiness in a child who doesn't want to be touched or looked at, consider *Croton tiglium,* especially if the skin feels very tight. ▮ If the child is very clingy, weepy, and thirstless, look at *Pulsatilla.*

Dosage

- Give three pellets of 30C every two to four hours until you see improvement.
- If there is no improvement after three doses, give a different medicine.
- After you first notice improvement, give another dose only if symptoms begin to return.
- Lower potencies (6X, 6C, 30X) may need to be given more often (every two to four hours).
- Higher potencies (200X, 200C, 1M) generally need to be given only once. Repeat only if symptoms return with intensity; give only infrequently in this case.

What to Expect from Homeopathic Self-Care

Homeopathic medicines help relieve the symptoms of chicken pox, particularly the itching and discomfort, and may shorten the course of the disease.

Other Self-Care Suggestions

Keep sores clean and avoid scratching. ▮ Apply cold compresses to the sores. ▮ Oatmeal bath: use Aveno (avoid the type that contains camphor) or place one cup of finely blended dry oatmeal in the bath to soothe the itching. ▮ To treat infected sores, apply a few drops of one part *Calendula* tincture diluted with three parts water and cover with bandages or gauze.

	Key Symptoms	Mind	Body	Worse	Better	Food & Drink
Antimonium crudum *(Antimony)*	**Sores have a honey-like discharge or thick, hard, honey-colored scabs** **Sores burn and itch, especially when warm in bed**	**Sulky and quite irritable** **Doesn't want to be looked at or touched**	**Tongue is coated white** Upset stomach	Heat Sour foods Cold water	Fresh air Rest Warm bath	Desire for sour food, cucumbers, or pickles
Antimonium tartaricum *(Tartar emetic)*	**Bluish eruptions or sores that crust over and leave a bluish-red mark** **Loose, rattling, gurgling cough**	**Desire to be left alone**	**Delayed or receding eruptions** **White, coated tongue**	Heat Warm room	Coughing up mucus	Desire for apples and other fruits Desire for sour foods, resulting in indigestion
Croton tiglium *(Croton seed oil)*	**Blister-like eruptions with intense itching** **Violent and painful itching** **Scratching is painful**	Very worried and anxious	**Skin feels painfully tight** **Burning, red skin** **Clusters of blisters that burst and form crusts** **Eruptions especially on the face and genitals** Rash alternating with diarrhea	Washing	Gentle rubbing	
Pulsatilla *(Windflower)*	**Itching sores that blister and crust** **Child is weepy, whiny, and clingy and wants to be carried and cuddled** **Very little thirst**	**Changeable emotions** **Wants company when sick**	**Itching is worse when the child becomes overheated**	Warm, stuffy room Rich food	Slow walking in the open air	Desire for butter, ice cream, creamy foods Aversion to fat, milk, and pork
Rhus toxicodendron *(Poison ivy)*	**Intense itching** **Squirmy; can't find a comfortable position because of the itching**	**Restless** Jovial	**Chilly, worse from cold damp or getting wet** Blisters are filled with clear liquid or pus	**At night** **From scratching** Warmth	Continued motion	**Desire for cold milk**

Cold Sores (Herpes simplex)

Description

Cold sores are caused by a virus, Herpes Simplex Virus I, which remains dormant in the nerve roots around the mouth. Episodes of outbreaks occur whenever stress levels are too high and the immune system is not strong enough to keep the virus in check. Exposure to the sun can also cause a recurrence.

Symptoms

Single or multiple blisters, which may be as large as a dime, usually occur on or around the lips. The blisters are often accompanied by swelling and are usually quite painful. Numbness and tingling may occur before the blisters appear, as well as fatigue.

Complications

Cold sores will usually disappear on their own in one to two weeks. There are usually no complications, although scarring may occur in some cases.

Look

How large are the blisters?
How many are there?
Where are they located?
Are they filled with fluid? Oozing?

Listen

"My lips just burn and burn." *Arsenicum album*
"The herpes came on right after my lover left me." *Natrum muriaticum*
"I got the herpes after being out in the sun and got a headache at the same time." *Natrum muriaticum*
"The sores are so painful that I can barely even touch them." *Hepar sulphuris*

Ask

Did you experience any stress before the outbreak? What kind?
Are there any mental or emotional symptoms associated with the outbreak?
When did the cold sores start?

How painful are they?
What makes the cold sores feel better or worse?
Is there any time when the cold sores feel worse?

Pointers for Finding the Homeopathic Medicine

Natrum muriaticum is the most frequently used medicine for cold sores. ■ For cold sores that come on from exposure to the sun in a sensitive person who easily gets her feelings hurt, the most common medicine is *Natrum muriaticum.* ■ Cold sores that burn in a chilly, anxious, restless person may require *Arsenicum album.* ■ People needing *Hepar sulphuris* are generally extremely chilly and their sensitivity to the pain of the cold sores seems out of proportion. ■ Cold sores that occur after exertion or exposure to cold, damp weather usually respond to *Rhus toxicodendron.*

Dosage

- Give three pellets of 30C every four hours until you see improvement.
- If there is no improvement within several days, give a different medicine.
- After you first notice improvement, give another dose only if symptoms begin to return.
- Lower potencies (6X, 6C, 30X) may need to be given more often (every two to four hours).
- Higher potencies (200X, 200C, 1M) generally need to be given only once. Repeat only if symptoms return with intensity; give only infrequently in this case.

What to Expect from Homeopathic Self-Care

Homeopathic medicines help the immune system fight the infection, reduce pain, and make the blisters go away faster. Herpes simplex usually responds best under the care of a qualified homeopath. Constitutional treatment between outbreaks may substantially reduce their frequency, or in some cases eliminate recurrences.

Other Self-Care Suggestions

Lysine: 500 mg three times a day. ■ Vitamin C: 1000 mg three times a day. ■ Beta-carotene: 50,000 IU a day. ■ Zinc: 30 mg a day. ■ One part *Calendula* tincture mixed with three parts water applied with a cotton swab three times a day.

	Key Symptoms	Mind	Body	Worse	Better	Food & Drink
Arsenicum album *(Arsenic)*	**Cold sores with intense burning pain of the lips** **Cold sores that are worse from sour or acid fruit** **Extreme anxiety about health, and fear of dying** **Chilly and thirsty for frequent sips of water**	**Restless and anxious** Needy and demanding Afraid of being alone Complains that he won't get well	**Bad breath** Bleeding gums	**Cold** After midnight, 1:00 to 2:00 A.M.	Heat, warm applications	Desire for fat
Hepar sulphuris *(Calcium sulfate)*	**Cold sores are very sensitive and painful, especially to touch** **Extreme sensitivity to cold air and applications**	**Extremely irritable and touchy** **Very sensitive to pain**	**Splinter-like pains anywhere in the body**	**Drafts** Uncovering	**Warmth** Covering up	
Natrum muriaticum *(Sodium chloride)*	**Cold sores on and near the lips** **The lips are dry and cracked, with a crack in the middle of the lower lip** **Outbreak after grief or disappointment in romance**	**Feelings hurt very easily** **Depressed, weepy, and withdrawn** **Wants to be left alone when sick**	**Cold sores from exposure to the sun** **May also have canker sores**	10:00 A.M. Heat By the ocean	Outside in the fresh air Sweating Cool bath	**Desire for pasta, bread, and salt**
Rhus toxicodendron *(Poison ivy)*	**Several small, intensely itching and burning blisters filled with watery, yellowish fluid** **Inflammation and swelling of the lips**	**Restless** Jovial	**Chilly, worse from cold, damp, or getting wet** **Worse after exertion**	**At night** **From scratching** **Cold baths or showers** At rest	Continued motion	**Desire for cold milk**

Colic

Description

Colic is a condition found in babies from just after birth until three or four months of age, with crying, irritability, and what seems to be pain or cramps in the abdomen. They usually seem quite hungry, eat and gain weight normally, and particularly like to suck. The actual cause and process by which colic happens are unknown.

Symptoms

Colicky babies cry and appear to be in pain or distress. Gas may be part of the problem. They may cry incessantly, or only at certain times. The crying can be very distressing to parents, who feel helpless to do anything about it.

Complications

Simple colic is not life-threatening, nor does it lead to any serious illness. It usually passes on its own in a matter of weeks. If the baby doesn't gain weight, vomits excessively, or has persistent diarrhea, medical attention should be sought to determine the cause of the problem.

Look

What position is the baby lying in?
Is the baby doubled over or curled up?
What does the stool look like?
Does the baby like to be rocked, carried, or cuddled?
What color is the baby's face?
Is there diarrhea or vomiting?

Listen

"She can't keep any milk down at all. The only time she's happy is when she lies next to our dog." *Aethusa*

"My baby seems so happy except when he's colicky, and he always sweats on his head." *Calcarea carbonica*

"I can't do anything to please him. I give him what he asks for and he throws it on the floor." *Chamomilla*

"She has lots of bloating and gets gas from anything that I eat before I nurse her. The only thing that helps is warm water." *Lycopodium*

"She is better if I rub her tummy and put her on a warmed-up blanket." *Magnesia phosphorica*

"My baby is so irritable. He wakes at 3:00 A.M. with the colic, but can't seem to burp." *Nux vomica*

"My baby just clings and wants to be cuddled. Her moods change every five minutes." *Pulsatilla*

Ask

When did the colic start?

What time of day or night does the colic come on?

Did the baby eat anything unusual?

What makes the colic better or worse?

Pointers for Finding the Homeopathic Medicine

If the baby can't seem to tolerate milk, first think of *Aethusa,* then *Magnesia phosphorica, Calcarea carbonica,* or *Lycopodium.* ▮ If there is a tendency toward frequent belching, and the baby seems to feel better after belching, *Carbo vegetabilis* is likely to be needed. ▮ For colic in extremely fussy, irritable babies, especially if they arch their backs and are inconsolable, consider *Chamomilla.* ▮ If a baby doubles over with the colic or brings his knees up to his chest, think of *Colocynthis* first then *Magnesia phosphorica.* ▮ For colic with excessive bloating and gas, particularly if the baby seems to be worse after ingesting milk, look at *Magnesia phosphorica.*

Dosage

- Give three pellets of 30C every four hours until you see improvement.
- If there is no improvement after three doses, give a different medicine.
- After you first notice improvement, give another dose only if symptoms begin to return.
- Lower potencies (6X, 6C, 30X) may need to be given more often (every two to four hours).
- Higher potencies (200X, 200C, 1M) generally need to be given only once. Repeat only if symptoms return with intensity; give only infrequently in this case.

What to Expect from Homeopathic Self-Care

Homeopathic medicines can resolve colic and stop the crying within a few minutes to an hour. Repeated doses may be needed if the symptoms return. Constitutional treatment by a qualified homeopath is recommended if the colic persists more than a few weeks or is not responding to acute treatment.

Other Self-Care Suggestions

Make sure the baby has been burped after eating. ▮ Rocking, carrying, or holding the baby may soothe him. ▮ Dill water: add one-half teaspoon dill to two cups boiling water, steep, and cool. Give up to three times a day. A British preparation called "Gripe water" is available in many East Indian grocery stores. ▮ Pacifiers may help with the urge to suck. ▮ Swaddling the baby fairly tightly and placing her on her stomach may help. ▮ A hot water bottle (not too hot) placed on the baby's abdomen may relieve discomfort.

	Key Symptoms	Mind	Body	Worse	Better	Food & Drink
Aethusa *(Fool's parsley)*	**Intolerance of milk** **Love of animals**	Awkward	**Babies vomit large curds of milk** **Vomiting and diarrhea in newborns** Colic followed by vomiting and dizziness Inability to hold up her head Bubbling sensation around the belly button Yellowish-green, slimy diarrhea	Evening 3:00 to 4:00 A.M.	Open air	Not thirsty
Calcarea carbonica *(Calcium carbonate)*	**Colic in chubby, happy babies who sweat on their heads** **Sour vomiting of curdled milk** **Milk not tolerated**	**Stubborn** Fearful Generally good-natured	**Sour burps** Diarrhea in babies who have a ravenous appetite	**Exposure to cold, damp weather** Becoming chilled after a bath	Lying on the painful side or on the back	**Desire for eggs,** ice cream, and salt Craves indigestible things like chalk, pencils, or dirt Thirsty for cold drinks
Carbo vegetabilis *(Charcoal)*	**Excessive amount of gas and burping** **Much relief after burping** **Very chilly, yet wants to be fanned or exposed to a draft**	Apathetic Irritable	**Very bloated and full of gas** **Loud, frequent burps or gas** Indigestion Appetite is usually decreased	Riding in the car Rich food	**Passing gas**	Desire for sweets and salt Aversion to rich foods and fat
Chamomilla *(Chamomile)*	**Great pain with irritability, impatience, and restlessness** **Child is inconsolable** **Child wants to be carried and rocked**	**Screaming and crying** **Nothing satisfies him** **Extremely fussy** **Capricious**	**Green diarrhea like chopped eggs or spinach** Abdominal pain is worse from touch Belching and diarrhea with an odor like rotten eggs	Anger Night	**Being carried**	Desire for cold drinks Aversion to warm drinks

continued on next page

	Key Symptoms	Mind	Body	Worse	Better	Food & Drink
Chamomilla *(Chamomile) continued*	**Symptoms are often worse during teething**	Arches his back, kicks, and hits Doesn't like to be touched One cheek may be red and hot, the other pale				
Colocynthis *(Bitter cucumber)*	**Agonizing, cutting pain that makes the child want to bend double** **Pain is better from pressure on the abdomen and from warmth**	**Oversensitive and easily irritated** Restless	**Baby lies on his abdomen and screams if he is moved** Colic is worse from eating, especially fruit Watery diarrhea with gas and pain Intestines feel like stones are grinding in them	Anger Intense emotions	Hard pressure Bending double	Desire for bread
Lycopodium *(Club moss)*	**Colic in babies that is relieved by warm drinks** **Abdominal bloating and gas worse 4:00 to 8:00 P.M.** **Can't handle the pressure of diapers or clothing around the abdomen**	Fear of strangers Timidity	**Lots of noisy gas** **Bloating after eating or drinking even the slightest amount** **Colic worse in the evening** Diarrhea from cold drinks Symptoms tend to be right-sided	**Pressure of clothing on the abdomen** **Beans, cabbage, cauliflower, broccoli, brussels sprouts (even when nursing mother eats them)** Warmth	Motion	

Magnesia phosphorica *(Magnesium phosphate)*	**Cramping pain that is relieved by bending double, rubbing, warmth, and pressure** **Pain is relieved by very hot applications and drinks** **Colicky pain with lots of gas**	Irritable Wants nurturing	**Burping doesn't relieve the colic** **Burps and passes gas** Abdomen looks bloated Trapped gas	Cold drafts or baths	**Warm bath** **Rubbing**	Desire for very cold drinks
Nux vomica *(Quaker's button)*	**Colic accompanied by constipation in an irritable baby** **Colic in nursing infants from stimulating food or drink ingested by mother** **Arching of the back with tense muscles** **Very irritable and impatient**	**Angry** **Easily frustrated** **Spasmodic crying**	**Constipated with terrible straining for a bowel movement** **Retching without vomiting** **Wakes up at 3:00 A.M. with colic** **Violent vomiting, after which he feels better**	**Cold** **Eating**	**Warmth** Warm drinks After a bowel movement	Desire for fat
Pulsatilla *(Windflower)*	**Colic in a sweet, clingy, mild baby who cries a lot** **Always wants to be close to her mother** **Wants to be held and fussed over** **Feels much better outdoors**	**Weepy and clingy** Gentle	**Changeable symptoms** Often plump Painful bloating of the abdomen with loud rumbling Diarrhea in infants Vomits what she ate or drank long before	**Warm, stuffy rooms** **Rich foods (even when eaten by nursing mother)** Getting the feet wet	**Gentle motion** **After crying**	**Not very thirsty** **Colic from fats and rich foods**

Common Cold

(See also Coughs and Flu.)

Description

The common cold is a viral infection associated with a large number of viruses that infect the nose, throat, and lungs.

Symptoms

Sore throat and stuffy nose, with a watery nasal discharge at first, then becoming thicker and colored. A low-grade fever and headaches are common. A loose or dry, hacking cough often occurs as the cold "goes into the chest," and may persist for up to several weeks.

Complications

Colds may be complicated by bacterial infections leading to sinusitis and ear infections, and may progress to bronchitis or, infrequently, pneumonia.

Look

Is the throat red, is the uvula swollen, or is there pus on the tonsils?
What color is the nasal discharge or coughed-up mucus?
Is the face red, pale, or otherwise discolored?
Is fever present?
Are the lymph glands along the throat swollen or hard?

Listen

"I felt fine until I went out to shovel snow yesterday. It came on so fast." *Aconite* or *Belladonna*
"My nose is running like a faucet!" *Allium cepa*
"I feel so much pressure in my head that I think it will burst." *Kali bichromicum*
"I've been working nonstop. This is the only way I'll slow down." *Nux vomica*
"Please stay with me. I have a bad cold," she says weepily. *Pulsatilla*
"It's cold in here. I need blankets and some hot tea right now. Do you think I will be all right?" *Arsenicum album*
"I can't seem to find a comfortable temperature. My sinuses are full of mucus and my partner can't stand my breath." *Mercurius*

Ask

When did the cold start?
What were the first symptoms?
What are the symptoms now?
Is the cold more in the head or the chest?
Is your throat sore on one side or the other? What does it feel like?
What makes your symptoms better or worse?
Are you hungry or thirsty?
Do you want anything in particular to eat or drink?
Are your muscles and joints painful?
Do you feel warm or chilly?
Do you have a headache? What kind of pain and where is it?

Pointers for Finding the Homeopathic Medicine

During the first twenty-four hours of a cold with a high fever, choose between *Aconite, Belladonna,* and *Ferrum phosphoricum.* ▮ If the symptoms fit *Belladonna* but it doesn't help, use *Ferrum phosphoricum.* ▮ *Allium cepa* is the most common medicine for colds in which the eyes and nose run or drip like a faucet. ▮ Give *Kali bichromicum* if the main symptom is pressing pain in the sinuses and root of nose. The discharge will usually be thick, greenish-yellow, and stringy. ▮ If the symptoms come on after overwork or anger, and if the person is very impatient and irritable, look at *Nux vomica.* ▮ *Pulsatilla* is good for a ripe cold with thick yellow-green discharge, changeable moods, and a whiny, clingy disposition. ▮ Give *Arsenicum album* for a cold with a watery, irritating nasal discharge in a chilly restless person who seems anxious and needy. ▮ People who need *Mercurius* are sensitive to both heat and cold, with yellow-green mucus and bad breath.

Dosage

- Give three pellets of 30C every four hours until you see improvement.
- If there is no improvement after three doses, give a different medicine.
- After you first notice improvement, give another dose only if symptoms begin to return.
- Lower potencies (6X, 6C, 30X) may need to be given more often (every two to four hours).
- Higher potencies (200X, 200C, 1M) generally need to be given only once. Repeat only if symptoms return with intensity; give only infrequently in this case.

What to Expect from Homeopathic Self-Care

Unlike conventional medicine, homeopathic medicines effectively treat the common cold, shortening the severity and duration of symptoms. Antibiotics are not recommended for colds, only for severe bacterial infections that have not responded to homeopathic treatment.

Other Self-Care Suggestions

Rest. ▮ Drink two to four cups of hot ginger tea. Boil three slices of fresh ginger in two cups of water for fifteen minutes. ▮ Avoid dairy products, wheat, bananas, and oatmeal because they increase mucus production. ▮ Vitamin C (500 mg every two hours, up to 3000 mg per day) in the first stage of the cold. ▮ Echinacea/goldenseal capsules or tincture. Take one dropper of tincture in warm water or two capsules every four hours. ▮ Beta-carotene: 50,000 IU per day. ▮ Zinc: 30 mg per day. ▮ Zinc lozenges if there is a sore throat. ▮ Garlic capsules, two every four hours. ▮ Nasal wash with one-fourth teaspoon salt to one cup warm water once or twice a day. For the nasal wash, snuff a small amount of salt water from a cupped hand into the nostrils. Tilt your head back closing the throat, let the water drain into your mouth and spit it out.

	Key Symptoms	Mind	Body	Worse	Better	Food & Drink
Aconite *(Monkshood)*	**The first stage of a cold that comes on suddenly and violently** **Colds that come on after exposure to a cold dry wind, or from fright or shock** **Usually needed within the first twenty-four hours after the illness begins** **High fever that comes on suddenly**	**Tremendously fearful, anxious, and restless** Afraid of death	**A croupy cough comes on suddenly** **One cheek red, the other pale, or both cheeks hot and red** Hot watery nasal discharge Nostrils hot and burning Throat red, dry, and hot, with swollen tonsils Choking sensation when swallowing	Fright or emotional shock Cold dry wind	Open air Sleep	**Intense, burning thirst for cold drinks** Everything tastes bitter except for water
Allium cepa *(Red onion)*	**A profuse watery nasal discharge that drips like a faucet** **Nasal discharge burns and irritates the nose and upper lip** **Eyes and nose run as if the person were peeling an onion**	Afraid that the pain will become unbearable	**Eyes run, but the discharge is non-irritating** Rawness in the throat and laryngitis Incessant hacking, tickling cough is worse from breathing in cold air	Warm room Damp, cold weather	Outdoors	Strong hunger and thirst Desire for onions Aversion to cucumbers
Arsenicum album *(Arsenic)*	**Thin, irritating, or burning watery nasal discharge with sneezing** **Nose feels stopped up while it runs** **Anxious, nervous, and restless** **Very chilly**	Needy and demanding Afraid of being alone Complaining that they won't get well	Right nostril runs Colds go to the chest Cough worse in the cold or outdoors	Cold After midnight, 1:00 to 2:00 A.M.	Heat	**Very thirsty for frequent sips of cold water** Desire for milk, fat on meat, sour foods

continued on next page

	Key Symptoms	Mind	Body	Worse	Better	Food & Drink
Belladonna *(Deadly nightshade)*	**Colds come on suddenly and violently** **Bright red flushed face, high fever, throbbing headache** **Throat is extremely red and very sore** **Symptoms are often right-sided** **Fever is often above 103°F**	**Child plays normally, even with a high fever** **Delirious with high fevers**	**Skin is hot and dry** **Eyes are glassy** Pupils are dilated Short, croupy, dry, barking cough	**Light** **Noise** **Jarring** **3:00 P.M.** Lying down Getting chilled or overheated	Sitting up in a quiet, dark room	**Desire for lemons or lemonade, sour food, and cold water** Either very thirsty or not thirsty at all
Ferrum phosphoricum *(Iron phosphate)*	**Useful in the very first stage of the cold, when he feels he is coming down with something but there are no clear symptoms** **High fever with flushed face, especially with round red spots on the cheeks, or very pale**	**Irritable** Talkative Excited	**Right-sided problems** **Inflammation of throat or lungs with fever, but few definite symptoms** Discharges may be blood-streaked Red and swollen tonsils Bruised soreness of the muscles Nosebleeds	Night 4:00 to 6:00 A.M.	Cold applications Bleeding Lying down	Desire for sour foods and cold drinks Aversion to meat and milk
Kali bichromicum *(Potassium bichromate)*	**Thick, stringy, yellow-green nasal discharge** **Pressure in the sinuses and pain at the root of the nose** **Thick postnasal drip** **Colds that develop into sinus infections**	**Explains symptoms in elaborate detail**	**Wandering aches and pains in small spots** Ripe or late-stage colds Croupy cough Coughs up thick, stringy, yellow-green mucus Nasal-sounding voice Laryngitis with hoarseness Sensation of a hair on the tongue	Cold, damp Beer, alcohol 1:00 A.M., 2:00 to 3:00 A.M.	Heat Motion Pressure	Desire for beer and sweets Aversion to meat
Mercurius *(Mercury)*	**Yellowish-green nasal discharge**	Suspicious Restless	**Nostrils raw and ulcerated** **Acrid nasal discharge**	**Night** Heat	**Moderate temperatures**	**Desire for bread and**

	Bad-smelling breath, perspiration, and discharges **Coated tongue** **Sensitivity to extremes of temperature, like the mercury in a thermometer** **Metallic taste in the mouth**	Hurried Reserved	**Nasal discharge runny or too thick to run** Cheeks swollen and red Frequent sneezing with runny nose	Drafts		
Natrum muriaticum *(Sodium chloride)*	**Thick nasal discharge like egg white** **Profusely runny nose for several days, then nose is stopped up** **Alternately dry and runny nose** **Cold sores on the lips while sick with a cold**	**Feelings hurt very easily** Depressed, weepy, and withdrawn Wants to be left alone when sick Doesn't like to cry in front of others	**Cold begins with sneezing** **The lips are dry and cracked, with a crack in the middle of the lower lip** **Headache in the forehead** Tiny sores in the nose Watery eyes when in the wind or outdoors Bitter, salty mucus from the throat	**10:00 A.M.** Heat Sun By the ocean	Outside in the fresh air Sweating Cool bath	**Desire for salt, pasta, and bread**
Nux vomica *(Quaker's button)*	**A cold that comes on from overwork** **A cold from overindulgence in rich foods or alcohol** **Sniffles** **Made worse by going outdoors**	**Irritable** **Impatient** **Obsessed with business** **Wants to be the first and the best** **Competitive and hard-driving, Type A** Easily offended Frustrated easily by little things	Nose runs during the day and is stopped up at night Nose feels plugged but there is a watery discharge Oversensitive to strong odors	**Anger** **Business worries** **Open air or drafts**	Rest Allowing the nose to run	**Desire for hot, spicy foods and meat** **Desire for stimulants and alcohol**
Pulsatilla *(Windflower)*	**A "ripe" cold with thick, bland, yellow-green mucus** **Child is weepy, whiny, and clingy, and wants to be carried and cuddled** **Lack of thirst**	**Changeable emotions** **Wants company when sick**	**Cold is better from going outdoors** **Nose is stuffed up; can't smell** **Loose cough in the morning, dry at night** Ears feel plugged	**Warm, stuffy room** **Rich food**	Slow walking in the open air	**Desire for butter, ice cream, and peanut butter** Aversion to fat and pork

Conjunctivitis (Pinkeye)

Description

Conjunctivitis, also known as "pinkeye," is an acute inflammation of the conjunctiva of the eye, which is a thin protective lining of the eyelids and eyeball. It is caused by bacterial or viral infection or an allergic sensitivity to an irritant.

Symptoms

The eye appears red and bloodshot, and there is often lots of watering and a clear or purulent (pus) discharge, depending on whether the infection is viral or bacterial. The eyelids are usually swollen. Intense itching occurs with allergic conjunctivitis. The eye feels irritated and painful, and there is a burning sensation or a feeling that something is in the eye.

Complications

Conjunctivitis may become chronic or may damage the eye if left untreated.

Look

Is the eye red?
Is there a discharge? What color? Thick or thin?
Are tears present?
Are the eyelids swollen?

Listen

"My eyes are all swollen and puffy, and they sting, too!" *Apis*
"My newborn baby has pinkeye." *Argentum nitricum*
"My eye is throbbing so much it's driving me crazy." *Belladonna*
"I can't stop my eyes from watering. I look like I'm crying, but I'm not sad." *Euphrasia*
"Mommy, wipe my eyes for me. They are all goopy." *Pulsatilla*
"My eye is burning like it has hot sand in it." *Sulphur*

Ask

Does anything may your eyes feel better or worse?
What kind of pain do you have?
Have there been any mental or emotional changes before or since you got sick?

Do you crave anything to eat or drink?
Do you feel warm or chilly?
Do you have a fever?

Pointers for Finding the Homeopathic Medicine

If the main symptom is puffy swelling of the eyelids, give *Apis*. ▮ For conjunctivitis in newborns, think of *Argentum nitricum*. ▮ When fever, redness, and throbbing pain are prominent, *Belladonna* is the medicine. ▮ If the main symptom is excessive, irritating tears, give *Euphrasia*. ▮ If the discharge is thick, creamy, and yellow-green in a whiny, moody person, give *Pulsatilla*. ▮ If burning in the eyes is prominent in a lazy, philosophical egotist, give *Sulphur*.

Dosage

- Give three pellets of 30C every four hours until you see improvement.
- If there is no improvement after three doses, give another medicine.
- After you first notice improvement, give another dose only if symptoms begin to return.
- Lower potencies (6X, 6C, 30X) may need to be given more often (every two to four hours).
- Higher potencies (200X, 200C, 1M) generally need to be given only once. Repeat only if symptoms return with intensity; give only infrequently in this case.

What to Expect from Homeopathic Treatment

Homeopathic medicines are able to relieve the pain and stimulate the body to heal the infection in twelve to twenty-four hours.

Other Self-Care Suggestions

Apply a clean washcloth that has been dipped in cold water and wrung out over the eyes. Replace it when it gets warm. ▮ Rub the hands together vigorously and place over the closed eyes for one minute. ▮ Do not touch the other eye after you have touched the infected eye, to avoid spreading the infection. ▮ Use sterile *Euphrasia* eyedrops to soothe the eyes, a few drops in each eye several times a day. ▮ Dissolve one-fourth teaspoon of salt in one cup of water. Use three cotton balls soaked in the water to swipe the edge of the eyelids from inside to outside. Discard after using once. Repeat four times a day. ▮ Take beta-carotene (50,000 IU per day) or Vitamin A (25,000 IU per day). ▮ Take Vitamin C (500 mg, six times per day).

	Key Symptoms	Mind	Body	Worse	Better	Food & Drink
Apis mellifica *(Honeybee)*	**Great swelling of the eyelids, which look red and puffy** **Stinging, burning pains** **The eyes are bright red, and very bloodshot** **Eyes are hot and made worse by heat; the tears are hot**	**Busy** Protective of family and children Jealous Does not like to be crossed	Sudden, piercing pains in the eyes Itching is intolerable at night Clear or pussy discharge from the eyes	Heat, hot drinks, or hot bath	**Cold cloth or ice pack** Cool air, cold baths Uncovering	Not usually thirsty
Argentum nitricum *(Silver nitrate)*	**Conjunctivitis in newborns** **Eye discharge is thick and purulent (pussy)** **Inner corners of the eyes are swollen and red** **Deep, splinter-like pains**	**Anxiety in crowds, closed rooms, elevators, theaters, airplanes** Hurried Impulsive Talks a lot	Flatulence	**Heat**	Cool air	**Strong desire for sweets and salt**
Belladonna *(Deadly nightshade)*	**Conjunctivitis comes on suddenly and violently, with a red face and fever** **Right-sided conjunctivitis** **The eye is quite red, hot, and very sensitive to light** **Throbbing pains are severe, and may include a throbbing headache**	Sudden outbursts of anger Children have high fever but play normally as if not sick at all	**Face fiery red, hot, and dry** **Fever is often above 103°F** Eyes glassy with fever	**Light** **Noise** **Jarring** **3:00 P.M.**	**Sitting up in a quiet, dark room**	Great thirst for cold water or no thirst at all Desire for lemons or lemonade, sour food

Euphrasia *(Eyebright)*	**Eye discharge is profuse, hot, and irritating, but the nasal discharge is bland** **Eyes water all the time**	**Hypochondriacal** **Indifferent** **Body or head seems large** Chaotic	**Lots of hot, irritating tears and blinking** **Feels like sand is in the eyes** Eyes are red Eyelids are red, itching, and burning Conjunctivitis from eye injuries or measles Eyes very sensitive to light	Sunlight Evening Smoke	Fresh air Blinking Wiping the eyes	
Pulsatilla *(Windflower)*	**Conjunctivitis with lots of thick, bland, yellow-green discharge** **Eyelids are stuck together in the morning upon waking up**	**Children are weepy, whiny, and clingy and want to be carried and cuddled** Feels abandoned, has changeable emotions, and cries very easily	**Conjunctivitis with a cold** Profuse tears Itching, burning eyes with a desire to rub them Eyes water in the wind or open air	**Warm, stuffy room** **Rich food**	**Slow walking in the open air**	**Desire for rich foods and creamy foods such as butter, ice cream, and peanut butter** Aversion to fat, milk, bread, and pork Aggravation from pork and rich foods
Sulphur *(Sulfur)*	**Red, hot, dry eyes** **Burning pain in the eyes and lids** **Eye discharge is yellow and sticky** **Sandy or gritty sensation in the eyes**	**Opinionated** **Philosophical** **Egotistical** Lazy Messy Impatient	Disgusted by the odors of others but can't smell his own	**Warmth, and the warmth of bed** Atmospheric changes 11:00 A.M. Left side	**Open air**	**Desire for alcohol, sweets, and spicy foods**

Constipation

Description

Constipation means difficulty passing stool, or the inability to have a bowel movement when desired. It can be caused by diseases affecting the bowel or nervous system, emotional stress, lack of bowel tone and peristalsis, insufficient fiber in the diet, dehydration, lack of exercise, drugs, and, rarely, obstruction of the bowel.

Symptoms

Hard, dry, or soft stool, pain on having a bowel movement, gas and bloating, and hemorrhoids are the main symptoms. Feelings of sluggishness, mental dullness, bad breath, and body odor often accompany constipation.

Complications

Acute constipation mainly causes discomfort. If it persists, impaction of the hard, dry stool can occur, blocking the rectum and requiring manual removal. Enlargement of segments of the colon may occur if constipation is chronic and severe.

Look

Does the person want to be in a particular position or posture when constipated?
What is the color and consistency of recent bowel movements?
Is the person straining at stool?
Are hemorrhoids present? What do they look like? (See Hemorrhoids.)

Listen

"I am so confused. I want to eat potatoes and rice." *Alumina*
"My rectum feels so dry." *Alumina, Bryonia,* or *Nux moschata*
"If I could just go home, I could have a bowel movement." *Bryonia*
"The constipation is my responsibility. I'll take care of it."
Calcarea carbonica
"I'm so sleepy and my mouth is dry." *Nux moschata*
"I get up at 3:00 A.M. with gas pains, and I just can't go, no matter how hard I try." *Nux vomica*

"The stool starts to come out, then it goes back in." *Silica*
"It feels like everything will fall out of my rectum if I try to go." *Sepia*

Ask

How long has it been since you had a bowel movement?
How often have you had bowel movements in the last week?
Was there anything unusual about your last bowel movement?
What was the stool like?
Any blood in the stool?
Is it painful to pass a stool?
What kind of foods have you been eating?
Are you drinking enough fluids?
Have you been getting any exercise?
Do you have any other illnesses going on now?

Pointers for Finding the Homeopathic Medicine

For constipation that is due to dryness with no urge, in a person who seems confused, consider *Alumina.* ▮ A person who needs *Bryonia* has large, hard stools with dryness, and a lot of thirst for cold drinks; many symptoms are worse from motion. ▮ For a stubborn, chilly, flabby person who sweats on his head and has stubborn constipation, try *Calcarea carbonica.* ▮ When there is dryness, and a dreamy, drowsy, dizzy state, give *Nux moschata.* ▮ When the person is an irritable businessperson, consider *Nux vomica* or *Bryonia.* ▮ If the person has constant urges but can't go, even with a lot of straining, try *Nux vomica.* ▮ For constipation during pregnancy and menstruation, and a feeling like a ball in the anus or that the rectum and uterus will fall out, consider *Sepia.* ▮ For bashful stool (comes out part way, then recedes) in a refined, shy person with sweaty feet, try *Silica.*

Dosage

- Give three pellets of 30C three times a day until you see improvement.
- If there is no improvement after three doses, give a different medicine.
- After you first notice improvement, give another dose only if symptoms begin to return.
- Lower potencies (6X, 6C, 30X) may need to be given more often (every four hours).
- Higher potencies (200X, 200C, 1M) usually only need to be given once. Repeat only if the symptoms definitely return after being better.

What to Expect from Homeopathic Self-Care

Homeopathic medicines stimulate the bowel to work normally, usually relieving constipation in a few hours to a couple of days. Homeopathic medicines can't, however, remove impacted stool, clear a bowel obstruction, or solve a problem that would require surgery or manual manipulation. If there is another disease process causing the constipation, it is necessary to treat the whole person homeopathically, not just the bowel. If there is chronic constipation, refer the person to a qualified homeopath.

Other Self-Care Suggestions

Drink eight glasses of water per day, starting with a glass of warm water with lemon immediately on rising in the morning. ▮ Eat lots of fresh fruits and vegetables, at least half of them raw. ▮ Eat whole grains and supplement with a tablespoon of bran stirred in juice or baked in muffins or in cereal. ▮ Take a one- to three-mile walk daily. ▮ Take one tablespoon flaxseed oil per day or one teaspoon ground flax seeds. ▮ Drink an eight-ounce glass of prune juice each morning. ▮ Take one tablespoon psyllium seed husks or powder per day. It is important to drink lots of water while taking psyllium.

	Key Symptoms	Mind	Body	Worse	Better	Food & Drink
Alumina *(Aluminum)*	**No urge to have a bowel movement** **Constipation so stubborn that the stool must be removed by hand** **Dryness of the mucous membranes**	**Dullness and slowness of mind**	**Constipation even with a soft stool** Constipation during pregnancy, with rectal dryness Newborns with constipation	**Potatoes** Morning, upon awakening Heat	Evening Open air Damp weather	**Desire for potatoes, rice, and dry foods** Desire for non-food items such as earth or coal Aversion to potatoes
Bryonia *(Wild hops)*	**Large, hard, dry stool** **Rectal dryness** **Dryness of the mucous membranes**	**Extremely irritable** **Talks of business** Wants to go home	**Dryness of mouth and lips, with extreme thirst for cold drinks**	**Worse from any motion** **Worse at 9:00 P.M.**	**Pressure** **Lying on the painful side** Warm drinks	
Calcarea carbonica *(Calcium carbonate)*	**Constipation in infants with large, sweaty heads and flabby bodies** **Constipation from low thyroid hormone** **No urge to have a bowel movement**	**Independent** **Stubborn** Worries about safety and security Sick from taking on too much responsibility	**Stubborn constipation** Doesn't feel bad while constipated Stool looks like clay Sour taste in the mouth and sour perspiration	**Cold damp weather** **Exertion** Teething	Dry weather	**Desire for eggs, sweets, and salty foods**
Nux moschata *(Nutmeg)*	**Dryness of the rectum** **Even soft stool must be removed by hand** **Very sleepy; can't stay awake** **Dizzy, drowsy, and dry** **Dry mouth and throat, but no thirst**	Confused	Extreme gas and bloating Fainting	Cold Pregnancy	Warmth Moist heat	

continued on next page

	Key Symptoms	Mind	Body	Worse	Better	Food & Drink
Nux vomica *(Quaker's button)*	**Constipated, with terrible straining for a bowel movement** **Constant urging, with unsuccessful attempts to pass stool** **Hard, painful stool** **Very irritable and impatient**	**Obsessed with business** **Wants to be the first and the best** **Competitive and hard-driving; Type A** Easily offended Frustrated easily by little things	**May have no urge whatsoever for a bowel movement** **Wakes up at 3:00 A.M. with gas pains** Nausea and vomiting Muscle tension	**Cold** Rich foods Eating Stimulants	**Warmth** Warm drinks After a bowel movement	**Desire for fat, spicy, rich foods, stimulants, and alcohol**
Sepia *(Cuttlefish ink)*	**No urge for stool for days** **Large, hard stools** **Feeling of a ball in the rectum or anus, not relieved by a bowel movement** **Constipation related to a hormonal imbalance**	**Aversion to her partner and to sex** Irritable Depressed and crying	**Constipation accompanied by other hormonal problems** **Constipation after childbirth, along with no sexual desire** Stools followed by mucus Prolapse of the rectum Crosses her legs to avoid the sensation that the uterus will fall out	**Vinegar** **Pregnancy** Too much sex Fasting or missing a meal Cold 4:00 to 6:00 P.M.	**Exercise, dancing** **Keeping busy** Warmth	**Desire for vinegar,** sour foods, and sweets Aversion to fat, salty foods
Silica *(Flint)*	**Bashful stool (comes out part way, then recedes)** **Strains to pass a hard stool** **Bowel movements feel incomplete**	Shy Perfectionist	**Constipated children** **Straining to have a bowel movement is exhausting** **Bad-smelling foot sweat** Refined and delicate features Constipation before or with the menstrual period Swollen lymph nodes	Cold, damp Touch Suppression of perspiration Vaccination	Warmth and heat	**Desire for eggs** and sweets Aversion to fat and milk

Coughs and Bronchitis

(See also Common Cold and Flu.)

Description

Acute bronchitis is an inflammation of the bronchial tubes of the lungs. It is often associated with a cold or upper respiratory infection, fever, sore throat, and a nasal discharge or postnasal drip. Although infection is the most common cause, it may also be caused by inhaling irritant substances, or it may be a complication of allergies and sinusitis. Bronchitis usually lasts three to five days, or up to several weeks.

Symptoms

Coughs may be dry or loose. The most common symptoms are a tickling feeling in the throat or chest, fits of uncontrollable coughing, excessive mucus, interrupted sleep due to the inability to lie down without coughing, hoarseness and pain in the throat, chest, or head.

Complications

Bronchitis may lead to pneumonia in serious cases. Patients with shortness of breath, weakness or exhaustion, persistent fever, and a thick yellow-green, brown, or bloody mucus from the lungs should see a qualified homeopath or other medical practitioner immediately.

Look

Blueness of the lips or under the nails.
Rapid pulse or breathing.
Posture while breathing or coughing.

Listen

"My chest is rattling and gurgling when I cough." *Antimonium tartaricum*
"Every time I move, I cough." *Bryonia*
"I feel like I'm choking to death when I cough because I have so much mucus." *Coccus cacti*
"My child vomits when he has a fit of coughing." *Drosera*
"I get so sick to my stomach that I feel like I'm going to throw up whenever I cough." *Ipecac*
"She has nosebleeds with her coughing fits." *Ipecac*
"I start coughing every time I lie down to go to sleep." *Rumex*

Ask

When did the cough start?
Was there any emotional trauma or stress that preceded the cough?
How severe is the coughing?
How frequently do you cough?
What makes you cough?
What makes your cough better or worse?
At what time is the cough better or worse?
What does the discharge from the lungs look like? How does it taste?
Is there any blood in the discharge?
How much appetite do you have? Do you have any desire for certain foods?
How thirsty are you? Is there any desire for certain drinks?
Do you have a fever?
Do you have any mental or emotional symptoms?
Are there any other symptoms since the cough started?

Pointers for Finding the Homeopathic Medicine

If the cough is extremely loose and rattly, think first of *Antimonium tartaricum,* then of *Ipecac* and *Pulsatilla.* ▮ If the person feels parched and is worse from any movement, give *Bryonia.* ▮ For bronchitis with fits of coughing, look at *Drosera, Hepar sulphuris, Spongia,* and *Rumex.* ▮ For dry, croupy coughs, think first of *Spongia, Drosera,* and *Hepar sulphuris.* ▮ For coughs that come from a tickle in the pit of the throat, look at *Rumex.*

Dosage

- Give three pellets of 30C every four hours until you see improvement.
- If there is no improvement after three doses, give a different medicine.
- After you first notice improvement, give another dose only if symptoms begin to return.
- Lower potencies (6X, 6C, 30X) may need to be given more often (every two to four hours).
- Higher potencies (200X, 200C, 1M) generally need to be given only once. Repeat only if symptoms return with intensity; give only infrequently in this case.

What to Expect from Homeopathic Self-Care

Bronchitis and coughs usually resolve in twenty-four to seventy-two hours with homeopathic treatment.

Other Self-Care Suggestions

For a wet cough, drink three to four cups a day of hot ginger tea. Boil three slices of fresh ginger in two cups of water for fifteen minutes. ▮ Hot water with plenty of freshly squeezed lemon juice and a little honey helps cut mucus. Drink three to four cups a day. ▮ Gargle with warm salt water. ▮ Vitamin C: 500 mg every four hours. ▮ Beta-carotene: 50,000 IU per day. ▮ Zinc: 30 mg per day. ▮ Drink licorice root tea, one cup three times a day, as an expectorant. ▮ Avoid dairy products, sweets, and heavy foods. ▮ Drink one to three glasses a day of freshly squeezed carrot juice. ▮ Wild cherry bark cough syrup: one-half teaspoon up to six times a day. Avoid cough syrups with eucalyptus, pine, camphor, or menthol while taking homeopathic medicines.

	Key Symptoms	Mind	Body	Worse	Better	Food & Drink
Antimonium tartaricum *(Tartar emetic)*	**Loose, rattling cough without much mucus coming up** **Bronchitis in infants and the elderly** **Child hates to be looked at or touched**	**Irritable and whining** **Wants to be left alone** Child desires to be carried	**Bronchial tubes are full of mucus** Overpowering sleepiness during bronchitis or cough Breathing is rapid, short, and difficult Lips may be blue	Warmth Anger Lying down	**Getting the mucus out** Belching Vomiting Cold, open air Sitting up	
Bryonia *(Wild hops)*	**Most symptoms are worse from any movement** **Extremely dry, chapped mouth and lips** **Great thirst for cold drinks** **Wants to go home**	**Irritable** **Overconcerned with business**	**Hard, dry cough that is worse from any movement** **Motion or cough causes pain in the chest and severe headache** **Holds onto chest to keep it from moving during the cough** Cough is dry at night Shortness of breath, with a great desire to take a deep breath but it makes the cough worse	**9:00 P.M.** Eating and drinking	**Lying on the painful side** **Pressure** Cool, open air Rest Warm drinks	**Gulps down large quantities of cold water** Desire for warm drinks, warm milk, and sometimes for cold drinks Desire for meat
Coccus cacti *(Cochineal)*	**Cough with which she almost chokes on thick, stringy mucus** **Constant clearing of the throat** **Fits of violent tickling** **Racking cough leading to vomiting**	Sad	**Accumulation of thick, stringy mucus in the nose and throat** **Profuse postnasal discharge** Vomiting from brushing teeth Feels like there is a thread hanging down the back of the throat Whooping cough	Heat Exposure to cold Lying down	Cold air Cold drinks Bathing in cold water	Desire for large quantities of water frequently
Drosera *(Sundew)*	**Violent fits of hard coughing with choking** **Can barely breathe while coughing** **Dry, barking, croupy, spasmodic cough that ends in**	Feels harassed	**Cough from a sensation of dryness and irritation in the larynx, like from crumbs or a feather** Nosebleed from the cough Painful cough Deep, hoarse voice; laryngitis	**Lying down in bed** **At night, after midnight** Getting warm in bed		

Hepar sulphuris *(Calcium sulfide)*	**Cough or laryngitis after exposure to cold** **Very chilly even to the point of shivering** **Croupy or barking cough** **Whooping cough** **Dry cough or a loose cough in which she can't bring anything up**	**Extreme hypersensitivity to pain** **Irritated and annoyed by everything**	**Recurrent bronchitis from every cold** **Chest tightens in cold air** **Nose is stopped up whenever she goes out in cold, dry air** **Very chilly** A lot of thick, yellow expectoration from the lungs Cough is worse from cold drinks or in the morning Very weak, with rattling in the chest	**Drafts** **Cold dry air** Evening until midnight	**Heat** **Bundling up**	**Desire for vinegar**
Ipecac *(Ipecac root)*	**Vomiting and nausea with coughing and nearly all problems** **Loose cough** **Nosebleeds and other conditions with bright red bleeding**	Hard to please Does not know what he wants Disgusted with everything	**Loose, gagging cough with rattling in the chest** **Great difficulty bringing up mucus from the chest** **Tongue is clear** Coughing up blood Severe cough makes breathing difficult Asthmatic bronchitis or croup Constant nausea not relieved by vomiting Sinking sensation in the stomach, and nausea at the smell or food	Warmth Eating or drinking Vomiting Lying down	Cold Fresh air	
Phosphorus	**Coughs or bronchitis with hoarseness** **Wants company when sick** **Very thirsty for cold and carbonated drinks**	**Outgoing** **Sympathetic** **Friendly** **Desires company** Afraid of the dark, thunderstorms, and ghosts	**Discharge from the lungs is rusty or bloody, thick, and frothy, and tastes salty or sweet** **Head colds that go to the lungs, causing bronchitis** **Cough first dry, then loose** Cough is hard, dry, painful, and hacking Comes on from a tickle in the throat Lingering coughs Breathing is difficult, and the chest feels tight and oppressed	Cold air Exertion Talking and laughing Change of temperature	**Lying on the right side** Sitting	**Desire for chocolate, ice cream, fish, and spicy foods**

continued on next page

	Key Symptoms	Mind	Body	Worse	Better	Food & Drink
Pulsatilla *(Windflower)*	**Bronchitis with thick yellow or green nasal discharge and expectoration** **Has to be propped up to sleep because of the cough** **Child is weepy, whiny, and clingy, and wants to be carried and cuddled** **Lack of thirst**	**Changeable emotions** **Wants company when sick**	**Cough is loose in the morning and dry in the evening or at night** **Feels better from going outdoors** **Loose cough in the morning, dry at night** Cough after measles Nose is stuffed up; can't smell Ears feel plugged	**Warm, stuffy room** **Rich food**	Slow walking in the open air	**Desire for butter, ice cream, and creamy foods** Aversion to fat and pork Aggravation from fat or rich food
Rumex *(Yellow dock)*	**Cough from a tickle in the pit of the throat or rawness in the larynx or trachea** **Cough is worse from uncovering the body or getting undressed**	Serious Indifferent to surroundings	**Dry, tickling cough that prevents sleep** Mucus in the throat	**Lying in bed; coughs as soon as the head touches the pillow** **Uncovering** 11:00 P.M. Morning upon awakening Inhaling cold air; change of temperature Touch or pressure on the throat Talking	Covering the mouth Sucking on a lozenge (don't use mentholated lozenges)	
Spongia *(Toasted sponge)*	**Hollow cough like a saw cutting through wood or a barking seal** **Cough is better from eating or drinking** **Croupy cough wakes him** **Dry cough worse from talking or singing**	Fearful of suffocation	**Hoarseness** **Feeling of a plug in the larynx with anxious, gasping breathing** **Suffocating feeling** **Cough is quite dry** Air passages feel dry Breathing is short and difficult	Warm room Lying down After midnight Exertion	Warm food Going down stairs or downhill	

Cuts, Scrapes, and Puncture Wounds

Description

A wound is caused by a sharp object piercing the skin. It may be a cut (laceration or incision), a puncture wound, or a scrape (abrasion).

Symptoms

Tissue damage, bleeding, bruising, inflammation, swelling, and pain are the most prominent symptoms of wounds. The seriousness of the wound depends on the amount of damage to underlying organs and tissues.

Complications

Superficial wounds are not serious, and usually heal rapidly on their own if they are kept clean and free of infection. Deep cuts may need stitches. If cuts or puncture wounds are deep, damage to organs, muscles, nerves, and bones needs to be assessed immediately by a qualified medical practitioner. A serious wound, such as a knife or gunshot wound, may be life-threatening.

Puncture wounds carry the risk of tetanus within two days to two months after a wound has been infected. Deep or dirty puncture wounds should have dirt and dead tissue removed by a qualified medical practitioner to help prevent tetanus. Early signs of tetanus include jaw stiffness, difficulty swallowing, and stiffness of the neck, arms, or legs after a wound. More advanced tetanus includes the inability to open the jaw (lockjaw), a fixed smile, and raised eyebrows, as well as spasms in the neck, back, and abdomen. Tetanus may be fatal if untreated. If the person has not had a tetanus immunization or booster in the last five years, a tetanus inoculation should be given immediately following the injury. A dose of homeopathic *Ledum* may be given immediately as well.

Look

Where is the wound? How large?

Is there discoloration of or around the area?

Is the wound bleeding?

Is swelling present?

Listen

"I stepped on a nail yesterday and now I have shooting pains up my leg."
Hypericum

"I cut my finger with a knife. It feels better if I run cold water on it." *Ledum*
"My son, Benny, fell on the pavement and scraped himself while running." *Arnica*

Ask

What happened to cause the wound?
Is there pain? If so, where?
What makes the pain better or worse?
Are there any other symptoms?
Is the area hot or cold to the touch?

Pointers for Finding the Homeopathic Medicine

The first medicines to consider for puncture wounds are *Ledum* and *Hypericum*. ▮ If the affected part is cold and cold to the touch, give *Ledum*. ▮ If there is numbness or shooting pains, use *Hypericum*. ▮ If there is bruising or bleeding, give *Arnica*.

Dosage

- Give three pellets of 30C every two to four hours until you see improvement.
- If there is no improvement after three doses, give a different medicine.
- After you first notice improvement, give another dose only if symptoms begin to return.
- Lower potencies (6X, 6C, 30X) may need to be given more often (every two to four hours).
- Higher potencies (200X, 200C, 1M) generally need to be given only once. Repeat only if symptoms return with intensity; give only infrequently in this case.

What to Expect from Homeopathic Self-Care

Wounds heal much more quickly with homeopathic treatment. Swelling, bleeding, and bruising are all reduced. Be sure to use the wound care suggestions that follow.

Other Self-Care Suggestions

For serious wounds: Apply direct pressure to stop bleeding. Get medical attention immediately.

For minor wounds: Apply direct pressure to stop bleeding. Clean the wound with soap and water. ▌ Apply *Calendula* gel, cream, or spray (for abrasions), or tincture, diluted one part tincture to three parts water. Dilute more if the tincture hurts when applied. *Calendula* prevents and heals infections. *Hypericum* tincture may be used, diluted one to three parts as well, especially for infected cuts or scrapes. Use the tinctures several times a day until there is definite healing, then once a day until healing is complete. ▌ Cover the wound with a bandage or gauze dressing. ▌ Change the dressing as needed.

For minor puncture wounds: Clean the wound with soap and water. ▌ Let the wound bleed freely to flush out dirt or debris unless bleeding is severe.

For severe bleeding: Apply direct pressure on the wound. Soak puncture wounds in warm water several times a day to remove more debris. ▌ Apply full-strength or diluted *Calendula* tincture to promote healing.

For general wound healing: Vitamin C (500 mg four times a day). ▌ Zinc (30 mg per day). ▌ Beta-carotene (50,000 IU per day). ▌ Bromelain (250 mg, two capsules three times a day) to reduce scarring. Must be taken immediately after injury for treatment to be effective. ▌ Echinacea and goldenseal tincture, thirty drops three times a day in water or juice, to stimulate the immune system to fight infection.

	Key Symptoms	Mind	Body	Worse	Better	Food & Drink
Arnica *(Leopard's bane)*	**Any trauma or wound resulting in bruising** **Shock of any kind**	**Says nothing is wrong** **Sends help away** Wants to be left alone	**Cuts bleed a lot or bruise** **Wants to lie down, but the bed feels too hard**	Touch Lying on a hard surface Motion	Lying down, especially with the head low	
Hypericum *(St. John's wort)*	**Lacerations or injuries to areas with lots of nerves, such as the tips of the fingers and toes** **Shooting pains** **Numbness and tingling**	Sad	Gaping wounds Wounds resulting in weakness from loss of blood	Jarring the injured area Touch	Rubbing the area Lying on the face Bending backwards	
Ledum *(Marsh tea)*	**Puncture wounds that feel cold to the touch and are better from cold cloth or ice pack** **Possibility of getting tetanus (also get a tetanus booster shot if needed)**	Bad-humored Dissatisfied	**Any puncture wound** Site of bite is purple and puffy	**Heat**	**Bathing, soaking, or applying cold**	

Diaper Rash

Description

Diaper rash is a skin irritation or infection which occurs when wet diapers stay in prolonged contact with the baby's skin.

Symptoms

The skin is moist, red, and raw. Red spots or patches may indicate a yeast infection due to *Candida*. Bacterial infection may cause blistering and pus.

Complications

Diaper rash rarely causes anything other than local inflammation or infection. If a high fever is present without another obvious cause and the lymph glands in the groin are swollen, seek medical attention to rule out an infection in the bloodstream.

Look

How does the skin look on the baby's bottom?
Is the skin red and somewhat shiny (indicating *Candida* infection)?
Is the skin blistering with pus present (indicating bacterial infection)?
Does the baby have a fever?
Does the baby have swollen lymph glands in the groin?

Listen

"My baby, Chrissy, has a very dry rash that oozes a thick, sticky, yellow discharge." *Graphites*
"Sammy was born with a bright red rash on his butt." *Medorrhinum*
"Little Carly scratches herself raw, especially after I bathe her." *Sulphur*
"Toby cries terribly from his diaper rash. He must be very sensitive to pain." *Hepar sulphuris*

Ask

How long has the diaper rash been present?
Where is the rash located?
Does the baby seem to be in pain?
Does anything make it better or worse?
Does the baby cry more than usual when wet or soiled?

Pointers for Finding the Homeopathic Medicine

Babies needing *Hepar sulphuris* are generally extremely chilly and very sensitive to uncovering. They have an infected diaper rash with pus that smells like rotten cheese. ▮ Infants who need *Graphites* have diaper rash in the folds of the skin, which is dry, red, cracked, and very itchy, with a honey-like discharge that crusts over. ▮ Babies needing *Medorrhinum* have a sharply demarcated red, sometimes shiny diaper rash often caused by *Candida* infection, called "thrush diaper rash." ▮ Infants who need *Sulphur* have a red, dry, itchy diaper rash around the anus that is worse from getting overheated and from a warm bath.

Dosage

- Give three pellets of 30C every four hours until you see improvement.
- If there is no improvement after three doses, give a different medicine.
- After you first notice improvement, give another dose only if symptoms begin to return.
- Lower potencies (6X, 6C, 30X) may need to be given more often (every two to four hours).
- Higher potencies (200X, 200C, 1M) generally need to be given only once. Repeat only if symptoms return with intensity; give only infrequently in this case.

What to Expect from Homeopathic Self-Care

Homeopathic medicines will help relieve the diaper rash within several days.

Other Self-Care Suggestions

Let the baby go without diapers whenever possible. ▮ Change diapers whenever they become wet or soiled. ▮ Cleanse the area with very mild soap and water. ▮ Dry the area carefully with a hairdryer on the lowest heat. ▮ Apply *Calendula* cream after every diaper change until diaper rash is gone. ▮ If yeast is present, take the baby off fruit juices and sweet foods. ▮ Cornstarch may be useful on the skin as a drying powder. ▮ Use all-cotton diapers instead of rubber pants.

	Key Symptoms	Mind	Body	Worse	Better	Food & Drink
Graphites *(Graphite)*	**Diaper rash with a thick, golden, honey-like discharge and yellow crusts** **Skin is dry, red, raw, and cracked** **Baby scratches until rash bleeds**	**Overly excitable** **Cries easily**		Warm covers in bed		**Aversion to sweets**
Hepar sulphuris *(Calcium sulfide)*	**Infected diaper rash with pus that smells like rotten cheese** **Area is extremely sensitive to the touch**	**Extremely irritable and touchy** **Very sensitive to pain**		**Cold** **Drafts** **Uncovering the body**	**Warmth** Covering up	
Medorrhinum *(Nosode)*	**Bright red diaper rash on the buttocks, with clear borders** **Sleeps on the tummy or in the knees-to-chest position**	**Restless** **Oversensitive** Cries easily	**Rashes, ear infections, or other symptoms from the moment of birth** Rash is itchy and sore Warts may also be present	**Cold damp weather** After urinating Sunrise to sunset	**Lying on abdomen**	**Desire for sour foods, unripe fruit, oranges, and ice**
Sulphur	**Bright red rash around the anus** **Very itchy, red diaper rash that is worse from a warm bath** **Child scratches rash until it bleeds**	**Critical** **Impatient** **Messy**		**Night** **Warmth** **Being in bed** Sweets		**Desire for sweets**

Diarrhea, Acute

(See also Amebiasis and Food Poisoning.)

Description

Acute diarrhea is usually due to infection by such bacteria as *Staphylococcus, E. coli, Salmonella,* or *Shigella* or such parasites as amebas or *Giardia lamblia*. Infection may come from eating or drinking contaminated food or water (see Amebic Dysentery). Some diarrhea is caused by emotional or digestive upset.

Symptoms

The stools are loose or watery, sometimes profuse or explosive, and may be foul-smelling. Food particles may be found in the stool.

Complications

Diarrhea often results in loss of fluids and electrolytes such as sodium and potassium, which must be replaced to prevent dangerous levels of dehydration and electrolyte imbalance. Homeopathic medicines can stop diarrhea, but rehydration is still important.

Look

Observe the stool if possible.
Note the color, consistency, and odor of the stool.
Are the eyes sunken?
Are the lips dry and chapped?
Get the stool tested for parasites if there is reason to suspect a parasitic infection.

Listen

"My stools are nearly all mucus. I feel like the stool's coming out all the time." *Aloe*

"My stools are very loose since I ate a pint of fresh cherries yesterday. Is it something serious?" *Arsenicum album*

"I got a rash on my scrotum at the same time as the diarrhea started." *Croton tiglium*

"Ever since I got back from Mexico last week, I have diarrhea that shoots out because of the gas. I also have lots of cramping and rumbling in my abdomen." *Podophyllum*

"I feel just terrible. Every time I sit on the toilet, the diarrhea just pours out, and I start shivering and sweating. The only thing that makes me feel better is ice." *Veratrum album*

Ask

When did the diarrhea start?
How long has it been going on?
What is the stool like?
Is there pain or cramping?
Is there gas?
What makes the diarrhea better or worse?
What time of day does it occur?
Are there any mental or emotional symptoms with the diarrhea?
Did any other physical symptoms start along with the diarrhea?
How are you sleeping?

Pointers to Finding the Homeopathic Medicine

If stool is like jelly or jello due to mucus, give *Aloe.* ▮ If the person is chilly, anxious, nervous, and restless, *Arsenicum album* is your best bet. ▮ If diarrhea comes immediately after eating or drinking, look at *Croton tiglium.* ▮ If the stool shoots into the toilet, think of *Podophyllum* first, then *Croton tiglium* and *Gambogia.* ▮ If there is a lot of rectal itching with the diarrhea, combined with urgency first thing in the morning, *Sulphur* is indicated. ▮ If the diarrhea is violent and is accompanied by profuse sweating and chills, give *Veratrum album.*

Dosage

- Give three pellets of 30C every two to four hours, depending on the severity, until you see improvement.
- If there is no improvement after three doses, give a different medicine.
- After you first notice improvement, give another dose only if symptoms begin to return.
- Lower potencies (6X, 6C, 30X) may need to be given more often (every one to four hours).
- Higher potencies (200X, 200C, 1M) generally need to be given only once. Repeat only if symptoms return with intensity; give only infrequently in this case.

Other Self-Care Suggestions

Drink plenty of fluids and replenish such electrolytes as sodium and potassium. Knudsen Recharge, Gatorade, Emergen-C, and electrolyte solutions available from pharmacies are useful. Clear liquids such as water, vegetable broth, and diluted fruit juice help replace fluids. ▮ The diet should be light and bland, including vegetable soup, whole-grain toast, brown rice, bananas, and applesauce. ▮ Applesauce with carob powder can be helpful for infants or children with diarrhea. ▮ A warm pack over the abdomen is soothing and may reduce cramping. Calcium (1000 mg per day) and Magnesium (500 mg per day) may also help to reduce cramping. ▮ One tablespoon psyllium seed husks per day often helps to firm up stools.

	Key Symptoms	Mind	Body	Worse	Better	Food & Drink
Aloe socotrina *(Aloe)*	**Feeling of insecurity in the rectum, as though stool would come out** **Stools are lumpy, gelatinous, slimy, bloody, and watery, and may be bright yellow** **Mucus and burning pain in the rectum after stool**	**Irritable, discontented, and angry, with abdominal pain or constipation** Doesn't want to be around people	**Feels like stool will come out while passing gas, and it does** **Rumbling and gurgling in the bowels; sudden urging to pass a watery, gushing stool** **Hemorrhoids protrude like a bunch of grapes and bleed** Beer and oysters cause diarrhea	Heat, summer, hot damp weather After eating or drinking	Cool, open air, cold bathing, cold applications Passing gas	
Arsenicum album *(Arsenic)*	**Food poisoning** **Nausea and vomiting after eating or drinking** **Severe abdominal cramping** **Burning pains in the abdomen and rectum** **Excessive anxiety and restlessness** **Chilly and thirsty for frequent sips of water**	**Nervous and anxious** **Needy and demanding** **Afraid of death** Afraid of being alone	**Diarrhea is worse after eating and drinking, especially sour foods, fruit, and cold food or drinks** **Stools are frequent, dark, watery, and bad-smelling, with blood and mucus**	**Midnight to 2:00 A.M.** **Cold food or drinks**	**Heat** **Warm drinks**	Desire for milk, sour food, and the fat on meat
Croton tiglium *(Croton oil seed)*	**Diarrhea gushing like a fire hydrant, combined with skin rash like poison ivy** **Diarrhea immediately after eating or drinking** **Diarrhea that shoots out explosively in one big gush**	**Anxious during diarrhea, as though something bad will happen**	**Gurgling in the intestines from drinking the least amount of liquid or from eating** **Strong urge to have a bowel movement with large quantities of watery diarrhea** **Sensation of sloshing in the intestines as if there is only water in them** Emptiness in the stomach Nausea with retching and vomiting Diarrhea along with skin rashes, particularly on the genitals	**Drinking or eating the least amount** Washing	After sleep Gentle rubbing	

continued on next page

	Key Symptoms	Mind	Body	Worse	Better	Food & Drink
Gambogia *(Gummi gutti tree)*	**Severe diarrhea** **Stools come out suddenly and in gushes**	Cheerful and talkative Depression alternating with diarrhea	**Stools come out in thin, prolonged gushes** **Rumbling and rolling in the abdomen** Diarrhea with vomiting Burning of anus Gurgling before stool Urine smells like onions	Toward evening and at night After stool (sometimes) Motion Open air	After stool (more often)	
Podophyllum *(May apple)*	**Diarrhea with sudden urgency** **Diarrhea drives her out of bed at 5:00 A.M.** **Exhausting diarrhea with abdominal cramping and rumbling** **Stools shoot all over the toilet**	Fidgety, restless, and whining Fear of becoming very ill or dying	**Rumbling and gurgling before the stool** **Diarrhea is often painless** Stools are frequent, profuse, liquid, gushing, and bad-smelling Yellowish-green stools Pain in the liver	**Sour fruit** **Hot weather** Eating Drinking Motion	Rubbing the liver area Lying on the abdomen or bending forward	
Sulphur *(Sulfur)*	**Sudden, explosive diarrhea makes her get out of bed in the morning 5:00 A.M.** **Worse at 11:00 A.M. in general**	**Opinionated and critical** **Thinking all the time, philosophical** **Lazy** Usually messy, but sometimes very neat	**Anus is red, sore, raw, and burning, and itches a lot** **Stool is loose and burning** **Rash on skin** **Very smelly diarrhea, gas, perspiration, and discharges** Diarrhea from beer	**Warmth, warmth of bed (sticks feet out from covers)** **Bathing** **Left side**	Open air	**Desire for alcohol, sweets, and spicy food** **Aversion to eggs, fish, and squash**
Veratrum album *(White hellebore)*	**Violent vomiting and diarrhea** **Icy cold, with cold sweat** **Strong craving for ice, cold drinks, juicy fruit, pickles, lemons, and salty food**	**Very active and busy** **Restless**	**Collapses, with bluish colored skin** **Diarrhea profuse, painful, and watery** **Diarrhea very forceful, followed by exhaustion and cold sweat**	**Cold** Menstrual period Fruit	**Warmth** Hot drinks Covering up	

Dizziness

Description

Dizziness is a symptom more than an illness, but it is nonetheless quite annoying and can be debilitating. Dizziness may accompany fever, headache, and nausea in acute illnesses. It is also present with fainting, motion sickness, and loss of balance.

Symptoms

Dizziness is often described as a loss of orientation, loss of balance, and visual disturbance, often with a "lightheaded" feeling or a sensation of the room spinning. Nausea and vomiting often accompany the dizzy feeling.

Complications

Dizziness may precede loss of consciousness and falling. It may be a symptom of more chronic, serious underlying problems with the endocrine or nervous system or the inner ear, such as hypothyroidism, multiple sclerosis, brain tumors, and Ménière's disease. Dizziness may also come from breathing chemical fumes or from alcohol intoxication. Prolonged or recurrent dizziness should be diagnosed by a qualified homeopath or other qualified healthcare practitioner.

Look

Is the person falling over or staggering?
Is there any paralysis?
What position does she prefer to be in?

Listen

"I'm so dizzy I want to go home." *Bryonia*
"How am I going to carry on my business without losing money?" *Bryonia*
"If everything would just stop moving I'd be all right." *Cocculus*
"I feel like I have been run over by a truck." *Gelsemium*
"I was so frightened." *Aconite*
"I feel like my legs are so weak I can't stand up." *Conium*
"Please hold me." *Pulsatilla*

Ask

What brought on the dizziness?
What makes the dizziness better or worse?

Is it accompanied by nausea? Vomiting?
Are there any mental or emotional symptoms with the dizziness?
Are you hungry or thirsty?
Are you desiring anything to eat or drink?
Do you feel too hot or too cold?

Pointers for Finding the Homeopathic Medicine

If the dizziness follows a fright or shock, give *Aconite.* ▮ Give *Gelsemium* for dizziness due to fright. ▮ When the dizziness is from motion or motion sickness, consider *Bryonia* or *Cocculus* first. ▮ Give *Bryonia* if the patient is very irritable, dry, and thirsty and talks of business or wants to go home. ▮ If the dizziness is definitely from riding in a car or airplane or watching moving objects, give *Cocculus.* ▮ If the dizziness is associated with paralysis or weakness of the legs, you can try *Conium* first, but also see a homeopath as soon as possible. ▮ If the dizziness is associated with overall weakness, exhaustion, and dullness of mind, give *Gelsemium.* ▮ If the dizziness is worse during the menstrual period, when looking upward, or from sitting down, in a weepy, clingy person who is worse in a warm, stuffy room, give *Pulsatilla.*

Dosage

- Give three pellets of 30C every two hours until you see improvement.
- If there is no improvement after three doses, give a different medicine.
- After you first notice improvement, give another dose only if symptoms begin to return.
- Lower potencies (6X, 6C, 30X) may need to be given more often (every one to two hours).
- Higher potencies (200X, 200C, 1M) often need to be given only once. Repeat infrequently only if the symptoms return with intensity.

What to Expect from Homeopathic Treatment

Both acute and chronic dizziness can be treated with homeopathic medicines. Acute dizziness should resolve within minutes to hours with the correct medicine. Chronic dizziness should be treated by a qualified homeopath or medical practitioner.

Other Self-Care Suggestions

Hold on to something to prevent falling. ▮ Do not drive or operate machinery while dizzy. ▮ Pick one point and look at it for orientation and balance. ▮ Sit or lie down; close your eyes.

	Key Symptoms	Mind	Body	Worse	Better	Food & Drink
Aconite *(Monkshood)*	**Dizziness from fright or shock** **Extreme anxiety and restlessness** **Fear of impending death** **Symptoms come on suddenly**	**Panic attacks** **Claustrophobia** **Fear of being alone** Fear of crowds, open spaces, and flying in airplanes	**Dizziness when standing up or rising from a seat** **Profuse perspiration with anxiety** **Rapid pulse** Violent heart palpitations Hot, heavy, burning sensation in the head	Chill	Rest	Very thirsty for cold drinks
Bryonia *(Wild hops)*	**Dizziness and most other symptoms are worse from any motion** **Dryness of mouth and lips, with extreme thirst for cold drinks** **Worse at 9:00 P.M.**	**Extremely irritable** Wants to go home Talks of business	**Dizziness when getting up from a seat or bed** **Dizziness when turning the head, or on bending over** Dizziness with headache in the back of the head Sensation of whirling Pain over left eye Bursting, splitting headache, worse from motion	Moving the eyes	Warm drinks	
Cocculus *(Indian cockle)*	**Any kind of motion sickness** **Seasickness, airsickness** **Dizziness from looking at moving objects or watching things out of the window of a moving vehicle** **Sick after caring for ill family member or from loss of sleep**	Very sensitive Anxiety about loved ones	**Room seems to spin** **Must lie down with the dizziness or gets nauseous** **Nausea from the sight or smell of food** **Headache, nausea, and vomiting with the dizziness**	**Emotional stress** **Loss of sleep** Open air Touch	Lying on the side	Aversion to food

continued on next page

	Key Symptoms	Mind	Body	Worse	Better	Food & Drink
Conium *(Hemlock)*	**Dizziness worse when lying or turning over in bed** **Dizziness from moving his eyes or head** **Feels like the room is whirling**	**Emotionally reserved** Doesn't want company	Feels sick with headache and can't urinate	**Beginning to move** Sexual abstinence	Continuing to move	
Gelsemium *(Yellow jasmine)*	**Dizziness following fright or from stage fright** **Dizzy, drowsy, droopy, and dull** **Muscle aching throughout body**	**Mind feels extremely dull** Thinking is an effort	**Dizziness, as if drunk, with heaviness of the eyelids** **Blurred vision** **Headache starts in the neck or back of head and goes to the forehead** **Head feels heavy and hard to lift** **Overall weakness** Wants to lie down and go to sleep	**Fright** Wine 10:00 A.M.	Bending forward Lying down with head held high Urination	**Lack of thirst**
Pulsatilla *(Windflower)*	**Dizziness while sitting, relieved by walking or sitting in the open air or by lying down** **Dizziness when looking upward** **Dizziness or fainting in a warm, stuffy room**	**Changeable emotions** **Clingy and weepy** **Wants company when sick**	**Warm, with desire for fresh air or open window** Dizziness during the menstrual period	**After eating** **Rich food** Evening	Slow walking in the open air	**Lack of thirst** **Desire for butter, ice cream, and creamy foods** Aversion to fat and pork Aggravation

Ear Infections
(Otitis media)

Description
Ear infections may be either internal or external. Otitis media, a middle ear infection, occurs behind the eardrum. Otitis externa, an outer ear infection, occurs in the ear canal outside the drum. Acute middle-ear infections are associated with bacteria. Chronic middle-ear inflammation may come from chronic bacterial infection or a buildup of fluid, usually caused by allergic reactions. Infants who are exposed to solid food and cow's milk (or in some cases soy milk) too early may develop significant food allergies which are directly correlated with chronic ear infections. The allergies often begin right after the child is weaned from breast-feeding.

Symptoms
Middle-ear infections cause acute pain, a clogged or blocked sensation in the ear with some temporary loss of hearing, and bulging of the eardrum. More rarely, the eardrum can rupture, discharging pus and fluid into the ear canal. Chronic ear infections cause redness of the eardrum and pressure and blockage in the ears with some, usually reversible, hearing loss.

Complications
Following a rupture, the eardrum will usually repair itself, but may leave scarring. Chronic ear infections may cause hearing loss, which usually resolves when the fluid drains or disappears. In chronic middle-ear inflammation with an allergic basis ("glue ear"), antibiotics are ineffective on a long-term basis, and the causative allergic responses must be addressed. Even in acute ear infections, antibiotics may not shorten the course of illness. Conventional physicians often recommend surgical insertion of tubes into the eardrums to drain off the fluid, in order to prevent chronic hearing loss which may interfere with language development in young children.

Look
Is the eardrum red (inflamed), bulging, or ruptured? (Requires an otoscope to look in the ear.)
Is fluid visible behind the eardrum?
Is there any discharge from the ears? What does it look like?

Is the child's face red or pale?
Is there mucus from the nose? What color?

Listen

"My baby suddenly got an ear infection after I took him for a walk in the stroller. I didn't realize how windy it was outside and I forgot his hat." *Aconite*

"My right ear is throbbing and my throat is terribly sore on the right side." *Belladonna*

"My ear hurts. Don't touch it!" *Chamomilla* or *Hepar sulphuris*

"My child has dragon breath with this ear infection, and is drooling like crazy." *Mercurius*

"My ear hurts! Will you hold me in your lap?" *Pulsatilla*

"The earache came on just after I developed a dental abscess." *Silica*

Ask

Is there pain? If so, what is it like?
Which ear hurts?
What does it feel like?
Are you drooling or do you have more saliva than usual?
Are there swollen glands in the neck or around the ear?
Has your hunger or thirst changed since the ear infection began?
Do you want anything in particular to eat? To drink?
Do you feel hot or cold?
Do you have a sore throat?
If the person is a child, does she tug on one or both ears, or bore her fingers into the ear?
Does the child have a fever? How high?
Is the child sweating?

Pointers for Finding the Homeopathic Medicine

If a child quickly develops an ear infection after playing in the cold air, she needs *Aconite*. ▮ If the child has intense, throbbing pain in the right ear, a bright red face, and a fever of 103°F or higher, give *Belladonna*. ▮ For fussy children whose ear infections are associated with teething, *Chamomilla* is best. ▮ Children who scream with pain during an ear infection may need *Hepar sulphuris, Belladonna,* or *Chamomilla*. ▮ If *Mercurius* is needed, there is likely to be bad breath, a coated tongue, excessive saliva, and bad-smelling perspiration. ■ Mild, moody children who cry easily and want to be held and caressed during an ear infection are likely to need *Pulsatilla*. ■ If *Silica* is needed, there will generally be a tendency to swollen glands, excessive bad-smelling perspiration, and possibly a history of dental problems.

Dosage

- Give three pellets of 30C every two to four hours until you see improvement.
- If there is no improvement after three doses, give a different medicine.
- After you first notice improvement, give another dose only if symptoms begin to return.
- Lower potencies (6X, 6C, 30X) may need to be given more often (every two to four hours).
- Higher potencies (200X, 200C, 1M) generally need to be given only once. Repeat only if symptoms return with intensity; give only infrequently in this case.

What to Expect with Homeopathic Treatment

Homeopathy is highly effective in treating both acute and chronic ear infections. Acute infections should resolve in one to several days. For chronic or recurrent ear infections, consult a qualified homeopath. Constitutional treatment will generally prevent any future ear infections or make them very infrequent.

Other Self-Care Suggestions

Mullein-garlic oil drops, three drops in the affected ear three times daily. Warm the oil bottle under the faucet first. Put a piece of cotton in the ear after inserting drops to prevent the oil from coming out. If there is a tendency for the infection to spread from one ear to the other, put the drops in both ears. ■ Alternating hot and cold compresses to the affected ear. ■ Beta-carotene: 50,000 units daily in acute cases; 25,000 units daily in chronic cases. ■ It is often helpful to remove milk products from the diet, at least temporarily. ■ Some practitioners recommend removing wheat and any other allergens from the diet. However, it is usually sufficient to temporarily remove only dairy products if the person receives constitutional homeopathic treatment, and sometimes even that dietary change is unnecessary. ■ Goat's milk is a good substitute for cow's milk.

	Key Symptoms	Mind	Body	Worse	Better	Food & Drink
Aconite *(Monkshood)*	**Very painful ear infections with a high fever** **Sudden onset of ear infection** **Ear infections that come on from exposure to a cold, dry wind** **Usually indicated within the first twenty-four hours of onset**	**Ailments from fright** **Anxious and restless** Great fear of death	**Ears bright red** **Extreme sensitivity to noise** Feels as if there's a drop of water in the ear	Cold dry weather Pressure or touch Teething Noise or light	Rest	
Belladonna *(Deadly nightshade)*	**Ear infections that come on suddenly and violently, with high fever and a bright red face** **The pain is intense and throbbing, and usually is worse in the right ear** **Sensitive to light, noise, and jarring** **Throbbing headache**	**Delirious if the fever becomes too high** Biting, striking rage Child often behaves as if he is perfectly healthy	**Right-sided ear infections** **Eyes are glassy** **Skin is hot and dry** **Mouth hot and dry with a red tongue** May also have an extremely sore throat that is worse on the right side Dilated pupils with staring	Drafts Touch Motion	**Propped up in a quiet, dark room** Bending backward Bed rest	**Great thirst for cold water or no thirst at all** **Desire for lemons and lemonade**
Chamomilla *(Chamomile)*	**Child is cross and contrary, especially during teething** **Child demands to be carried or rocked** **One cheek may be red and hot, the other pale**	**Quarrelsome** **Can't bear to be touched or examined** **Inconsolable** Doesn't want anyone near Asks for something, then, when he receives it, wants something else	**Great pain with red-hot ears** **Ear infection, especially during teething** **Child is inconsolable with ear pain** **Tremendous hypersensitivity to pain** Hearing may be lost during the infection Can't stand to listen to music Greenish diarrhea, like chopped spinach, during teething	**Teething** Cold wind Night 9:00 P.M.	**Being carried**	
Hepar sulphuris *(Calcium sulfide)*	**Extremely painful ear infection** **Child wakes at night screaming inconsolably with pain** **Oversensitive and annoyed by every little thing**	**Constantly complaining**	**Thick pus behind the eardrum** **Discharge from ears is offensive and smells sour or like rotten cheese** Darting pains in the ears Perforation of the eardrum	**Drafts** **Uncovering the body** **Wind**	**Heat**	**Desire for vinegar** Desire for sour foods and fat

	Hypersensitive to pain **Ears are very sensitive to the wind and cold air** **Extreme chilliness**	**Dissatisfied with everything**	Mastoiditis (painful inflammation of the mastoid bone behind the ear) Head is extremely sensitive to being uncovered Swollen tonsils and neck glands	**Cold air and applications** Touch		
Mercurius *(Mercury)*	**Increased saliva or drooling with ear infection** **Bad breath and bad-smelling perspiration** **Like the mercury in a thermometer, very sensitive to both heat and cold**	**Suspicious** Hurried Restless Emotionally reserved	**Ears are quite painful, with sharp or stinging pains** **Discharge of offensive yellow-green pus or a thin, irritating, bloody discharge** Pain extends to the ear from the teeth Dental abscesses Gums can be spongy and painful Ear pain is worse from swallowing and blowing the nose Tongue often has a white coating	**Night** Sweating Damp cold Drafts	**Moderate temperature** Rest	**Desire for bread and butter** Desire for cold drinks Aversion to sweets and salty foods
Pulsatilla *(Windflower)*	**Ears that feel stopped up or full with symptoms of a "ripe" cold (profuse, thick nasal discharge)** **Thick, bland, yellow-green discharge from the nose, ears, and lungs** **Weepy, whiny, clingy child who wants to be carried and cuddled** **Lack of thirst**	Changeable emotions Can't make up her mind	**Ears feel stopped up** **Aching of ears worse at night** Discharge of offensive pus or blood from the ears (only with a ruptured eardrum) External ear red and swollen	**Warmth** **Warm, stuffy room** **Getting the feet wet** Rich food, pork	Slow walking in the open air	**Desire for butter, ice cream, and creamy foods** Aversion to fat, pork, and warm foods and drinks Aggravation from fats and rich food
Silica *(Flint)*	**Chronic ear infections** **Swollen lymph nodes** **Low stamina and energy** **Bad-smelling foot sweat** **Delicate features**	**Shy** **Timid** **Refined**	**Eardrum can rupture; ear is filled with offensive-smelling pus** Irritating, thin, foul-smelling discharge from the ear Ears feel blocked; better from yawning or swallowing Perforated eardrum Sensitivity to noise Mastoiditis (painful inflammation of the mastoid bone behind the ear) Infections slow to heal	Cold, damp Touch	Warmth and heat	**Desire for eggs** **Aversion to milk**

Fainting

Description

Fainting is a sudden brief loss of consciousness caused by a lowering of blood pressure to the brain. Fainting may result from physical or emotional causes. Common causative factors are blood loss, dehydration, pain, fright, shock, becoming overheated, exhaustion, arrhythmias of the heart, overexertion, and hyperventilation.

Symptoms

Sudden loss of consciousness with collapse.

Complications

Fainting is usually brief and causes no harm other than the trauma from falling. Fainting may be a symptom of a more serious problem such as shock, head injury, heart attack, stroke, or brain tumor. If pulse or breathing are absent, perform CPR (cardio-pulmonary resuscitation) immediately and have someone call 911 for emergency medical assistance. If pulse and respiration are normal, but the person doesn't regain consciousness within a few minutes, seek immediate medical attention.

Look

Is the person breathing? Is the chest rising and falling?
What color is the person's face? Lips? Nails?
Look around to observe the circumstances.

Listen

"I fell off my bicycle and took a really hard fall. I somehow just got up and walked away. Then, for some reason, I fainted." *Arnica*
"A robber came in with a gun. I was so scared that I fainted." *Aconite*
"I got a cramp while swimming. I started to drown. When they pulled me out I was blue and shivering." *Carbo vegetabilis*
"I was getting my blood drawn, and I just keeled over." *China*
"I was so happy to get my college acceptance letter that I fainted." *Coffea*
"I was supposed to give a violin concert to three hundred people. I was so nervous that I fainted dead away right before the performance." *Gelsemium*

"After I found out that my sister died, I was so shocked and grief-stricken that I fainted." *Ignatia*

Ask

What happened just before the person fainted?
Was there a trauma?
Is there a friend or relative present? Can he explain the situation?
Is there injury or blood loss?
Did she fall suddenly, or did she slump down gradually?
Did she say anything before she fainted?
Is the room unusually warm or chilly?

Pointers for Finding the Homeopathic Medicine

In cases of fainting due to an extreme fright, give *Aconite* first. ▪ For fainting following an accident or trauma, always give *Arnica* first. ▪ For fainting from hypothermia or drowning, give *Carbo vegetabilis* first, then consider *Veratrum album*. ▪ If the person has fainted following donating or losing blood, give *China*. ▪ If the fainting follows excitement, give *Coffea*. ▪ For fainting from stage fright, *Gelsemium* is the best choice. ▪ Fainting from grief requires *Ignatia*. ▪ Hysterical fainting calls for *Moschus*.

MEDICAL CONDITIONS

Dosage

- Give three pellets of 30C every five minutes until you see improvement.
- If no improvement after two to three doses, give a different medicine.
- After you first notice improvement, give another dose only if symptoms begin to return.
- Lower potencies (6X, 6C, 30X) may need to be given more often (every five minutes).
- Higher potencies (200X, 200C, 1M) generally need to be given only once. Repeat only if symptoms return with intensity; give only infrequently in this case.

What to Expect with Homeopathic Self-Care

Homeopathic medicines work very quickly in cases of fainting. You should see a response within seconds to minutes if the medicine is correct. Place one pellet under the tongue (be sure the person does not choke on it), or dissolve it in a small amount of water and moisten the person's lips and tongue with it.

Other Self-Care Suggestions

Make sure the person has a clear airway. ▮ A cold washcloth on the forehead may help revive the person. ▮ Moisten the lips or tongue with a few drops of Bach Flower Essence Rescue Remedy; it will often work quickly to help revive the person. ▮ Make sure the person has fainted, rather than having suffered a serious injury or heart attack, before moving him.

	Key Symptoms	Mind	Body	Worse	Better	Food & Drink
Aconite *(Monkshood)*	**Ailments from fright or shock** **Extreme anxiety and restlessness** **Fear of impending death** **Symptoms come on suddenly**	Claustrophobia Fear of crowds, air-planes, and earthquakes Agoraphobia Panic attacks Fear of being alone	**Fainting from fear, fright, or anxiety** **Hot, heavy, burning sensation in the head** **Violent heart palpitations** **Profuse perspiration with anxiety** **Rapid pulse**	Chill	Rest Fresh air	Desire for cold drinks
Arnica *(Leopard's bane)*	**Fainting from blood loss or shock** **Fainting after an accident or traumatic injury** **Shocks of any kind** **Trauma, injuries, falls, sprains, or strains** **Any trauma with bruising** **Bleeding anywhere in the body**	Wants to be left alone Insists that nothing is wrong	Sore, bruised feeling anywhere in the body Feels like the bed is too hard	Touch Overexertion	Lying down with the head low	
Carbo vegetabilis *(Charcoal)*	**Acute episodes of fainting** **Collapsed, weak, or exhausted with difficulty breathing** **Wants to be fanned** **Fainting from indigestion**	**Apathetic** Irritable	**Excessive gas and belching** **Pale with bluish skin** **Great coldness in general and in parts of the body** **Cold breath**	**Loss of body fluids** **Warmth** Rich food	**Being fanned** **Cool air** **Belching**	Desire for sweets and salty foods

continued on next page

Remedy	Key Symptoms	Mind	Body	Worse	Better	Food & Drink
China *(Peruvian bark)*	**Faints from loss of bodily fluids, especially blood loss** **Periodic fevers**	**Irritable, sensitive, and moody** **Fantasies about great things he'd like to do** **Feeling of persecution**	**Intermittent fever with chills, weakness, drenching sweats, and exhaustion** Oversensitive to light, noise, odors, and pain	Touch Drafts Noise Fruit	Hard pressure	Desire for sips of cold water Desire for cherries, sweets, salty food, and spicy food Aversion to hot food, fats and rich food, fruit, and meat
Coffea *(Unroasted coffee)*	**Fainting from joy or excitement** **Hypersensitivity to all emotions**	**Can't tolerate noise** **Overactive mind**	**Hypersensitivity to pain** **Becomes wide awake at 3:00 A.M.** Trembling	Noise Strong smells	Sleep Warmth	
Gelsemium *(Yellow jasmine)*	**Fainting from stage fright** **Dull, drowsy, droopy feeling** Wants to lie down	**Anxiety before a performance** Confusion	**Dizzy as if drunk** **Eyelids heavy** Weakness Headache in forehead and the back of the head	Fright	Bending forward Lying with the head up	Not thirsty Poor appetite
Ignatia *(St. Ignatius bean)*	**Fainting from grief, loss, or profound disappointment** **Uncontrollable sobbing** **Frequent sighing**	**Contradictory** **Overly sensitive** Erratic Excitable	**Lump in the throat** **Chest feels tight** **Muscle cramping** **Numbness and tingling**	**Grief** Touch Coffee and tobacco	**Deep breathing** Swallowing	**Desire for, or aversion to, fruit**

Moschus *(Musk)*	**Hysterical fainting with diffi-cult breathing** **Face turns blue**	Scolding Anger Complaining Anxiety with the fear of death	Fainting: **from the least excitement** **from asthma** **from lack of oxygen** **while eating** **during the menstrual period** Sudden, intense asthma attacks Sensation of a lump in the throat	**Excitement** Cold	Fresh air Rubbing Smell of musk	Desire for cheese
Veratrum album *(White hellebore)*	**Collapse, with bluish color of face and cold sweat** **Vomiting and diarrhea** **Feels icy cold**	**Restless** Constantly busy	Fainting: from emotions, from the least exertion from slight injuries from bleeding after a bowel movement after vomiting	**Cold** **Cold drinks** **Menstrual period**	**Warmth** Hot drinks Covering up	**Desire for very cold drinks, ice, juicy fruits, lemons, pick-les, sour foods, and salty foods**

Fear of Flying

Description

Fear of flying in an airplane is a common phobia which often keeps people out of the air and in cars, ships, and trains for their long-distance travel needs.

Symptoms

Acute panic, claustrophobia, and fear of dying are the most common states found in this syndrome. The physical symptoms are common to all phobias and panic attacks: muscle tension, cold sweat, heart palpitations, rapid pulse, and hyperventilation. The symptoms can occur before the flight or while on the airplane. If the airplane encounters sudden altitude changes, turbulence, storms, engine failure, a near collision, hijacking, or other unusual circumstances that might provoke a normal fear response in passengers, the response of the airplane-phobic person will be much more severe and long-lasting. Even hearing of the possibility of such conditions will make the phobic person cancel his air travel plans.

Complications

Acute fear can induce fainting, shock, and heart attack in susceptible individuals.

Look

Does the person appear frightened?
Is he hyperventilating?
Is his pulse rapid?
Is he sweating?
Is he trembling?

Listen

"The plane is going to crash and we are all going to die!" *Aconite*
"If I fly tonight I'm afraid I'm not going to make it; come with me!" *Arsenicum*
"I wonder if there are any parachutes on this thing." *Argentum nitricum*
"I feel responsible until we all get home safe and sound on the ground." *Calcarea carbonica*

Ask

Have you or a relative had any bad experiences with an airplane flight?
What exactly are you afraid of?
How do you feel when thinking of the airplane flight?
Does anything make you feel better or worse?
Is there anything you can do to calm yourself down?
Are you hungry or thirsty?
Do you desire anything in particular to eat or drink when you are afraid?
Are you feeling warm or chilly?
Do you want to be in any particular position or posture?

Pointers to Finding the Homeopathic Medicine

If the fear of flying is sudden or intense, or precipitated by a frightening event, give *Aconite*. ▮ When the fear is self-centered and the person wants support to calm his anxiety and can't sleep before the flight, consider *Arsenicum*. ▮ If the person is full of anxiety and apprehension before the flight and seems impulsive, consider *Argentum nitricum*. ▮ If the person feels responsible for everyone's safety and is afraid of heights, think of *Calcarea carbonica*.

Dosage

- Give three pellets of 30C every fifteen minutes until you see improvement.
- If no improvement after two to three doses, give a different medicine.
- After you first notice improvement, give another dose only if symptoms begin to return.
- Lower potencies (6X, 6C, 30X) may need to be given more often (every five minutes).
- Higher potencies (200X, 200C, 1M) generally need to be given only once. Repeat only if symptoms return with intensity; give only infrequently in this case.

What to Expect from Homeopathic Self-Care

The correct homeopathic medicine can help the phobic person to calm down very quickly and be able to enjoy the planned or current airplane flight.

Other Self-Care Suggestions

▮ Close your eyes and concentrate on your breath. ▮ Take Bach Flower Essence Rescue Remedy, five drops under the tongue every fifteen minutes.

	Key Symptoms	Mind	Body	Worse	Better	Food & Drink
Aconite *(Monkshood)*	**Fear of airplanes and crowds** **Sudden fright and emotional shock about the airplane flight** **Very afraid of death or sure that they will die, even predicting the time when the plane will crash** **Extreme anxiety** **Tremendous restlessness**	Anguish Claustrophobia (fear of enclosed or narrow places) Agoraphobia (fear of wide open spaces, leaving the house) Desire for the company of others	**Rapid heartbeat and violent heart palpitations** **Profuse perspiration with anxiety** Shortness of breath Flushing or paleness of the face Hot, heavy, burning sensation in the head	Chill	Fresh air Rest Wine	Strong thirst for lots of cold water
Argentum nitricum *(Silver nitrate)*	**Anticipation, apprehension, and fear before the flight** **Fear of heights** **Feeling of being trapped (claustrophobia) during the flight** **Anxiety about getting to the plane on time**	**Impulsive; impulse to jump out of the airplane** Anxious	Bloated with gas Diarrhea from fear Sore throat and hoarseness	**Anxiety before an event** Crowds Heat Sugar	Cool air Open air	
Arsenicum album *(Arsenic)*	**Tremendous anxiety before and during the flight** **Fear of dying when the plane crashes** **Restlessness**	**Very anxious about health** **Insomnia after midnight, 1:00 to 2:00 A.M.** Wants to have company and fears being left alone Needy and demanding	**Burning pains** **Very chilly** Palpitations	Midnight to 2:00 A.M. Cold food or drinks	Heat Warm drinks	Wants to sip cold drinks frequently Desire for milk, the fat on meat, sour food, and warm food
Calcarea carbonica *(Calcium carbonate)*	**Worry about airplane and other safety and security issues** **Fear of flying, heights, mice, insanity** **Feels responsible for the safety of her family**	**Independent** **Obstinate** **Overwhelmed** **Anxious about health**	**Large, sweaty head and flabby body** **Calf, foot, and thigh cramps** Pains in the bones and joints from cold damp weather Sour perspiration Low thyroid	**Cold damp weather** Exertion Going uphill Teething		**Desire for eggs,** sweets, and salt

Fever

Description

Fever is a symptom, not a disease in itself. The body raises its temperature in order to fight infection when the immune system is in the process of responding to foreign invaders such as bacteria and viruses.

Symptoms

When your body temperature rises over 100°F, you have a fever. Fever is a beneficial reaction of the body to illness, and as such should be allowed to run its course unless it is very high. Chills often precede or accompany fever, and sweats occur when the fever is going down or "breaking." Fever may occur in the absence of infection, and in some cases it may be of unknown origin.

Complications

Fever rarely goes above 105°F, but it may induce febrile seizures at that point. A high fever with a severely stiff neck may be caused by meningitis, a life-threatening disease that requires immediate medical attention. Homeopathy is quite effective in dealing with the bacterial or viral infections that cause fever, even in cases in which antibiotics have failed. However, in serious infections with high fevers that do not respond to homeopathy, medical attention should be sought.

Look

What is the person's temperature?
Is the person flushed or pale?
Is the pulse rapid?
Is the person sweating?
Are chills present?

Listen

"My fever started after the bomb threat, when we had to leave the plane in the cold and wind." *Aconite*
"The fever shot up so fast. When I looked in the mirror my face was flushed, and my head hurts like a jackhammer is pounding it." *Belladonna*
"My fever goes up and down like clockwork, but it's the chills and sweats that are the worst part." *China*

"I have a fever, but nothing much else yet. My cheeks are so rosy that I look healthier than usual." *Ferrum phosphoricum*

Ask

When did the fever start?
How high is the fever?
How do you feel with the fever?
Do you feel any pain?
Are there any other symptoms with the fever?
Does anything make the fever go up or down?
Have you felt any different mentally or emotionally before or during the fever?
Is there anything you particularly want to eat or drink?

Pointers for Finding the Homeopathic Medicine

Use *Aconite* or *Belladonna* for fevers that come on suddenly and violently. ▮ Fevers that need *Aconite* often start after a shock or fright, or exposure to a cold dry wind. ▮ *Belladonna* is useful when the fever is high, the person's face is red, and the fever is accompanied by a throbbing headache. ▮ When the fever is intermittent or comes at the same time every day, consider *China*. ▮ Give *Ferrum phosphoricum* for fevers in the first stage of illness with few other symptoms than red cheeks.

Dosage

- Give three pellets of 30C every four hours until you see improvement.
- If there is no improvement after three doses, give a different medicine.
- After you first notice improvement, give another dose only if symptoms begin to return.
- Lower potencies (6X, 6C, 30X) may need to be given more often (every two to four hours).
- Higher potencies (200X, 200C, 1M) generally need to be given only once. Repeat only if symptoms return with intensity; give only infrequently in this case.

What to Expect from Homeopathic Self-Care

Homeopathic medicine treats the whole person, not just a fever, but when fever is the primary symptom, particularly at the beginning of an illness, these medicines will often cure the illness that is the source of the fever in twelve to forty-eight hours.

Other Self-Care Suggestions

Soak in a tepid bath, then dry completely. ▮ Drink two cups of hot yarrow or sage tea, take a hot bath, wrap up in plenty of blankets, and go to sleep. This promotes sweating, which allows the fever to break. ▮ Take a hot bath, put on cold wet socks, wrap up under lots of blankets, and go to sleep. ▮ Take a tepid sponge bath with water or diluted apple cider vinegar. ▮ Make sure that the fever is not an indicator of a deeper problem that needs attention.

	Key Symptoms	Mind	Body	Worse	Better	Food & Drink
Aconite *(Monkshood)*	**High fevers that come on suddenly and violently** **Fevers that come on after a shock, fright, or exposure to a cold dry wind** **Symptoms in general that come on suddenly**	**Fear and anxiety** Panic attacks Restlessness Feeling as though they would die	**Dry, croupy cough comes on suddenly** **Skin and mouth are dry** **Pupils are contracted** **Violent heart palpitations** **Profuse perspiration with anxiety** **Rapid pulse** One cheek may be red, the other pale Hot, heavy, burning sensation in the head	Cold Cold dry wind	Fresh air Rest Wine	Great thirst for cold drinks
Belladonna *(Deadly nightshade)*	**Fevers come on suddenly and violently** **Bright red flushed face, high fever, and throbbing headache** **Very red, very sore throat** **Symptoms are often right-sided** **Very sensitive to light, noise, and being jarred**	Can become delirious High fever	**Pupils are dilated**	Any motion at all	**Quiet, dark room** **Sitting up**	**Desire for lemons or lemonade and cold water** Not much thirst
China *(Cinchona officinalis)*	**Fevers that are intermittent or periodic** **Fevers with chills, weakness, drenching sweats, and exhaustion** **Loss of bodily fluids (blood loss, diarrhea, or excessive sweating)**	Sense of persecution Irritable, sensitive, moody Active fantasy life Fear of animals, dogs	**Fever rises and falls as though on a schedule** Liver pain under the right ribs Diarrhea is frothy and yellow, and made worse by fruit, fat, beer, and milk	Touch Drafts Noise Fruit	Hard pressure	Desire for sweets, salty food, and spicy food Desire for sips of cold water Aversion to hot food, fats and rich food, fruit, and meat
Ferrum phosphoricum *(Iron phosphate)*	**First stage of an acute illness without clear, differentiating symptoms** **High fever with flushed face, especially with round red spots on the cheeks** **State is less intense than for *Belladonna* or *Aconite***	Talkative, excited Not restless, fearful, or delirious	**Right-sided problems** **Inflammation of throat or lungs with fever, but few definite symptoms** **Face bright red or very pale** Discharges may be blood streaked Bruised soreness of the muscles Nosebleeds	Night 4:00 to 6:00 A.M.	Cold applications Bleeding Lying down	Desire for sour foods Thirst for cold drinks Aversion to meat and milk

Flu
(Influenza)

Description

Flu, or influenza is an acute illness caused by the body's response to viral infection by influenza viruses, types A, B, or C. It often comes in the form of epidemics in the winter.

Symptoms

People with the flu complain of headache, fever and chills, aching muscles and joints, fatigue, sore throat, and cough. There is less nasal secretion and more fatigue than with the common cold. Flu sufferers often feel "wiped out," and just want to stay in bed. Some influenza has a gastrointestinal component with nausea, vomiting, and diarrhea.

MEDICAL CONDITIONS

Complications

Conventional medicine has no effective treatment for the flu. Babies and the elderly sometimes succumb to the flu if it is very severe or complicated by secondary bacterial infections, particularly pneumonia.

Look

Is there fever present? Take the temperature.
What color is the person's face?
Does the person want the room dark or quiet?
Is the person shivering with chills?
What body position is preferred?

Listen

"My flu just started out of the blue." *Ferrum phosphoricum, Oscillococcinum*
"It hurts whenever I move." *Bryonia*
"I want to go home." *Bryonia*
"I feel like my bones are broken." *Eupatorium*
"My bones and muscles ache." *Eupatorium, Gelsemium*
"I feel like I've been run over by a truck." *Gelsemium, Eupatorium*
"I feel exhausted and dizzy and I have to go lie down." *Gelsemium*

"I need to go wash my hands." *Oscillococcinum*
"All my joints feel stiff." *Rhus toxicodendron*

Ask

What makes you feel worse?
What makes you feel better?
Are you worse at a particular time?
Are there any mental or emotional changes?
What do you want to eat or drink?

Pointers for Finding the Homeopathic Medicine

If the flu is just starting and there are no definite symptoms yet, choose between *Oscillococcinum* (also called "Flu Solution") and *Ferrum Phosphoricum*. ▮ *Oscillococcinum* is available over the counter in many pharmacies, health food stores, and supermarkets, and is our first choice at this stage unless high fever and red cheeks are prominent symptoms. ▮ After symptoms have developed, consider *Bryonia* if all the symptoms are made worse by movement and the person is very irritable and thirsty. ▮ Think about *Gelsemium* if the person is dizzy, drowsy, droopy, and dull, feels totally exhausted, and is not thirsty. ▮ Consider *Eupatorium* if the person feels deep aching in the bones and muscles and feels like his bones are broken. (See material following for specific symptoms). ▮ Give *Rhus toxicodendron* when stiffness is the main symptom, and it is made worse by cold damp weather or exertion, and better by stretching or moving around for a while.

Dosage

- Give three pellets of 30C every four hours until you see improvement.
- If there is no improvement after three doses, give another medicine.
- After you first notice improvement, give another dose only if symptoms begin to return.
- Lower potencies (6X, 6C, 30X) may need to be given more often (every two to four hours).
- Higher potencies (200X, 200C, 1M) generally need to be given only once. Repeat only if symptoms return with intensity; give only infrequently in this case.

What to Expect from Homeopathic Self-Care

Homeopathic medicines can stop the flu in the very beginning or shorten its course by days or weeks. The medicines usually act within two to twenty-four hours to produce an improvement.

Other Self-Care Suggestions

Rest. ▮ Drink plenty of fluids. ▮ If it is an upper respiratory flu, follow suggestions for Common Cold, Coughs and Bronchitis, and Fever. ▮ If it is a gastrointestinal flu, follow suggestions for Acute Diarrhea.

	Key Symptoms	Mind	Body	Worse	Better	Food & Drink
Bryonia *(Wild hops)*	**Most symptoms made worse by any movement** **Extremely dry, chapped mouth and lips** **A great thirst for large amounts of cold drinks** Wants to go home Worse at 9:00 P.M.	**Very irritable** **Wants to be left alone** **Talks of business and money**	**Hard, dry cough made worse by any movement** **Motion or cough causes pain in the chest and severe headache** Bursting, splitting headache made worse by motion	Eating and drinking Coughing	**Pressure** **Lying on the painful side** **Warm drinks**	**Desire for warm drinks or warm milk**
Eupatorium perfoliatum *(Boneset)*	**Deep aching in the bones and muscles** **Sore and bruised, like their bones are broken**	Very restless, but they would rather keep still because it hurts to move	**Eyeballs feel sore** Sneezing and a runny nose Chills occur especially between 7:00 and 9:00 A.M., and make them feel better Headache in the back of the head and heaviness after lying down Cough with soreness in the chest Hoarseness	Cold air Coughing Sight or smell of food	Conversation Perspiration	Desire for cold foods and ice cream Great thirst for cold drinks, especially before or during a chill
Ferrum phosphoricum *(Iron phosphate)*	**The very first stage of the flu when there are no clear symptoms** **High fever with flushed face, especially with round red spots on the cheeks**	Talkative, excited	**Right-sided problems** **Inflammation of throat or lungs with fever, but few definite symptoms** **Very red checks or pale face** Discharges may be blood-streaked Bruised soreness of the muscles Nosebleeds	Night 4:00 to 6:00 A.M.	Cold applications Bleeding Lying down	Desire for sour foods Thirst for cold drinks Aversion to meat and milk

Gelsemium *(Yellow jasmine)*	**Dizzy, drowsy, droopy, and dull** **Exhausting flu** **Muscle aches throughout body** **Illness following fright (stage fright)**	**Mind feels extremely dull** Thinking is an effort Flu after bad news or worry	**Dizziness, as if drunk, with heaviness of the eyelids** **Blurred vision** **Dull pain and chills up and down the spine** **Wants to lie down and go to sleep** Feel like they have been run over by a truck Pressing headache across forehead and back of head		Fright	Bending forward Lying down with head held high
Oscillococcinum *(Wild duck liver and heart; also called Flu Solution)*	**The first sign of the flu, when specific symptoms have not yet appeared**	Desire to wash the hands Fear of contagious disease	Bursting, throbbing headache Earache like needles Eye inflammation Nose stuffed up, sneezing; clear followed by thick discharge Hoarse Loose cough with thick mucus Fever and chills Muscle aches	Milk Eggs	Heat Rest	
Rhus toxicodendron *(Poison ivy)*	**lu with extreme muscle aching and stiffness** **A constant desire to stretch and move around to find a comfortable position** **Flus that come on from overexertion or getting cold and wet**	Restless Anxious	**Muscles ache but feel better with continued motion** Especially achy on getting out of bed in the morning or rising from a seat	Staying in one position for two long Cold bath or applications	Stretching or continuing to move Heat, hot shower, warm applications	Desire for cold milk

Food Poisoning

Description

Food poisoning occurs by eating contaminated food that contains toxins, chemicals, or bacteria to which the body reacts violently.

Symptoms

Loss of appetite, nausea, abdominal cramping, diarrhea, vomiting, sweating, and fever are common symptoms of food poisoning.

Complications

Severe dehydration, electrolyte imbalance, kidney failure, and shock are possible complications of any food poisoning, caused by prolonged or excessive vomiting and diarrhea. Medical attention should be sought immediately if vomiting and diarrhea cannot be stopped within a few hours, or if food poisoning occurs after eating canned food, which can be contaminated with *Clostridium botulinum,* which causes botulism, a potentially fatal illness that can also cause paralysis. Get immediate emergency medical help if you develop symptoms after eating unknown mushrooms.

Look

Observe the color and consistency of the stool.
Are the eyes sunken?
Are the lips dry and chapped?
Is there sweating? Fever?
Is there vomiting? How often? Dry heaves?
Get the stool tested for parasites or bacteria if symptoms do not resolve quickly.

Listen

"I feel high, but my feet feel frozen and I'm twitching." *Agaricus*
"I feel so sick after what I ate. I'm afraid I'll die." *Arsenicum album*
"I never should have eaten that canned hash." *Botulinum*
"The nausea is terrible and I can't stop vomiting." *Ipecac*
"We closed the deal, but the dinner made me sick." *Nux Vomica*
"My bowels were rumbling and the stool gushed out all over the toilet." *Podophyllum*
"I'm sure it was the nachos. Please help me get better." *Pulsatilla*"
"The meat smelled bad when I took it out of the refrigerator." *Pyrogen*
"Those spoiled clams and oysters gave me diarrhea and hives." *Urtica urens*

"I'm freezing and sweating, with terrible cramping and vomiting."
Veratrum album

Ask

When did the diarrhea and/or vomiting start? How long has it been going on?
What is your stool like?
Do you have pain or cramping? Gas?
What makes the vomiting or diarrhea better or worse?
What time of day does does the vomiting and diarrhea occur?
Are there any mental or emotional symptoms with the food poisoning?
Have any other physical symptoms occurred?
Do you have any desires for particular foods or drinks?

Pointers

If the person feels excessively anxious, give *Arsenicum album.* ▮ With vomiting, consider *Ipecac* and *Veratrum album.* ▮ For illness after rich foods, consider *Nux vomica* and *Pulsatilla*.▮ For severe diarrhea and abdominal cramping, think of *Podophyllum* and *Veratrum album.* ▮ For mushroom poisoning, give *Agaricus*.

Dosage

- Give three pellets of 30C every hour, depending on the severity, until you see improvement.
- If no improvement after three doses, give a different medicine.
- After you first notice improvement, give another dose only if symptoms begin to return.
- Lower potencies (6X, 6C, 30X) may need to be given more often (every one to four hours).
- Higher potencies (200X, 200C, 1M) generally need to be given only once. Repeat infrequently only if the symptoms return with intensity.

What to Expect from Homeopathic Treatment

Homeopathic medicines can stop food poisoning symptoms within a few hours to a day. If symptoms persist or are severe, seek medical attention.

Other Self-Care Suggestions

Drink plenty of fluids, especially those that replace electrolytes such as Recharge, Gatorade, or V8 juice. ▮ If hungry, eat a bland diet including bananas, rice, applesauce, and toast. ▮ A small amount of unflavored yogurt or acidophilus can help replenish healthy intestinal flora. ▮ Rest.

	Key Symptoms	Mind	Body	Worse	Better	Food & Drink
Agaricus *(Fly agaric)*	**Mushroom poisoning** **Twitching, jerking, or convulsions**	Looks intoxicated Delirious or ecstatic states	**Awkward clumsiness** **Icy coldness in the extremities** **Feeling of burning and itching like being frostbitten**	Freezing cold air	Gentle motion	
Arsenicum album *(Arsenic)*	**Nausea and vomiting after eating or drinking** **Severe abdominal cramping** **Tremendous anxiety** **Fear of death** **Restlessness** **Burning pains** **Chilly and thirsty for sips of warm water**	**Very anxious about health** Fear of germs and contagion Despairs of recovering Needy and demanding	**Burning pains in the abdomen and rectum** Diarrhea is worse after eating and drinking, especially sour foods, fruit, and cold food or drinks Stools are frequent, dark, watery, and bad-smelling, with blood and mucus	**Midnight to 2:00 A.M.** Cold food or drinks	Heat Warm drinks	Desire for milk and the fat on meat Wants to sip cold drinks frequently
Botulinum *(Nosode)*	**Food poisoning from canned food** **Cramping pain in stomach** **Difficulty in swallowing and breathing** **Weakness of facial muscles** **Weak, with staggering gait, dizziness, and slurred speech**		Vision is double or blurred Choking sensation Paralysis of respiration, speech, and legs Severe constipation			

		Hard to please Does not know what he wants	**vomiting** **Sinking sensation in the stomach and nausea at the smell of food** Cutting, clawing, cramping pains in the abdomen, especially around the navel Strain at stool very painfully until they have nausea Stool is slimy and dark, grass green, or like frothy molasses with lumps of mucus	drinking Overeating, especially rich food Vomiting		
Nux vomica *(Quaker's button)*	**Heartburn, burping, nausea, unproductive vomiting** **Sick after eating too much rich food or drinking too much alcohol**	**Irritable** **Impatient** Worries excessively about business	**Constipation without any urge for a bowel movement** Sour burping Headache and constipation with digestive symptoms Very chilly	**Over-indulging** Anger	Warmth and warm applications	**Desire for spicy and fatty foods** **Desire for coffee and other stimulants**
Podophyllum *(May apple)*	**Abdominal cramping with rumbling, explosive diarrhea and exhaustion** **Yellowish-green diarrhea that shoots out all over the toilet** **Diarrhea forcing them from bed at 5:00 A.M.** Pain in the liver	Imagines he is going to die or be very ill Fidgety, restless, and whining Delirious and talkative during fever and chills	**Rumbling and gurgling before the stool** Stools are frequent, profuse, liquid, gushing, and bad-smelling Diarrhea is often painless Liver problems	**Sour fruit** **Eating** **Drinking** Motion Early morning Hot weather	Rubbing over the liver Lying on the abdomen or bending forward	
Pulsatilla *(Windflower)*	**Indigestion from eating rich or fatty foods, ice cream, or pork** **Feeling of heaviness in the abdomen** **Symptoms are changeable** **Not thirsty at all**	**Changeable moods** **Cries easily** **Wants to be comforted when sick**	Bloating of the abdomen Belching and gas Bad taste stays in the mouth for a long time Vomits food she ate a long time ago	**Warm stuffy room**	**Open air**	**Desire for creamy and rich oods, ice cream** **Aversion to fats, milk, and warm foods and drinks**

continued on next page

	Key Symptoms	Mind	Body	Worse	Better	Food & Drink
Pyrogen *(Decomposed beef)*	**Food poisoning after eating rotten meat** **Septic state, with fever and very bad-smelling discharges**		**Bloating and cramping with horribly offensive black diarrhea or constipation** Vomit can be like coffee grounds Pulse is disproportionate to the fever (fast pulse with moderate fever or slow pulse with high fever)	Cold	Heat Hot drinks	Desire for cold drinks, but vomits them after they become warm in the stomach
Urtica urens *(Stinging nettle)*	**Food poisoning or allergic reaction from shellfish** **Intensely itching, stinging, burning hives like stinging nettle rash**		**Hives, made worse by bathing, warmth, and exercise** **Burning, itching skin** Diarrhea or vomiting after the hives have been treated with drugs Stools have mucus mixed with white specks like boiled egg white	Cool, moist air Cold bathing	Rubbing Lying down	
Veratrum album *(White hellebore)*	**Violent abdominal cramping with vomiting and diarrhea** **Icy cold with cold sweat**	Very active and busy Restless	**Collapses with bluish color** **Diarrhea profuse, painful, watery** **Diarrhea very forceful, followed by exhaustion and cold sweat** Stools like rice water (as in cholera)	**Cold** Cold drinks Menstrual period Fruit	Warmth Hot drinks Covering up	**Desire for sour foods, sour fruit, pickles, lemons, salt, and ice**

Fractures

Description

Fractures are breaks in the bones.

Symptoms

Different kinds of fractures include simple breaks, compound fractures (in which the bone ends protrude through the skin), greenstick (incomplete) fractures, splintering fractures, and compression fractures, usually from osteoporosis. After an injury, if you are not sure if a bone has been broken, get an X ray. Get medical attention right away for a fracture.

Look

Is the skin broken at the fracture site?
Is there bleeding or bruising?
Is the bone displaced? (If so, get medical attention.)
Has the fracture been set and casted?

Listen

"Go away, there is nothing wrong with me." *Arnica*
"My leg just isn't healing fast enough." *Calcarea phosphorica, Symphytum*
"My bones ache like they are broken." *Eupatorium perfoliatum*

Ask

What caused the injury?
Is there any previous history of fracture?
What does the pain feel like?
What makes the fracture feel better or worse?
Has the fracture been properly set?
Are there any mental or emotional symptoms since the fracture?
Are there any desires for food or drink since the fracture?

Pointers for Finding the Homeopathic Medicine

Give *Arnica* right away. ▮ If deep aching is present give *Eupatorium.* ▮ When the soreness and bruised feeling improves give *Symphytum* after the fracture is set. ▮ If it still doesn't heal properly after six weeks, give *Calcarea phosphorica*.

Dosage

- Three pellets of 30C every four hours for the first few days, or give it whenever the pain returns after being lessened.
- If the first medicine does not work within twelve hours, give a different one.
- After initial improvement, give another dose only if symptoms begin to return.
- Lower potencies (6X, 6C, 30X) may need to be given more often (every one to two hours).
- Higher potencies (200X, 200C, 1M) may need to be given only once, but they may be repeated if the symptoms definitely return after having improved.

What to Expect from Homeopathic Self-Care

Homeopathic medicines can help the bones mend more quickly and with less pain, but they are not a substitute for proper setting of the bone (splinting and casting). The homeopathic medicines discussed next are useful either immediately when a fracture occurs or for long-term healing of the fractured bone after it has been set.

Other Self-Care Suggestions

Do not manipulate or move the bone unnecessarily, to avoid causing further damage to the tissues. ▮ Get the bone X-rayed, set, and properly casted or splinted by a medical professional. ▮ Calcium (1500 mg) and Magnesium (750 mg) per day.

	Key Symptoms	Mind	Body	Worse	Better	Food & Drink
Arnica *(Leopard's bane)*	**Bleeding, bruising, pain, and trauma** **Sore, bruised feelings in the muscles as if beaten, and bluish-black discoloration under the skin**	**Wants to be left alone** Insists that nothing is wrong Tells the doctor to go away	**Wants to lie down, but the bed feels too hard; looks for a softer spot** **Compound fractures that bleed**	Touch Lying on hard surfaces Motion	Lying down, especially with the head low	
Calcarea phosphorica *(Calcium phosphate)*	**Fractures that do not heal well after a long time**	Wants change Dissatisfaction Likes to travel	Non-union of fractured bones Bones are soft, thin, or brittle	Change of weather Lifting Cold and dampness, especially melting snow	Warm, dry weather Lying down	Desire for smoked meats
Eupatorium perfoliatum *(Boneset)*	**Deep aching in the bones** **Sore and bruised feeling in the muscles**	Very restless, but she would rather keep still because it hurts to move	**Deep aching in the bones**	Cold air Sight or smell of food	Conversation Perspiration	**Strong thirst for cold drinks** Desire for cold foods and ice cream
Symphytum *(Comfrey)*	**Fracture (use after the bruise soreness has resolved with *Arnica* and after the bone is set properly)** **Fractures that are slow to heal**		**Pains persist long after the injury** Phantom limb pain after amputation Sensation of the rough end of bones poking into the flesh After-effects of fractures and injuries to the periosteum, the outermost covering of the bone	Injuries Trauma from blunt instruments	Warmth	

Fright

Description

Fright occurs when there is a sudden shock or extreme fear as a result of witnessing or experiencing horrible or frightening events, or having nearly been injured or killed, such as in a collision, earthquake, assault, or combat situation.

Symptoms

The immediate effects of fright are rapid heartbeat, shortness of breath or hyperventilation, shock, cold perspiration, trembling, diarrhea, nausea, dizziness, and possibly fainting.

Complications

Fright may become chronic and recurrent, either from continued exposure to frightening events or from re-experiencing the events through memories and nightmares. People who have been subjected to frightening experiences may also faint, develop panic attacks, or even suffer heart attacks.

Look

Does the person look frightened?
Is the pulse very rapid?
Is the breathing rapid and shallow?

Listen

"I will die by tonight." *Aconite*
"I am afraid I am going to die." *Aconite* or *Arsenicum*
"I have been afraid ever since the accident." *Aconite* or *Arnica*
"I am afraid of crowds." *Arnica*
"I am afraid someone is going to break in the house." *Arsenicum*
"I am afraid to perform tonight." *Gelsemium*
"There are wolves out there." *Stramonium*
"I am going to kill you." *Stramonium*
"I am afraid of the dark." *Stramonium*

Ask

Did the fright occur suddenly?
Were you in a collision?
What kind of fear do you have?
Have you been ill since you were frightened?

Dosage

- Three pellets of 30C every thirty minutes as needed for the first two to three hours.
- Give it whenever the fear returns after being better.
- If the first medicine does not work in two hours, give a different one.
- After initial improvement, give another dose only if symptoms begin to return.
- Lower potencies (6X, 6C, 30X) may need to be given more often (every fifteen to thirty minutes).
- Higher potencies (200X, 200C, 1M) may need to be given only once. Repeat only if symptoms return with intensity; give only infrequently in this case.

What to Expect from Homeopathic Self-Care

Homeopathic medicines may be very helpful in treating an acute fright. Usually they will work in minutes to a few hours. The person will calm down and feel a lot less frightened. For recurring or severe fears consult a qualified homeopath for constitutional treatment.

	Key Symptoms	Mind	Body	Worse	Better	Food & Drink
Aconite *(Monkshood)*	**Sudden fright, fear, and emotional shock** **Very afraid of death or sure that she will die, even predicting the time of death** **Extreme anxiety** **Illnesses after a fright** **Symptoms that come on suddenly** **Tremendous restlessness**	**Terror-stricken** **Anguished** Claustrophobic (afraid of enclosed or narrow places) Agoraphobic (afraid of wide open spaces, leaving the house) Afraid of crowds, airplanes, and ghosts Wants the company of others	**Rapid heartbeat and violent heart palpitations** **Shortness of breath** **Flushing or paleness of the face** Hot, heavy, burning sensation in the head Profuse perspiration with anxiety	Chill	Fresh air Rest Wine	**Strong thirst for lots of cold water**
Arnica *(Leopard's bane)*	Shock of any kind Fright due to traumatic injury Fear of crowds and public places	**Wants to be left alone; insists that nothing is wrong** **Fears being touched** Afraid of heart symptoms Afraid of sickness and death.	**Black and blue areas following injury** **Sore, bruised feeling anywhere in the body** Feels like the bed is too hard	Touch Overexertion	Lying down with the head low	
Arsenicum album *(Arsenic)*	**Tremendous anxiety; anxious about health** **Fear of death** **Restlessness** **Fear of robbers**	**Insomnia after midnight or at 3:00 A.M.** Hypochondriacal Fear of germs and contagion Wants to have company and fears being left alone	**Very chilly** **Burning pains** Palpitations Heartburn	**Midnight to 2:00 A.M.** Cold food or drinks	Heat Warm drinks	Wants to sip cold drinks frequently Desires milk, fat on meat, sour foods

Gelsemium *(Yellow jasmine)*	**Dizzy, drowsy, droopy, and dull** **Muscle aching throughout body** **Stage fright** **Illnesses following fright, bad news, or worry**	Mind feels extremely dull Thinking is an effort	**Diarrhea from fright or stage fright** **Wants to lay down and go to sleep** Pressing headache across forehead and back of head Dizziness, as if drunk, with heaviness of the eyelids Blurred vision Dull pain and chills up and down the spine Overall weakness	Fright	Bending forward Lying down with head held high	**Lack of thirst**
Stramonium *(Thorn apple)*	**Very frightened, like being alone in a dark jungle filled with wild animals or in a graveyard at night** **Biggest fear is of the dark** **Child wants to cling to someone for security**	**Fear of running water and bright objects such as mirrors** **Rage and violence if he is attacked or provoked** Fear of animals, death, ghosts, and nightmares	Convulsions Heart palpitations	**Darkness**	Light Company Warmth	Great thirst Desire for sweets Aversion to water

Frostbite

Description
Frostbite is the freezing of a part of the body from exposure to cold.

Symptoms
The affected body part becomes cold, hard, and white as it is actually frozen, and is usually not painful until it warms up again. The part may become red, itching, and throbbing on rewarming, and blistering may occur.

Complications
If severe, frostbite may lead to gangrene, in which the tissue becomes black and eventually sloughs off. The limb (or part of it) may require amputation as a result of the gangrene. If the frostbitten area is black, seek medical attention immediately.

Look
What is the appearance of the frostbitten area? Color?
Is there any swelling?
Is the person's appearance or behavior out of the ordinary?

Listen
"My feet are burning, itching, and red. I tried to warm them by a campfire. I also feel a bit disoriented." *Agaricus*
"My fingers are cracked and it feels like I have splinters in them." *Nitric acid*
"My toes are kind of a bluish red color since skiing yesterday. I was afraid my friend would leave without me and that I would be stranded on the mountain." *Pulsatilla*
"My hands got frostbitten during a winter hike and it really hurts to rub them. I also feel unusually restless, especially my feet." *Zincum metallicum*

Ask
What were the circumstances of the frostbite?
Which parts are affected?
Is there pain? Numbness?

What makes the pain or numbness better or worse?
Are there any other sensations?
Has the mental state changed?

Pointers for Finding the Homeopathic Medicine

Agaricus is always the first medicine to consider for frostbite. ▮ In mild frostbite with splinter-like pains, *Nitric acid* is the best choice. ▮ If there is bluish-red discoloration, itching, and pain, especially in the feet, consider *Pulsatilla*. ▮ If the frostbitten area feels worse from rubbing and the person has restless legs, give *Zincum metallicum*.

Dosage

- Give three pellets of 30C every one to four hours until you see improvement.
- If there is no improvement after three doses, give a different medicine.
- After you first notice improvement, give another dose only if symptoms begin to return.
- Lower potencies (6X, 6C, 30X) may need to be given more often (every two to four hours).
- Higher potencies (200X, 200C, 1M) generally need to be given only once. Repeat only if symptoms return with intensity; give only infrequently in this case.

What to Expect from Homeopathic Self-Care

Homeopathic medicines are used to help prevent tissue damage and to speed healing. They are not a substitute for rewarming, which must be done as well.

Other Self-Care Suggestions

Do not apply ice or snow to the frozen part. ▮ Rewarm the part as soon as possible, preferably with circulating warm water or contact with warmth, but not with excessive heat.

	Key Symptoms	Mind	Body	Worse	Better	Food & Drink
Agaricus *(Fly agaric)*	**Itching of toes and feet** **Intoxicated appearance with awkward clumsiness**	**Very anxious about health** Delirious or ecstatic states	**Burning, itching, redness, and swelling of the skin and ears, nose, and extremities** **Skin is painful when cold** **Hands and feet feel frozen** Legs feel heavy and limbs feel as if they belong to someone else	**Cold or freezing air** Open air Stormy weather	Gentle slow motion	
Nitric acid	**Mild frostbite** **Pains can be splinter-like**	**Irritable, negative, and pessimistic** **Great anxiety about health**	**Inflamed, itching, painful fingers and toes with cracked skin** **Skin is delicate and turns red easily**	Cold Touch Jarring	Slow riding in a car	Desire for fat and salty foods
Pulsatilla *(Windflower)*	**Burning, sticking, itching pains in the frozen parts** **Parts are swollen and bluish-red and can be very painful** **Mild, gentle, weepy, changeable emotions, and wants to be consoled** **Changeable symptoms**	**Clingy** **Indecisive** **Highly emotional**	**Frostbitten limbs with dark red, bluish swelling** **Severe burning pain in frostbitten toes** **Frostbitten part is hot to the touch with lack of sensation** Burning, sticking pain with itching in frostbitten limbs, especially the ball of the heel	**Warm stuffy rooms** Warmth Fats and rich foods	Slow walking in the open air	**Lack of thirst** **Desire for creamy foods like butter, cheese, and ice cream** Aversion to pork Aggravation from fats and rich foods
Zincum metallicum *(Zinc)*	**Frostbite that feels worse from rubbing** **Very restless legs, particularly in bed at night**	Complains a lot Feels like the police are after him	**Nose is often affected and remains red for a long time** **Toes are the other main frostbite site** Limbs may twitch and jerk	**Cold** **Cold bathing** Wine and other alcoholic drinks		

Gas

Description

Gas is a byproduct of fermentation or rotting of food in the digestive tract by yeast and bacteria. It may be odorless or foul smelling. Fermentation produces carbon dioxide, which has no smell. Bacteria often produce methane and hydrogen sulfide, which do have a foul smell.

Symptoms

Belching, passing gas, and abdominal bloating with rumbling sounds are the most common symptoms of gas.

Complications

Gas may be painful if it is trapped in the stomach or intestines. More serious abdominal problems are sometimes mistaken for simple gas pains. If gas doesn't resolve within six to twelve hours, or is very severe or accompanied by fever, nausea, and vomiting, seek medical attention to get a proper diagnosis of the abdominal pain. (See Stomach Aches and Abdominal Pain.)

Look

Does the person appear to be in pain?
What position seems to be the most comfortable?

Listen

"I want to have the fan to get air." *Carbo vegetabilis*
"I have gas after eating too much rich food." *Carbo vegetabilis, Nux vomica* or *Pulsatilla*
"When I bend over I feel better." *Colocynthis*
"I am so full of gas I can't eat another bite." *Lycopodium*
"I have to get better right away; I can't wait any longer." *Nux vomica*
"Please hold me and take care of me." *Pulsatilla*

Ask

How long have you had the gas?
Was there any event that seemed to precede the gas?

What did you eat before the gas came on?
Is it painful? If so, where?
Is there any rumbling or other noises in the abdomen?
Does any position make the pain feel better or worse?
What else makes the gas better or worse?
Do you want anything special to eat or drink?
Are there any mental or emotional symptoms with the gas?
Do you feel warm or chilly?

Pointers for Finding the Homeopathic Medicine

If bloating is extreme or if the person is exhausted or collapsed and wants to be fanned, give *Carbo vegetabilis.* ■ If the person is doubled over in pain, and doubling over makes him feel better, give *Colocynthis.* ■ When gas and bloating take away the appetite, and the person lacks confidence and is worse from 4:00 to 8:00 P.M., give *Lycopodium.* ■ If the person is chilly, irritable, and impatient and can't seem to pass the gas without straining, give *Nux vomica.* ■ When the person is weepy, changeable, and clingy, and has eaten too much fat or rich food, give her *Pulsatilla.*

Dosage

- Give three pellets of 30C every two to four hours until you see improvement.
- If there is no improvement after three doses, give a different medicine.
- After you first notice improvement, give another dose only if symptoms begin to return.
- Lower potencies (6X, 6C, 30X) may need to be given more often (every two to four hours).
- Higher potencies (200X, 200C, 1M) generally need to be given only once. Repeat only if symptoms return with intensity; give only infrequently in this case.

What to Expect from Homeopathic Self-Care

Homeopathic medicines rapidly relieve gas and bloating within minutes to hours. The gas will pass or disappear.

Other Self-Care Suggestions

Charcoal capsules are helpful in relieving gas. Take two capsules every four hours. ■ Lying on the back and bringing the knees to the chest may cause gas to pass. ▮ Squatting helps relieve gas. ▮ Massaging the abdomen in a clockwise direction helps the lower bowel gas to pass. ▮ Babies may be burped over the shoulder. ▮ Treat constipation to relieve chronic gas. ▮ Eliminate gas-forming foods from the diet, such as beans, potatoes, sweets, and carbonated drinks. ▮ Follow the principles of food combining for better digestion. Avoid combining proteins and carbohydrates at the same meal, and eat fruit by itself, not as a dessert.

	Key Symptoms	Mind	Body	Worse	Better	Food & Drink
Carbo vegetabilis *(Charcoal)*	**Tremendously bloated with gas** **Collapsed, weak, or exhausted with difficulty breathing** **Wants to be fanned**	**Apathetic** Irritable	**Excessive gas and belching** **Fainting from indigestion and passing gas** **Indigestion** **Great coldness in general and in parts of the body** Pale with bluish skin Cold breath	**Warmth** **Rich food** Loss of body fluids	**Being fanned** **Cool air** **Belching**	Desire for sweets and salty food
Colocynthis *(Bitter cucumber)*	**Agonizing, cutting gas pains that make her want to bend over double** **Pain is alleviated by pressure on the abdomen and by warmth**	**Angry** **Everything annoys her** **Offended easily** Restless	**Gas is worse from eating, especially fruit** **Watery diarrhea with gas and pain** Intestines feel like stones are grinding inside	**Anger or indignation** Intense emotions	**Hard pressure** **Bending double**	Desire for bread
Lycopodium *(Club moss)*	**Gas and bloating like a drum** **Lacks confidence** **Worse 4:00 to 8:00 P.M.**	**Fearful inside, but may seem bossy** **Illnesses from performance anxiety**	**Gas and bloating, right after a meal** **Abdomen is sensitive to pressure** **Aggravated by gas-forming foods such as beans and cabbage** **Pain in the liver area under the rib cage** **Pain goes from right to left, across the abdomen**	Pressure of clothes Eating	**Warm drinks** Belching	**Desire for sweets and warm or room-temperature drinks**

Nux vomica *(Quaker's button)*	**Unsuccessful attempts to pass the gas, with a lot of straining** **Arching of the back and a lot of muscle tension** **Very irritable and impatient**	**Obsessed with business** **Wants to be the first and the best** **Competitive and hard-driving, Type A** Easily offended Frustrated easily by little things	**Wakes at 3:00 A.M. with gas pains** **Constipated with terrible straining for a bowel movement** Nausea and vomiting	**Eating** **Cold** **Rich foods** **Stimulants**	Warmth Warm drinks After a bowel movement	**Desire for fatty, spicy, rich foods and stimulants**
Pulsatilla *(Windflower)*	**Indigestion from eating ice cream, pork, fats, and rich foods** **Abdominal bloating from gas** **Temperament and symptoms change very quickly** **Wants others around, especially when sick**	Soft, affectionate, and wants attention Clingy and weepy Highly emotional, changeable	**Dry mouth but no thirst** **Diarrhea in children** **Gas with the menstrual period**	**Heat; hot stuffy rooms** **Rich foods**	Open air Cold applications, food, or drink	**Usually has desire for ice cream, rich foods, and peanut butter** May have aversion to fats, meat, and pork Meat, fats and rich foods do not agree with them

Grief, Acute

Description

Grief is an emotional reaction to loss and disappointment, such as the loss of a loved one, the breaking up of a relationship, or losing a job.

Symptoms

Grief is characterized by weeping, wailing, sobbing, sighing, withdrawal, and depression. Rational thinking is usually overcome by emotion during acute grief.

Complications

People who are grief-stricken may become seriously depressed and even suicidal. If the person makes serious statements about suicide or makes any plans or attempts, emergency psychiatric intervention may be necessary.

Look

How does the person look?
Has her appearance changed?
Is she crying? Withdrawn?

Listen

"My dog died yesterday. We were together for fifteen years and I can't stop crying." *Ignatia*

"My girlfriend broke up with me last week. I've been holed up in my apartment. I don't want anyone to see how broken-hearted I feel." *Natrum muriaticum*

"Since my father died, I haven't gone anywhere or done anything. I can't even think straight." *Phosphoric acid*

Ask

How are you feeling?
What happened? When?
Do you need help?
Are you experiencing any physical symptoms?
Would anything make you feel better or worse?

Do you have someone who can be with you?
In cases of extreme grief: Do you think you'll be okay? Do you need a counselor?
Would you like me to do anything for you?

Pointers to Finding the Homeopathic Medicine

Ignatia is the first medicine to think of in acute grief. If there is lots of sobbing and sighing and the person is hysterical give *Ignatia*. ▮ *Natrum muriaticum* is useful when the person is withdrawn, hides her tears from others, and desires salty food. ▮ *Phosphoric acid* should be given when the person is completely exhausted and apathetic after grief or hearing bad news.

Dosage

- Give three pellets of 30C every four hours until you see improvement.
- If there is no improvement after three doses or several days, give a different medicine.
- After you first notice improvement, give another dose only if symptoms begin to return.
- Lower potencies (6X, 6C, 30X) may need to be given more often (every two to four hours).
- Higher potencies (200X, 200C, 1M) generally need to be given only once, and may be the most effective for acute grief. Repeat only if symptoms return with intensity; administer only infrequently in this case.

What to Expect from Homeopathic Self-Care

Homeopathic medicines are very helpful for acute grief, often allowing the acute crisis to pass within hours or days.

Other Self-Care Suggestions

Confide your feelings to friends and family or a qualified therapist or spiritual counselor. ▮ Do not spend too much time alone. ▮ Let yourself cry until it passes on its own. ▮ Try not to dwell too much on the past, guilt, and regrets. ▮ Let the person or situation go, and move on with your life as soon as you are ready. ▮ Do something special for yourself to get your mind off your grief for a time. ▮ Do something to help someone else who needs it. ▮ For intense grief that has not yet responded to homeopathy, try Bach Flower Essence Rescue Remedy.

	Key Symptoms	Mind	Body	Worse	Better	Food & Drink
Ignatia *(St. Ignatius bean)*	**Immediately following grief or loss** **Uncontrollable crying, loss of appetite, and extreme sadness** **Great mood swings** **Frequent sighing**	**High-strung and emotionally reactive** **Upset after hurt or disappointment** Says or does the opposite of what you would expect	**Numbness and cramping anywhere in the body** **Sensation of a lump in the throat** **A feeling or pressure or tightness in the chest** Symptoms that are just the opposite of what you would expect	Disappointment	**Deep breathing** Changing positions	**Strong desire for or dislike of fruit** Desire for cheese
Natrum muriaticum *(Sodium chloride)*	**Grief or disappointment in relationships** **Wants to be left alone** **Feelings hurt very easily**	**Very sensitive to the slightest reprimand or insult** **Pouty, sulky** **Deeply affected by music**	**Withdraws and isolates herself after grief** **Says she'll never be in a relationship again** **Introspective** Headaches, canker sores, or herpes after grief	10:00 A.M. Heat In the sunlight By the ocean	Open air	**Desire for salty food, pasta, bread, and lemons** Aversion to slimy food
Phosphoric acid	**Exhaustion and apathy from grief, emotional shock, sudden loss or disappointed love** **Strong desire for large quantities of cold or carbonated beverages**	**Depressed** Withdrawn Homesick	**Extremely tired and burned out** **Painless diarrhea after grief** **Diarrhea doesn't cause exhaustion**	**Bad news** **Dehydration from loss of body fluids due to bleeding, diarrhea, and vomiting** Cold	Warmth Naps	**Desire for fruit, refreshing food, and carbonated drinks**

Hay Fever

Description

Hay fever, or acute allergic rhinitis, is a reaction to pollens from grasses, trees, and flowers. Bouts of hay fever often occur annually when pollens are released, generally in the spring, summer, or fall.

Symptoms

Runny nose with clear watery discharge, sneezing, and itchy eyes, nose, and mouth are the common symptoms. Headache and irritability often accompany hay fever. People who have it often feel miserable. Many hay fever sufferers also have allergies at other times of the year.

Look

Are the eyes watery? Red?
Is the nose running?
What kind of discharge is there?

Listen

"My nose is running like a faucet." *Allium cepa*
"My palate and nose itch." *Arundo, Wyethia*
"My eyes are watering intensely." *Euphrasia*
"I have a cold sore." *Natrum muriaticum*

Ask

Does anything itch?
How much are you sneezing?
How much is your nose running?
Do you have any food desires or aversions?

Pointers for Finding the Homeopathic Medicine

The most common medicine for hay fever with watery eyes, watery nasal discharge and sneezing is *Allium cepa*. ▮ If there is an irritating discharge from the nose and a bland discharge from the eyes, consider *Allium cepa*. ▮ If itching of the nose and palate is the primary symptom, give *Arundo* or *Wyethia*. ▮ When eye symptoms, especially watering, are the most significant symptoms, give *Euphrasia*. ▮ When the eye discharge is irritating but the nasal discharge is bland, give *Euphrasia.* ▮ When the discharge is like egg white and the person has cold sores or canker sores, a headache, and perhaps a recent disappointment, rejection, or grief, *Natrum muriaticum* is the medicine. ▮ If sneezing is the most prominent symptom, strongly consider *Sabadilla.*

Dosage

- Give three pellets of 30C every four hours until you see improvement.
- If there is no improvement after three doses, give another medicine.
- After you first notice improvement, give another dose only if symptoms begin to return.
- Lower potencies (6X, 6C, 30X) may need to be given more often (every two to four hours).
- Higher potencies (200X, 200C, 1M) generally need to be given only once. Repeat only if symptoms return with intensity; administer only infrequently in this case.

What to Expect from Homeopathic Self-Care

Luckily, homeopathy is very effective for hay fever symptoms. It will often keep them under control during the acute phase. Constitutional treatment in the off-season will greatly reduce allergic response during the hay fever season.

Other Self-Care Suggestions

Use an air purifier indoors to remove pollens from the air. ▮ Vacuum your living and work areas more often during hay fever season. ▮ Bioflavonoids (1000 mg one to two times a day) can be helpful. ▮ Some people find nettles to be of benefit, either in tea, capsule, or tincture form. ▮ Sip a glass of one to two Alka-Seltzer Gold tablets dissolved in water. ▮ Drink one teaspoon of baking soda dissolved in a glass of water. ▮ Take 500 mg of buffered Vitamin C every two hours until symptoms pass (up to 3000 mg per day).

	Key Symptoms	Mind	Body	Worse	Better	Food & Drink
Allium cepa *(Red onion)*	**Thin, watery, irritating nasal discharge, pouring like a faucet** **Eyes and nose run as if person were peeling an onion**	Fear that the pain will become unbearable	**Burning nasal discharge, especially from the left nostril, irritating the upper lip** **Red, burning, very watery eyes with a non-irritating discharge** Hacking, tickling cough, worse from breathing cold air Sneezing when entering a warm room	**Warm room**	**Cool, open air**	Strong hunger and thirst **Desire for onions** Aversion to cucumbers
Arundo *(Reed)*	**Strong itching of the palate and inside the nose, which causes sneezing**		**Runny nose** **Profuse salivation when the nose runs** **Burning and itching ear canals** Bluish mucus			Desire for sour foods
Euphrasia *(Eyebright)*	**Hay fever centers on the eyes** **Hot, irritating discharge from the eyes, but a bland nasal discharge (the reverse of symptoms that call for *Allium cepa*)**	**Hypochondriacal** **Indifferent** **Body or head feels large** Chaotic	**Eyes are constantly sensitive to light and water** **Frequent sneezing** **Frontal headache**	Sunlight Wind Warm room	Open air Blinking Wiping the eyes	
Natrum muriaticum *(Sodium chloride)*	**Watery or egg-white-like discharges** **Cold sores** **Crack in the middle of the lower lip** **Illness after grief or disappointment in romance**	**Depressed, withdrawn, and sad** Feelings hurt very easily Wants to be left alone when sick Doesn't like to cry in front of others	**Watery eyes with swollen lids** **Loses sense of smell and taste** **Nose alternates between lots of discharge and being stopped up** **Headaches**	**10:00 A.M.** **Sunlight** **Heat** At the ocean	**Outside in the fresh air** Sweating Cool bath	**Desire for salt, pasta, bread, lemons** Aversion to slimy food

continued on next page

	Key Symptoms	Mind	Body	Worse	Better	Food & Drink
Nux vomica *(Quaker's button)*	**Runny nose in the daytime and outdoors; dry nose at night** **Violent sneezing**	**Irritable** **Impatient** **Obsessed with business** **Wants to be the first and the best** **Competitive and hard-driving, Type A** Easily offended Frustrated easily by little things	**Sniffles** **Intense crawling sensation in the nostrils** **Acute sense of smell** **Nose feels blocked, but there is watery nasal discharge through one nostril** Spring conjunctivitis (pinkeye) Photophobia Bloodshot eyes	**Being outside** **Cold air or drafts** Rich foods, high living, being sedentary Coffee and other stimulants Overwork	**Staying indoors** Warmth Hot drinks	**Desire for spicy foods, fat, coffee, alcohol, and tobacco**
Sabadilla *(Mexican grass)*	**Violent sneezing that comes in attacks** **Watery nasal discharge, worse from the smell or even the thought of flowers**	**Imaginary diseases** Imagines his body to be some way it is not	**Itching and tickling in the nose with a thin, irritating discharge** Nose is dry Sensitive smell One nostril is stuffy Face feels hot and bright red Lips are hot and burning	**Open air** Cold air Cold drinks	Warmth Warm drinks	Desire for warm drinks, lemons, onions Aversion to onions
Sulphur	**Watery, burning nasal discharge when outside** **Nose is plugged when indoors**	**Lazy** **Messy** **Opinionated** Irritable, Impatient Thinking all the time	**Frequent sneezing** **Nose is blocked on alternate sides** Tip of nose is red and swollen Disgusted by the odors of others but can't smell his own	**Warmth, and warmth of bed** Atmospheric changes 11:00 A.M. Left side of the	**Open air**	**Desire for alcohol, sweets, and spicy food**

Wyethia *(Poison weed)*	**Extreme itching in the throat, palate, and nose** **Terrible itching at the back of the sinuses** **Desire to scratch his palate with his tongue** **Throat feels swollen** **Back of the throat is dry and burning**	Depressed	**Violent sneezing** **Sensation as if something were in the nasal passages** Constant desire to swallow saliva to relieve dryness in throat, but it doesn't help	Eating Motion Exercise Afternoon

Headache

Description

Headache is simply pain in the head. It is more a symptom than a disease. Various kinds of headaches can occur, including tension headaches, migraine headaches, and cluster headaches.

Symptoms

The pain of headaches may be localized, or may involve the entire head. It often begins in one place and extends to another. Many types of pain may occur, such as throbbing, bursting, aching, hammering, and so on. Migraine headaches are often one-sided; they arise from a circulatory problem, and involve visual disturbances, vomiting, and great sensitivity to noise, light, and jarring. Tension headaches often result from increased stress. Headaches in women may have a hormonal component.

Complications

Most headaches resolve on their own over time. Headaches that are very painful, persistent, or recurrent may indicate a more serious underlying condition such as a brain tumor or brain aneurysm. Headaches may accompany serious acute illnesses, such as meningitis, strep throat, or other conditions with high fever. If you have very severe or persistent headaches, see a medical professional so that your condition may be properly diagnosed.

Look

Is the face red?
Is the pulse throbbing?
Is the person sensitive to light, noise, or jarring?

Listen

"I have been out in the sunlight too long." *Glonoine, Natrum muriaticum, Sanguinaria*
"My head feels like it is going to burst." *Bryonia, Glonoine*
"It feels like hammers beating on my skull." *Natrum muriaticum*
"I feel like throwing up." *Iris, Sanguinaria*
"I feel like a hot poker is sticking into my left eye." *Spigelia*

"The pain is worse whenever I move." *Bryonia*
"I feel totally wasted." *Gelsemium*
"I get a headache right before I go on stage." *Gelsemium*

Ask

What makes the headache better or worse?
What do you want to eat or drink when you have a headache?
Are there any mental or emotional changes with the headache?
Did the headache come on suddenly or gradually?
Are there any changes in your vision?

Pointers for Finding the Homeopathic Medicine

Headaches that are worse from the sun: *Belladonna, Glonoine, Natrum muriaticum, Sanguinaria.* ▮ Lack of thirst with the headache: *Belladonna, Gelsemium.* ▮ Right-sided headaches: *Belladonna, Iris, Sanguinaria.* ▮ Migraine headaches: *Belladonna, Natrum muriaticum, Iris, Sanguinaria.* ▮ Throbbing headaches: *Belladonna, Glonoine, Sanguinaria.* ▮ Sensitivity to light, noise, jarring: *Belladonna, Sanguinaria.* ▮ Very thirsty with the headache: *Belladonna, Bryonia.* ▮ Left-sided headaches: *Bryonia.* ▮ Headaches made worse by motion: *Bryonia.* ▮ Bursting headaches: *Bryonia, Glonoine.* ▮ Dizzy, drowsy, droopy, and dull: *Gelsemium.* ▮ Migraine headaches with visual disturbances: *Iris.* ▮ Headaches from stomach problems: *Iris, Sanguinaria.* ▮ Headaches with a lot of vomiting: *Iris, Sanguinaria.* ▮ Migraines with herpes: *Natrum muriaticum, Iris.* ▮ Burning headaches like a hot wire or poker: *Spigelia.*

Dosage

- Give three pellets of 30C every two to four hours, depending on the severity of the pain, until you see improvement.
- If there is no improvement after three doses, give a different medicine.
- After you first notice improvement, give another dose only if symptoms begin to return.
- Lower potencies (6X, 6C, 30X) may need to be given more often (every two to four hours).
- Higher potencies (200X, 200C, 1M) generally need to be given only once. Repeat only if symptoms return with intensity; give only infrequently in this case.

What to Expect from Homeopathic Self-Care

Homeopathic medicines often work quickly on an acute headache, usually in minutes to hours. Constitutional treatment can be very effective in treating and preventing chronic or recurrent headaches.

Other Self-Care Suggestions

Wrap a cold, wet cloth around your head or use an ice pack while you put your hands and feet in hot water. ▮ Lie down in a dark, quiet place. ▮ Play soft, soothing music. ▮ Do deep, slow breathing. ▮ Take a hot bath with one cup of Epsom salts. ▮ Massage your scalp and the trigger points on your neck and shoulders. ▮ Press deeply on the two points just below the flat bone at the back of the skull about two inches to either side of the center. Release when the pain goes away.

	Key Symptoms	Mind	Body	Worse	Better	Food & Drink
Belladonna *(Deadly nightshade)*	**Maddening, violent headaches** **Right-sided headaches with severe throbbing pain** **Migraines made worse by the least movement or jarring** **Extreme sensitivity to noise, light, and being jarred** **Right-sided symptoms** **Sudden onset of symptoms**	Sudden outbursts of anger	**Headaches from sunstroke** **Headaches at 3:00 P.M.** **Glassy eyes** **Fiery red, hot, dry face**	**Touch** **Being jarred** **Exposure to sun**	**Lying perfectly still in a dark room** Bending backward in a semi-erect position Sitting up	**Great thirst for cold water or no thirst at all** Desire for lemons and lemonade
Bryonia *(Wild hops)*	**Bursting, splitting headache that is made worse by motion** **All symptoms made worse by any motion** **Extremely irritable** **Worse at 9:00 P.M.**	Wants to go home Talks about business	**Dry mouth and lips** **Holds the head to keep it from moving** Pain over left eye Headache worse on the left side Headache extends from over left eye to back of head or whole head	**Moving the eyes** Coughing Morning Constipation	**Closing the eyes** **Pressure** **Lying on the painful side** Warm drinks	**Extreme thirst for large quantities of cold drinks**
Gelsemium *(Yellow jasmine)*	**Headache following fright or from stage fright** **Dizzy, drowsy, droopy, and dull** **Muscle aching throughout body**	**Mind feels extremely dull** Thinking is an effort	**Headache starts in the neck or back of the head and goes to the forehead** **Head feels heavy and hard to lift** **Pressing headache across forehead and back of head** Dizziness, as if drunk, with heaviness of the eyelids Blurred vision Dull pain and chills up and down the spine Overall weakness Wants to lie down and go to sleep	Fright Wine 10:00 A.M.	Bending forward Lying down with head elevated Urination	**Lack of thirst**

continued on next page

	Key Symptoms	Mind	Body	Worse	Better	Food & Drink
Glonoine *(Nitroglycerin)*	**Terrible bursting, pounding headache, especially after exposure to the sun** **Sunstroke**	**Confused and bewildered** Disoriented	**Face flushed and hot** **Violent throbbing headache with rushing of blood** Hot sensation down the spine	**Direct sun, especially on the head**	Open air Cold applications	
Iris *(Blue flag)*	**Headaches with visual disturbances** **Migraine headaches with a visual aura, pain on one side of the head, and a lot of nausea and vomiting** **Migraines that are worse on the right side or that change from side to side** **Blurred vision before the headache**	**Afraid of illness** Depressed Nervous Has difficulty studying	**Headaches above or below the eye or in the temple** **Headaches on the weekend, especially Sundays** **Migraines along with herpes or psoriasis** Vomiting sour bile with the headache Lots of urination after the headache is over	Sweets Weekly	Gentle motion Cold cloth on the head	
Natrum muriaticum *(Sodium chloride)*	**Headaches after grief or disappointment** **Headaches from exposure to the heat or sun** **Headache in the forehead** **Desire to be left alone when not feeling well**	**Very sensitive to the slightest reprimand or insult** **Feelings hurt very easily** Pouty, sulky Deeply affected by music	**Headaches that throb or feel like hammers knocking on the brain** **Headaches over the eyes** **Migraine headache** **Headache from grief**	**10:00 A.M. or from 10:00 A.M. to 3:00 P.M.** **Heat** **Sunlight** **Reading**	Open air Lying in a dark, quiet room Cold cloth on the head Perspiration	**Desire for salty food, pasta, bread, and lemons** Aversion to slimy food

Sanguinaria *(Bloodroot)*	**Migraine on the right side, extends from the neck or upper back to the right forehead and eye** **Right-sided symptoms**	**Hot-tempered** Depressed Anxious before vomiting	**Headaches at menopause** **Headache from indigestion with burning pain in the stomach** **Hot flashes with burning heat** Sensitivity to odors	**Sun** Heat Light Noise Jarring	Vomiting Sleep Passing gas or belching	**Desire for spicy food**
Spigelia *(Pinkroot)*	**Left-sided pain affecting nerves, particularly the facial nerve** **Violent, burning pains** **A sensation of a hot needle, poker, or wire in or above the left eye** **Extreme sensitivity to touch**	**Afraid of pins and needles** Anxious Gloomy	**Parts touched feel bruised** Pain from the left side of the back of the head to over the left eye Headache is worse when looking down, so she must look straight ahead	**Touch** **Sunlight** **Smoke** Motion Stooping	**Lying on the right side** **Steady pressure**	

Head Injury

Description
Head injuries result from a blow to the head or a fall.

Symptoms
Head injuries can cause bleeding, bruising, skull fracture, concussion, brain injury, and loss of consciousness.

Complications
Seek medical attention immediately for any severe head injury, especially if there is disorientation, loss of consciousness, dilated pupils, severe pain, or a fracture. Head injuries may result in brain damage, which can affect the functioning of many parts of the body. For excessive sleepiness, confusion, stupor, or coma after a head injury, consult a homeopath for treatment after emergency medical attention has been given.

Look
Are there any visible signs of a head injury?
Are there any visible indications of trauma to other parts of the body?
Is the person walking, lying down, conscious? Staggering?
Is there bleeding?
Are the pupils of the eyes normal or abnormal?

Listen
"I'm just fine. Please go away. I don't need any help at all." *Arnica*
"My son, Billy, has been acting so silly since his bike accident." *Cicuta*
"I feel so out of it since my car accident. I can't even think straight." *Helleborus*
"I've been having shooting pains up my spine since I hit my head." *Hypericum*
"I've felt terribly depressed since my head injury." *Natrum sulphuricum*

Ask
What were the circumstances of the injury?
How do you feel?
Are you in pain?

If so, where is the pain?
Describe the pain.
Does anything make the pain better or worse?
Are there any problems with your speech, vision, or thinking?
Is there any bleeding?

Pointers for Finding the Homeopathic Medicine

The first medicine to give, unless another medicine is more specifically indicated, is *Arnica.* ▮ For extreme dullness, slowness, and mental confusion after head injury or concussion, give *Helleborus.* ▮ For injuries to the spinal cord and nervous system, head injury, or concussion, especially if the spinal nerves are also involved, give *Hypericum.* ▮ To treat the after-effects of head injury, especially convulsions or headaches, consider *Natrum sulphuricum* or *Cicuta.*

MEDICAL CONDITIONS

Dosage

- Give three pellets of 30C every one to four hours until you see improvement.
- If there is no improvement after three doses, give a different medicine.
- After you first notice improvement, give another dose only if symptoms begin to return.
- Lower potencies (6X, 6C, 30X) may need to be given more often (every two to four hours).
- Higher potencies (200X, 200C, 1M) generally need to be given only once. Repeat only if symptoms return with intensity; give only infrequently in this case.

What to Expect from Homeopathic Self-Care

If the injury is recent, improvement should be noticeable in a matter of days or weeks. If the injury occurred months or years ago, constitutional treatment is required and the improvement may be more gradual. In either case, homeopathy can be tremendously helpful in treating head injuries.

Other Self-Care Suggestions (for minor head injuries)

Apply an ice pack to a closed head injury to reduce swelling. ▮ Give clear fluids unless the person is unconscious or vomiting. ▮ Treat open wounds (see Cuts, Scrapes, and Puncture Wounds). ▮ Treat for shock if necessary (see Shock).

	Key Symptoms	Mind	Body	Worse,	Better	Food & Drink
Arnica *(Leopard's bane)*	**Any serious head trauma, especially with bruising** **Shock**	**Wants to be left alone** **Refuses help** **Says nothing is wrong with her**	**Concussion and bleeding, and bruising of the tissues and the brain** **Black eyes** **Sore, bruised feelings as if beaten** **Bluish-black discoloration under the skin** Wants to lie down, but the bed feels too hard	**Touch** **Lying on hard surfaces** Motion	**Lying down, especially with the head low**	
Cicuta *(Water hemlock)*	**Neurological problems after head injury, especially convulsions and developmental disability due to brain damage**	**Childish; feels like a child** **Excitable** Shrieking Doesn't remember what has happened Doesn't recognize anybody	**Very severe convulsions with twitching and jerking** **Tremendous spasms with severe arching of the back**	Cold Touch Jarring	Heat	Desire for inedible things such as dirt and charcoal
Helleborus *(Black hellebore)*	**Dullness and mental confusion after head injury or** **Stupefied or bewildered** **Seems as if she is not really present**	**Slow to respond to the senses and in answering questions** **Information has difficulty getting in and out** **Indifferent to surroundings and loved ones** **Staring** **Anguish**	**Headache with dullness of mind after head injury** **Furrowed brow, especially when trying to think or concentrate** Rolls the head from side to side or burrows it into the pillow Cold sweat	**4:00 to 8:00 P.M.** Cold		

Hypericum *(St. John's wort)*	**Head injury and concussion, especially if the spinal nerves are also involved** **Injuries to the spinal cord and nervous system** **Shooting pains**	**Dull and forgetful after head injury** Sad	**Head feels as if touched by an icy cold hand** **Dizziness, headache, and convulsions after injury to the head or spine** **Numbness and tingling**	Jarring the injured area Touch Cold air Fog, cold damp weather	Rubbing the area Lying on the abdomen Bending backward	Desire for wine, pickles, and cold drinks
Natrum sulphuricum *(Sodium sulfate)*	**After-effects of head injury, especially convulsions or headaches** **Severe depression following a head injury** **Profound sadness, even feeling suicidal, after injury to the head**	**Overly sensitive to criticism or scorn** **Concerned about his family**	**Indigestion with headache** Crushing pain in the back of head Light sensitive during headache Scalp sensitive to combing hair	3:00 to 6:00 A.M. Noise Stooping Light Eating	Dark room vomiting	Desire for yogurt and sour foods, especially during a headache

Hemorrhoids

Description

Hemorrhoids are varicose veins of the rectum. They may be inside the rectum, or they may protrude outward through the anus. They most commonly result from constipation or pregnancy, and may also be associated with liver problems.

Symptoms

The most annoying symptom associated with hemorrhoids is pain due to inflammation and swelling. This may range from a mild discomfort with or without itching, to pain so severe that sitting or having a bowel movement is excruciating. Hemorrhoids often bleed.

Complications

Blood clots may become lodged in the hemorrhoidal veins surrounding the hemorrhoid. The hemorrhoids may ulcerate and bleed profusely. Other possible causes of rectal bleeding should be investigated, including colitis, polyps, and tumors.

Look

If the hemorrhoids are visible, what color are they?
Is there one hemorrhoid, or are there several?
How much swelling is there?
Is there blood in the stool?

Listen

"My hemorrhoids are purple. The only thing that relieves the pain is when they bleed." *Aesculus*
"I feel a sticking pain in my rectum when the hemorrhoids flare up." *Aesculus* and *Collinsonia*
"My stool is all mucus." *Aloe*
"My hemorrhoids are so swollen, and they bleed terribly." *Hamamelis*
"The worst thing about my hemorrhoids is that my butt itches so much." *Sulphur*
"I get hemorrhoids whenever I'm really constipated or after I drink wine." *Nux vomica*

Ask

When did the hemorrhoids begin?
Was there any particular cause?
What is most distressing about the hemorrhoids?
What does the pain or sensation feel like?
When does the pain occur?
How much do they hurt?
What makes the hemorrhoids feel better or worse?
Is there anything unusual about bowel movements?
Are there any unusual sensations in the anus or rectum?
Have any other symptoms occurred since the hemorrhoids began?
Were there any mental or emotional changes or stress that led up to the hemorrhoids?

Pointers for Finding the Homeopathic Medicine

If the main symptom is pain like small sharp sticks in the rectum, consider *Aesculus* and *Collinsonia*. ▮ If swelling and bleeding are prominent, think first of *Hamamelis*. ▮ If the person is chilly, over-stressed, and drinks too much alcohol, consider *Nux vomica*. ▮ In a warm-blooded person with lots of rectal itching and rectal spasms, give *Sulphur*.

Dosage

- Give three pellets of 30C every four hours until you see improvement.
- If there is no improvement after three doses, give a different medicine.
- After you first notice improvement, give another dose only if symptoms begin to return.
- Lower potencies (6X, 6C, 30X) may need to be given more often (every two to four hours).
- Higher potencies (200X, 200C, 1M) generally need to be given only once. Repeat only if symptoms return with intensity; give only infrequently in this case.

What to Expect with Homeopathic Self-Care

You should notice a significant decrease in the pain within twenty-four hours. If your hemorrhoids are chronic, allow at least several days. Do not continue using a particular homeopathic medicine if you see no improvement after several days.

Other Self-Care Suggestions

Take a sitz bath. Fill the bathtub with hot water to two inches below the navel. Sit with knees bent. Stay in the tub for five minutes. Then squat in a tub of cold water for one minute. Repeat the cycle two to three times. ▮ Take 1000 milligrams of bioflavonoids daily to strengthen the capillaries. ▮ Keep the rectal area clean. ▮ If you are constipated, drink plenty of water and take one tablespoon of bran, flaxseed oil, or psyllium seed one to two times daily until the constipation is relieved. ▮ Avoid spicy foods; they may aggravate the hemorrhoids. ▮ Get exercise to increase circulation in the pelvic area. ▮ Peel a garlic clove, scratch its surface several times and insert in the rectum as a suppository. Remove after eight hours or when the stool is passed. ▮ Use homeopathic rectal astringent suppositories. They contain one or more of the medicines listed in the chart that follows. ▮ If the hemorrhoids are due to constipation, one to two glycerine suppositories a day rectally may be helpful. ▮ Witch hazel applied externally to the hemorrhoids may help them to shrink.

Note: Hemorrhoids are one of the few conditions for which homeopathic ointments or suppositories can be just as helpful as oral medications. Homeopathic medicines are also available in a topical preparation or suppository from homeopathic manufacturers, usually in combination.

	Key Symptoms	Mind	Body	Worse	Better	Food & Drink
Aesculus *(Horse chestnut)*	**Feels better when the hemorrhoids are bleeding** **Hemorrhoids are external, purple, and painful** **Rectum feels full of small sticks**	Gloomy Irritable Confused and bewildered upon awakening	**Pain persists long after having a bowel movement** Stools are dry, hard, and knotty Burning in the anus Chills and sharp, shooting pains up the back	**After urination or stool** During sleep 'tea	Cool, open air Bathing	
Aloe *(Aloe socotrina)*	**Feeling of insecurity in the rectum as though stool would come out** **Hemorrhoids like a bunch of grapes** **Stools contain gelatinous lumps of mucus**	Irritable, discontented, and angry, with abdominal pain or constipation Doesn't want to be around people	**Hemorrhoids are filled with blood and feel congested** **Stool comes out while passing gas** Rumbling and gurgling in bowels, with sudden, gushing watery stool Gushing stool is worse early morning in bed Diarrhea after beer or oysters	Heat and summer Hot damp weather After eating or drinking Beer	Cool, open air, cold bathing, and cold applications Passing gas	Desires beer
Collinsonia *(Stone-root)*	**Sensation of sharp sticks or sand in the rectum** **Hemorrhoids combined with heart palpitations or constricted feeling in the heart** **Hemorrhoids with swelling of the face or lips**	**Ailments from emotional excitement** **Excited, with heart palpitations**	**Hemorrhoids are painful and bleed** **Chronic constipation alternating with diarrhea** Heaviness in rectum Anus itches and may prolapse	Cold Pregnancy	Warmth	Desire for or aversion to cheese

continued on next page

	Key Symptoms	Mind	Body	Worse	Better	Food & Drink
Hamamelis *(Witch hazel)*	Weakness of veins leading to congestive fullness, bleeding, and a sore, bruised feeling Hemorrhoids are swollen, purple, and filled with blood Hemorrhoids and nosebleeds may occur together	Irritable	**Throbbing in the rectum** **Pain often lasts for hours after a bowel movement** **Considerable bleeding** Anus feels sore, raw, and as if full of sticks Back pain; sharp shooting pains up the back or into the sacroiliac joints or hips Burning and chills up and down the back	Injuries		Aversion to water
Nux vomica *(Quaker's button)*	**Hemorrhoids after too much stress, rich food, drugs, alcohol, or stimulants** **Hemorrhoids from chronic constipation** **Unsuccessful efforts to have a stool, with great urging and straining**	**Irritable** **Impatient** **Type A personality** Competitive and hard-driving Easily offended Frustrated easily by little things	**Itching, painful hemorrhoids** **May not even have the urge for a bowel movement** **Rectum feels constricted** May also have indigestion and heartburn Wakes with pain or discomfort at 3:00 A.M.	**Cold, drafts** **Rich foods, high living** **Sedentary lifestyle** **Coffee and other stimulants** Pressure of clothing	Warmth Hot drinks After stool	**Desire for stimulants, rich food, and fat**
Sulphur *(Sulfur)*	**Hemorrhoids both internal and external** **Very large hemorrhoids, in bunches** **Hemorrhoids itching, tender, and bleeding**	**Opinionated and critical** **Thinking all the time, philosophical** **Lazy** Usually messy, but	**Diarrhea drives him out of bed in the morning around 5:00 A.M.** **Anus is red, sore, raw, burning, and very itchy** Stool is loose and burning Spasms in the rectum	**Warmth, and warmth of bed** **Bathing** Left side	Open air	**Desire for alcohol, sweets, and spicy foods**

Hepatitis, Acute
(Hepatitis A)

Description

Hepatitis is an inflammation of the liver, usually of viral origin, but it may also be caused by drugs or alcoholism. Hepatitis A is transmitted by contact with contaminated water or food, stool, blood, or secretions. Hepatitis B is transmitted primarily through blood transfusions or contaminated needles. Hepatitis C occurs mostly after blood transfusions, causing acute hepatitis that may become chronic. Legally it is necessary to call the local health department to report a newly diagnosed case of hepatitis.

Symptoms

Overall weakness or discomfort, nausea and vomiting, diarrhea, poor appetite, and fever are the main symptoms. Jaundice may be marked, depending on the stage of the hepatitis. Hives and joint pains may also occur.

Complications

Hepatitis causes severe liver dysfunction with jaundice, bloating, and diarrhea, and may be fatal in extreme cases. Hepatitis may become chronic, causing long-term liver damage that can be fatal.

Look

Is the person jaundiced (yellowish coloration to skin and whites of the eyes)?

Is the liver enlarged, projecting more than one inch below the ribs on the right side?

Is the liver tender when you touch it?

Listen

"My right shoulder blade is killing me." *Chelidonium*

"I feel bloated after I eat anything at all." *Lycopodium* or *China*

"The hepatitis started after I used a lot of marijuana." *Natrum sulphuricum*

"My liver is sore to the touch. I'm sweating like crazy and my breath is awful." *Mercurius*

"My liver feels much better after I drink pop." *Phosphorus*

Ask

What are the symptoms of the hepatitis?
When did the symptoms begin?
How severe are the symptoms?
Are you weak and exhausted?
Were you exposed to anyone with hepatitis? How?
Are there any mental or emotional symptoms?
Is there any specific time of the day or night that you feel better or worse?
What kind of pain is there?
What makes you feel better or worse?
How is your appetite? Do you have any food cravings or aversions?
Are there any changes in your urine or stool?

Pointers for Finding the Homeopathic Medicine

The most common medicines are *Chelidonium, China,* and *Lycopodium.* ■ If there is considerable right-shoulder-blade pain, give *Chelidonium.* ■ If the person has a history of gonorrhea or chlamydia, he probably needs *Natrum sulphuricum.* ■ If perspiration and the breath smell bad and there is excessive saliva, give *Mercurius.* ■ If the person has a strong craving for cold drinks, look at *Phosphorus.*

Dosage

- Give three pellets of 30C twice a day until you see improvement.
- If there is no improvement after three doses, give a different medicine.
- After you first notice improvement, give another dose only if symptoms begin to return.
- Lower potencies (6X, 6C, 30X) may need to be given more often (every two to four hours).
- Higher potencies (200X, 200C, 1M) generally need to be given only once. Repeat only if symptoms return with intensity; give only infrequently in this case.

What to Expect from Homeopathic Self-Care

After the condition has been properly diagnosed by a physician and confirmed by a blood test, it can be very helpful to consult a homeopath for treatment of hepatitis. Although homeopathy offers effective treatment, acute hepatitis is a serious, communicable illness. If improvement is not rapid with homeopathic treatment, medical attention should be sought in a timely manner to avoid complications. Expect improvement in Hepatitis A within a few days if you are using the correct homeopathic medicine. If the first medicine you try doesn't work, see a homeopath as soon as possible. Hepatitis B and Hepatitis C are much more complicated and should be treated by a qualified homeopath or qualified medical practitioner.

Other Self-Care Suggestions

Get a hepatitis screen to determine the type of hepatitis you have. ▮ Make sure that the local public health department has been contacted. ▮ Eat a light, low-fat diet with lots of fruits and vegetables, especially beets. ▮ Take Vitamin C, 1000 mg three times a day. ▮ Take liver herbs, including dandelion root, milk thistle, or beet greens. ▮ Take lipotropic factors, including cysteine, methionine, and inositol, to help the liver break down fat. ▮ Do not share dishes with family members or cook for them until you are completely well. ▮ Practice safe sex with your partner; some hepatitis is sexually transmitted. ▮ Drug users should not share needles.

	Key Symptoms	Mind	Body	Worse	Better	Food & Drink
Chelidonium *(Celandine)*	**Liver enlarged and tender** **Pain extending from the liver backward to the lower angle of the right shoulder blade** **Right-sided symptoms**	**Doesn't want to talk or to exert himself mentally** **Worries that he has ruined his health**	**Jaundiced (yellowish skin and whites of eyes)** **Nausea and vomiting that are lessened drinking hot water** **Bright yellow or clay-colored stool, in hard balls or diarrhea** Head feels heavy, often with headache over the right eye Dirty yellow color of the whites of the eyes Bitter taste in the mouth Urine bright yellow and foamy Icy cold fingertips	Motion Change of weather	Hot food	Desire for cheese, milk, and hot food and drinks
China *(Cinchona officinalis)*	**Liver pain under the right ribs** **Jaundice and bloating** **Tremendous sweating, especially at night** **Symptoms that are worse after loss of bodily fluids**	**Irritable, sensitive, and moody** **Fantasies about great things he'd like to do** **Feeling of persecution**	**Liver and spleen are swollen and enlarged** **Bitter belching, which gives no relief** Gas pains are lessened by bending double Diarrhea is frothy and yellow, especially after fruit, fat, beer, or milk	Losing blood or other bodily fluids		Desire for sips of cold water Desire for cherries, sweets, salty food, and spicy food Aversion to hot food, fats and rich food, fruit, and meat
Lycopodium *(Club moss)*	**Lots of bloating of the abdomen** **Pain in the liver area under the rib cage** **Pain goes from right to left, across the**	**Insecurity or lack of courage, which the person tries to cover up** **Fearful inside but may seem bossy**	Can't tolerate tight clothing around the abdomen Aggravated by gas-forming foods such as beans and cabbage	**Eating**	**Warm drinks** **Belching**	**Desire for sweets and warm or room-temperature drinks**

	Gas and bloating even after eating a small amount **Worse 4:00 to 8:00 P.M.**	Desire to have someone in the next room				
Mercurius *(Mercury)*	**Enlarged liver that is very sore to touch and pressure** **Sharp pains in the liver extending to the spine**	**Suspicious** Hurried Hesitant	**Small amounts of dark, bloody urine** **Stool is greenish and slimy** Trembling, sweating, and salivating Bad-smelling breath, perspiration, and discharges Coated tongue, imprinted along the edges with the teeth Metallic, sweetish taste in the mouth	**Heat and cold** **Night** Perspiring	**Desire for bread and butter** Aversion to sweets	
Natrum Sulphuricum *(Sodium sulfate)*	**Liver is sore to the touch** **Sharp, stitching pains in the liver** **May have history of heavy use of street drugs** **Worse in cold, damp weather**	**Depressed, even suicidal** Overly sensitive to criticism or scorn	**Can't stand to have tight clothing around the waist** **Passes gas** **Jaundice and vomiting of bile** **Diarrhea is watery and yellow** **After-effects of head injury** Tongue is coated brown, with a bitter taste	Tight clothing around the abdomen Lying on the left side 3:00 to 6:00 A.M.	Lying on the right side with the legs curled up	**Desire for yogurt and sour foods**
Phosphorus	**Full feeling in the liver** **Liver is large and hard** **Jaundice** **Great thirst for cold or carbonated drinks**	**Outgoing** **Sympathetic** **Friendly** **Desires company** Afraid of the dark, thunderstorms, and ghosts	**Craves cold drinks but vomits them up as soon as they become warm in the stomach** **Stomach pain relieved by cold drinks** Burning pain in the stomach Empty, hollow pain in the stomach Large yellow spots on the abdomen	**Lying on the left side** **Warm food or drinks**	**Lying on the right side** **Cold food or drinks** Sleep	**Great thirst for cold or carbonated drinks** **Desire for salty food, chocolate, ice cream, and spicy food** Spicy food doesn't agree with her

Hives

(See also Allergic Reactions and Insect Bites and Stings.)

Description

Hives appear on the skin as part of an allergic reaction to a food or an environmental allergen such as pollen, dust mites, or wool. Hives may also occur due to exercise or from becoming cold.

Symptoms

Hives are red, raised welts that are often quite itchy, hot, and swollen.

Complications

In a serious case of acute hives, anaphylaxis (characterized by intense itching, swelling, and difficulty breathing due to constriction of the bronchioles) can be life-threatening and requires emergency medical attention. Hives may become chronic or may occur repeatedly if the allergen that causes the body to react is not eliminated.

Look

What is the appearance of the hives? How many are there? How big? What color are they?
Where are the hives located?
Is there any significant swelling?
Are there any other visible symptoms?

Listen

"I feel like my whole face is swollen." *Apis*
"Ever since I got the hives, my joints feel really stiff." *Rhus toxicodendron*
"The hives began right after I ate some prawns." *Urtica urens*

Ask

What seemed to cause the hives?
What is bothering you the most?
Are you in pain?
Are there any other symptoms?
What makes the itching and other symptoms better or worse?
Do you have any difficulty breathing?

Pointers for Finding the Homeopathic Medicine

If there is tremendous swelling, give *Apis* first. ▮ For hives due to bee stings, give *Apis*. ▮ If itching is the main symptom and the person is very restless, give *Rhus toxicodendron*. ▮ If the hives sting and there is not significant swelling, consider *Urtica urens*.

Dosage

- Give three pellets of 30C twice daily until you see improvement.
- If there is no improvement after three doses, give a different medicine.
- After you first notice improvement, give another dose only if symptoms begin to return.
- Lower potencies (6X, 6C, 30X) may need to be given more often (every two to four hours).
- Higher potencies (200X, 200C, 1M) generally need to be given only once. Repeat only if symptoms return with intensity; give only infrequently in this case.

What to Expect from Homeopathic Self-Care

Homeopathic medicines are capable of rapidly relieving hives in a few minutes to a few hours. People with chronic hives should consult a qualified homeopath.

Other Self-Care Suggestions

For itching: soak in a bathtub of warm water with one cup of baking soda or one cup of raw oatmeal. ▮ For swelling: ice pack or cold wet compresses. ▮ Sip a glass of one to two Alka-Seltzer Gold tablets dissolved in water. ▮ Drink one teaspoonful of baking soda dissolved in a glass of water. ▮ Take 500 mg of buffered Vitamin C every two hours until symptoms pass (up to 3000 mg per day).

	Key Symptoms	Mind	Body	Worse	Better	Food & Drink
Apis *(Honeybee)*	**Hives that are swollen and red with stinging and burning** **Intolerable itching at night** **Swelling and puffiness of the face and eyelids or any affected part of the body**	**Busy** **Irritable if crossed** Jealous'	**Hives feel better with cold applications** **Large hives** **Stinging pains**	**Heat and hot applications**	Uncovering	**Not very thirsty**
Rhus toxicodendron *(Poison ivy)*	**Hives from getting wet or chilled** **Hives during chills and fever** **Hives accompanied by joint stiffness**	**Jovial** **Restless**	**Hives with intense itching** **Hot, burning pain with the hives**	**Cold, damp** Overexertion Becoming chilled when hot and sweaty	**Heat** Warm dry weather	**Desire for cold milk**
Urtica urens *(Stinging nettle)*	**Hives from shellfish** **Hives itch, burn, and sting**		**Sensation like prickly heat** **Itchy, raised, red blotches** **Nettle rash** Hives with joint pain	**Cool wet air** **Cold bathing**	**Warmth**	

Indigestion and Heartburn

Description

Indigestion and heartburn are common conditions following eating too much or not being able to digest food properly.

Symptoms

Indigestion can include nausea, gas, belching, stomach pain, and heartburn. It usually occurs in the two hours immediately after eating. Heartburn is burning pain in the chest behind the sternum, which is associated with the reflux of acidic or caustic stomach fluids into the esophagus. Heartburn may occur after eating any food which stimulates acid production in the stomach, such as proteins, spicy foods, or chocolate.

Complications

Indigestion and heartburn are usually uncomplicated, and respond easily to change in diet, antacids, or homeopathic treatment. The symptoms may be confused with symptoms of a stomach ulcer, a hiatal hernia, or angina. If indigestion is severe or persistent, medical attention should be sought to determine the cause of the problem.

Look

Is the person passing gas?
Is she in a particular position to relieve the pain or discomfort?
Is the discomfort worse when lying down?

Listen

"My indigestion came on after I ate some fruit. I'm really afraid it's an ulcer." *Arsenicum*
"I'm so full of gas that even burping doesn't help." *Carbo vegetabilis*
"No matter what I eat, I get bloating, gas, and indigestion." *Lycopodium*
"I got terrible heartburn because of a hangover." *Nux vomica*
"I just can't handle rich foods." *Pulsatilla*
"The worst part of the indigestion is that I wake up with diarrhea every morning." *Sulphur*

Ask

What brought on the indigestion?
What kinds of foods are difficult for you to digest?
What are your symptoms?
Is there pain? If so, describe it.
How severe is the pain?
Does the pain stay in one place or does it radiate? If so, to where?
What makes the pain better or worse?
Are there any other symptoms that came with the indigestion?
Are there any changes in your mental or emotional state?

Pointers for Finding the Homeopathic Medicine

When extreme burning pain is the main symptom, along with a lot of anxiety and restlessness, think of *Arsenicum,* especially in a self-centered person who wants support and has many fears. ▮ *Lycopodium* is the medicine if the person is insecure yet bossy and full of false bravado, gets lots of gas from just a little food, and is worse from 4:00 to 8:00 P.M. ▮ When the person is irritable, impatient, and hard-driving, and suffers from too much rich food, coffee, and alcohol, give *Nux vomica.* ▮ Conversely, when the person suffers from rich food, but is mild, gentle, changeable, and weepy and wants to be taken care of, think of *Pulsatilla.* ▮ If the person is lazy, intellectual, egotistical, and sloppy and suffers from heartburn and morning diarrhea, give *Sulphur.*

Dosage

- Give three pellets of 30C every four hours until you see improvement.
- If there is no improvement after three doses, give a different medicine.
- After you first notice improvement, give another dose only if symptoms begin to return.
- Lower potencies (6X, 6C, 30X) may need to be given more often (every two to four hours).
- Higher potencies (200X, 200C, 1M) generally need to be given only once. Repeat only if symptoms return with intensity; give only infrequently in this case.

What to Expect from Homeopathic Self-Care

Homeopathic medicines quickly relieve symptoms of acute indigestion or heartburn. If indigestion is chronic, constitutional treatment by a homeopath and a diagnostic workup are recommended.

Other Self-Care Suggestions

Avoid overeating, especially heavy or rich foods. ▮ Avoid fats, spicy foods, alcohol, coffee, and chocolate. ▮ Commercial antacids may provide temporary relief. ▮ Charcoal capsules are helpful in relieving gas. Take two capsules every four hours. ▮ Lying on the back and bringing the knees to the chest may cause gas to pass. ▮ Squatting helps gas to pass. ▮ Eliminate gas-producing foods from the diet, such as beans, potatoes, sweets, and carbonated drinks. ▮ Follow the principles of food combining for better digestion. Do not combine proteins and carbohydrates at the same meal, and eat fruit alone and not as a dessert. ▮ Elevate the head of the bed six inches to reduce heartburn.

	Key Symptoms	Mind	Body	Worse	Better	Food & Drink
Arsenicum album *(Arsenic)*	**Extreme burning pains in the stomach and esophagus** **Very anxious, with fear of dying** **Chilly and thirsty for sips of cold water**	**Restless and anxious** **Needy and demanding** Afraid of being alone Complains that he won't get well	**Stomach pains are lessened by drinking milk** **Stomach pain at 2:00 A.M.** **Severe abdominal cramping** **Indigestion is worse after eating and drinking, especially fruit and cold food or drinks** Vomiting after drinking	**After midnight, 1:00 to 2:00 A.M.** **Cold** Cold drinks	**Heat** Warm food and drinks	Desire for milk, sour food, and the fat on meat
Carbo vegetabilis *(Charcoal)*	**Tremendous bloating and gas** **Collapsed, weak, or exhausted, with difficulty breathing** **Wants to be fanned**	**Apathetic** Irritable	**Excessive gas and belching** **Fainting from indigestion and passing gas** **Indigestion** **Pale with bluish skin** **Great coldness in general and in parts of the body** Cold breath	**Warmth** **Rich food** Loss of body fluids	**Being fanned** **Cool air** **Belching**	Desire for sweets and salty food
Lycopodium *(Club moss)*	**Gas, belching, and bloating like a drum** **Lacks confidence** **Worse from 4:00 to 8:00 P.M.** **Gets full too quickly after only a small amount of food**	**Indigestion from performance anxiety** **Fearful inside but may seem bossy** Wants someone in the next room	**Abdomen is sensitive to pressure** **Worse from gas-producing foods such as beans, onions, and cabbage** Pain in the liver area under the rib cage Pain goes from right to left, across the abdomen	**Tight clothes** Eating	**Warm drinks** **Belching**	**Desire for sweets and warm or room-temperature drinks**

Nux vomica *(Quăker's button)*	**Heartburn after eating fats and sour foods** **Wakes up at 3:00 A.M. with indigestion** **Very irritable and impatient**	**Obsessed with business** **Wants to be the first and the best** **Competitive and hard-driving, Type A** Easily offended Frustrated easily by little things	**Constipation with terrible straining for a bowel movement** Abdominal cramping Nausea and vomiting Sour or bitter belching and taste in the mouth	**Anger** **Becoming chilled** **Rich foods** **Stimulants** **Alcohol**	**Warmth** Warm drinks After a bowel movement	**Desire for fat, spicy, rich foods and stimulants**
Pulsatilla *(Windflower)*	**Heartburn after eating fats and rich foods** **Indigestion from ice cream, pork, fats, and rich foods** **Abdominal bloating from gas** **Quickly changing temperament and symptoms**	**Soft, affectionate, and wants attention** **Clingy and weepy** **Highly emotional; changeable** **Wants others around, especially when sick**	**Stomach aches in children** Rancid belches Slow digestion with poor assimilation Can't digest fat well Craves food that she can't digest	**Rich foods** **Heat; hot stuffy rooms**	Open air Cold applications, food, or drinks	**Lack of thirst** **Desire for creamy, rich foods, peanut butter** **Aversion to fat, milk, bread, meat, and pork** **Aggravation from pork, fat, and rich foods**
Sulphur *(Sulfur)*	**Heartburn after overeating or eating wrong foods** **Hungry at 11:00 A.M.** **Sudden, explosive diarrhea makes him get out of bed in the morning (5:00 A.M.)**	**Opinionated and critical** **Thinking all the time, philosophical** **Lazy** Usually messy, but sometimes very neat	**Burning pain in the stomach and esophagus** **Belching, with a bad taste in the mouth** **Loose, burning stool** **Skin rashes** **Very smelly diarrhea (like rotten eggs), gas, perspiration, and discharges**	**Warmth; warmth of bed (sticks feet out)** Bathing Lying on left side	Open air	**Desire for alcohol, sweets, spicy food, and cold drinks** Aversion to eggs, fish, and squash

Insect Bites and Stings

Description

Everyone has had the experience of a bee sting or an insect bite. It is usually just annoying, painful, or inconvenient, putting a damper on a perfect outing or picnic. Sometimes it can cause a severe allergic reaction or anaphylactic shock.

Symptoms

Redness, swelling, and itching occur after the bite, sometimes with burning or stinging pain. Hives, difficulty breathing, and shock may occur with severe anaphylactic reactions. Signs of anaphylactic shock are paleness, perspiration, confusion or unconsciousness, rapid pulse, and shallow, irregular breathing.

Complications

Occasionally the person who is bitten or stung can have a severe allergic or anaphylactic reaction, which can be life-threatening. This may occur from a second bite or sting when there was not much reaction to the first one. Get medical attention immediately if the bite is from a poisonous insect or spider, or if there is difficulty breathing, severe swelling, or loss of consciousness. Consult a physician if you think the person may have been exposed to Lyme disease; a red circle resembling a target around the site of a deer tick bite is one early symptom. Antibiotics may be necessary to avoid later complications of heart and muscle or joint disease.

Look

What is the appearance of the area that has been affected?
What is the location of the affected area?
What is the color at or around the area of the bite or sting?

Listen

"Everything is swollen." *Apis*
"I itch like crazy and I can't stop scratching. I can't stand smoke." *Caladium*
"My throat is closing up and I'm having trouble breathing." *Carbolic acid*
"I'm covered with flea bites. They're quite annoying." *Ledum*

"It's worse than a bee sting. I was up near the roof. I don't remember being stung, but I think it may have been a wasp." *Vespa*

Ask

When did the bite or sting occur?
What is the area of the body affected?
What are the symptoms?
Is there pain? If so, how severe and where?
What does the pain feel like?
Does anything make it feel better or worse?
Is the pain lessened by heat or cold?
Does the site feel cold or hot?
Are there any emotional changes since the bite?

MEDICAL CONDITIONS

Pointers to Finding the Homeopathic Medicine

The first medicine to give if there is swelling is *Apis.* ▮ For bee stings, give *Apis.* ▮ For bites with terrific itching, consider *Caladium.* ▮ In the case of anaphylactic shock, call 911 and give *Carbolic acid* or *Apis.* ▮ For most insect bites, first try *Ledum.* ▮ For wasp stings, *Vespa* is the first choice. Use *Apis* if *Vespa* is not available.

Dosage

- Give three pellets of 30C every thirty minutes to four hours, depending on the intensity of the bite or sting, until you see improvement. Only give the medicine more than every two hours if the bite or sting or the reaction to it is very severe.
- If there is no improvement after three doses, give a different medicine.
- After you first notice improvement, give another dose only if symptoms begin to return.
- Lower potencies (6X, 6C, 30X) may need to be given more often (every two to four hours).
- Higher potencies (200X, 200C, 1M) generally need to be given only once. Repeat only if symptoms return with intensity; give only infrequently in this case.

What to Expect from Homeopathic Self-Care

Reduces inflammation, relieves pain and itching, helps the bite or sting heal more rapidly.

Other Self-Care Suggestions

Remove the stinger with a flicking motion using a fingernail or a sterilized needle. Pulling it straight out may release additional venom. ▮ Apply an ice pack or a cold, moist pack to reduce swelling and circulation, and to prevent the spread of the venom. ▮ Cleanse the area with soap and water. ▮ *Calendula* (Marigold flower) cream can ease itching and irritation. ▮ Baking soda mixed with water applied to the area can reduce swelling. ▮ If nothing else is available, put a dab of toothpaste on the bite.

	Key Symptoms	Mind	Body	Worse	Better	Food & Drink
Apis mellifica *(Honeybee)*	**Bee stings** **Stinging pain that is lessened by cold applications**	**Busy** **Active** Irritable if crossed	**Heat, redness, and stinging pain, with lots of swelling** **Site of the sting is hot and worse from heat, and better from cold applications** **Hives with burning, stinging, and itching after a bite or sting** Anaphylactic shock Itching that is intolerable at night	**Heat, hot drinks, or a hot bath**	**Cool air, cold baths, and uncovering**	**Not usually thirsty**
Caladium *(American arum)*	**Mosquito, flea, and fly bites that burn and itch intensely**	Nervous and excitable Fearful of catching disease Restless after smoking		**Smoking** Motion	Cold air	
Carbolic acid	**Anaphylactic reaction and collapse following a bee or wasp sting** **Hives all over the body**	Illnesses from mental exertion Does not feel like working	**Swelling of face and tongue from bee stings** **Ears and throat feel swollen as if they are closing** **Difficulty breathing** **Water-filled blisters that burn and itch** Pale, collapsed, bathed in cold sweat Sense of smell increased	Jarring Reading	Smoking Strong tea	

continued on next page

	Key Symptoms	Mind	Body	Worse	Better	Food & Drink
Ledum *(Marsh tea)*	**Insect bites, like mosquito or flea bites or stings** **Affected part feels cold; feels better from cold applications or cold bathing**	Averse to company and friends Dissatisfied	Site of bite is purple and puffy Deer tick bites that could result in Lyme disease	Heat	Cold applica-tions or bathing	
Vespa *(Wasp)*	**Stinging, burning pains as if pierced by red hot needles**	**No recollection of having been bitten**	**Redness and swelling** **Convulsions following wasp stings with loss of consciousness and star-ing into space** Chilly, cold sensation around the sting	Heat Closed room	Washing the hands in cold water Bathing with vinegar	

Insomnia

Description
Insomnia is difficulty falling asleep or staying asleep, to the point that it interferes with getting adequate rest. Insomnia may be caused by emotional distress, worry, nervous tension, too much thinking, pain, drugs, caffeine, overeating, or environments that are not conducive to sleeping.

Symptoms
People with insomnia either can't get to sleep, or they sleep too lightly and awaken too early or too frequently. They often feel tired in the morning upon waking, and do not dream normally.

Lack of sleep contributes to irritability, stress, poor performance at school or work, and a greater tendency to make mistakes or have accidents. People with chronic insomnia may become irritable or depressed.

Complications
An occasional lost night of sleep will not cause much difficulty, but chronic insomnia can take its toll on one's health. Sleep deprivation impacts the proper functioning of the immune system and decreases overall alertness and mental functioning.

Look
Does the person look fatigued?
Does the person have dark circles under the eyes?

Listen
"I can't sleep since I was so badly frightened." *Aconite*
"I am so worried that I can't get to sleep. If I don't get to sleep, I'll die!" *Arsenicum album*
"I feel really alert and I can't shut my mind off." *Coffea*
"I can't sleep because of the pain." *Coffea, Chamomilla*
"I am very tired, but I am so excited about my performance tomorrow that I can't sleep!" *Gelsemium*
"I just can't sleep since my father died. Sigh!" *Ignatia*
"It's 3:00 A.M. and I can't get to sleep. All I can think of is my business!" *Nux vomica*

Ask

Is the insomnia occasional, or is it chronic?
Do you have trouble getting to sleep or staying asleep?
Do you wake at a particular time of night?
Are any mental or emotional things bothering you?
Are you too warm or chilly?
Do you need the window open or closed?
How does noise or light affect your sleep?
Do you have any nighttime worries or fears?
Do you crave anything to eat or drink at night?
Are you hungry or thirsty in bed?
What position do you like to sleep in?

Pointers for Finding the Homeopathic Medicine

If the person can't sleep following a terrifying experience, the medicine is *Aconite.* ▮ For insomnia that begins right after a financial crisis, give *Arsenicum album.* ▮ For someone who sits up in bed wide awake at 3:00 A.M., think of *Coffea.* ▮ *Coffea* and *Chamomilla* can be helpful for sleeplessness due to hypersensitivity to pain. ▮ For inability to sleep because of anticipation or stage fright, *Gelsemium* fits best. ▮ If the insomnia began during a period of grieving after the death of a loved one, the best medicine is *Ignatia.* ▮ People who wake at 3:00 A.M. worrying about business often benefit from *Nux vomica.*

Dosage

- Give three pellets of 30C twice a day until you see improvement.
- If there is no improvement after three doses, give a different medicine.
- After you first notice improvement, give another dose only if symptoms begin to return.
- Lower potencies (6X, 6C, 30X) may need to be given more often (every two to four hours).
- Higher potencies (200X, 200C, 1M) generally need to be given only once. Repeat only if symptoms return with intensity; give only infrequently in this case.

What to Expect from Homeopathic Self-Care

Homeopathic medicines can provide a short-term solution to a sleepless night by rapidly helping people to get a good night's sleep. Chronic insomnia should be treated constitutionally by a homeopathic practitioner.

Other Self-Care Suggestions

Drink a cup of warm milk, containing the amino acid tryptophan, one-half hour before bedtime. ▮ Equal parts of valerian root, skullcap, passionflower, and hops is a useful herbal sleep formula. Take thirty drops of tincture in warm water one-half hour before bedtime or every two hours as needed. ▮ Take an hour of quiet time or relaxation without noise or entertainment before going to bed. ▮ Lie on the right side with arm outstretched to induce sleep more rapidly. ▮ Do alternate nostril breathing for five minutes at bedtime. Close the right nostril with your thumb pressed to the side of your nose. Inhale slowly through the left nostril. With your middle finger close the left nostril, release your thumb to open the right and exhale. Inhale through the right. Then close the right nostril and exhale through the left. Inhale slowly through the left and switch again, exhaling through the right. Continue for three to ten minutes.

	Key Symptoms	Mind	Body	Worse	Better	Food & Drink
Aconite *(Monkshood)*	**Insomnia due to fright or shock** **Extreme anxiety** **Tremendous restlessness** **Fear of impending death**	Claustrophobia Panic attacks Wants company	**Violent heart palpitations** **Profuse perspiration with anxiety** **Rapid pulse**	Chill	Rest	Very thirsty for cold drinks
Arsenicum album *(Arsenic)*	**Insomnia due to worry and anxiety** **Insomnia worse from midnight to 2:00 A.M.** **Restlessness**	**Very anxious about health** Hypochondriacal Wants someone close by for support Complains that she'll never sleep	**Burning pains** **Very chilly**	Cold food or drinks	Heat Warm drinks	Desire for sips of water frequently Desire for milk
Chamomilla *(Chamomile)*	**Insomnia due to pain, including teething** **Tremendous hypersensitivity to pain**	**Child is cross and contrary (especially infants during teething)** **Child demands to be carried or rocked**	**Child is inconsolable with ear or teething pain** Painful colic of infants prevents sleep	Cold wind Night 9:00 P.M.	Being carried	
Coffea *(Unroasted coffee)*	**Insomnia; wide awake at 3:00 A.M. with mind full of thoughts** **Overstimulation, hypersensitivity, and hyperexcitability** **Nervous agitation and restlessness**	**Unusual activity of body and mind** Overreaction to all emotions, even joy and surprise Abundance of ideas	**Exquisite sensitivity to pain** **Hypersensitivity to noise, light, and touch**	**Excessive emotions, including joy** Strong odors Noise Touch	Lying down Sleep	

Gelsemium *(Yellow jasmine)*	**Insomnia following fright or from stage fright**	Mind feels extremely dull Thinking is an effort	**Wants to lie down and go to sleep, but can't** **Diarrhea from stage fright** **Dizzy, drowsy, droopy, and dull**	**Fright**	Bending forward Lying down with the head up	Lack of thirst
Ignatia *(St. Ignatius bean)*	**Insomnia following grief or loss** **Uncontrollable crying, loss of appetite, and extreme sadness** **Pronounced mood swings**	High-strung and emotionally reactive Upset after hurt or disappointment	**Frequent sighing** **Numbness and cramping anywhere in the body** Sensation of a lump in the throat, especially after grief Symptoms that are just the opposite of what you would expect, such as an injury with no pain or feeling cold in a hot room	**Grief or disappointment**	Deep breathing Changing positions	**Strong desire for or dislike for fruit** Desire for cheese
Nux vomica *(Quaker's button)*	**Waking at 3:00 A.M. with thoughts of business** **Highly irritable and impatient** **Chilly**	**Obsessed with business** **Wants to be the first and the best** **Competitive and hard-driving, Type A** Easily offended Frustrated easily by little things	**Insomnia due to heightened sensitivity to light, noise, sound, and other stimuli** **Insomnia after too much rich or spicy food or alcohol**	Early morning Cold dry air	Rest	**Desire for spicy food, fat, coffee, alcohol, and tobacco**

Leg Cramps and Growing Pains

Description

Leg cramps are painful spasms of the muscles in the calf or thigh. Growing pains are unpleasant sensations in the muscles, bones, or joints of growing children and adolescents.

Symptoms

Leg cramps or "charley horses" are felt as painful cramps that will not release for seconds to minutes. Growing pains are felt in the tendons, muscles, joints, or long parts of the bones as a deep aching pain. Both conditions can be quite painful.

Complications

Cramps and growing pains resolve on their own with time. Neither is serious, but the pain may be considerable.

Look

Is there anything visible about the leg cramps?
Can you observe any position that makes the cramping more comfortable?

Listen

"I get cramps in my calves from walking uphill." *Calcarea carbonica*
"My daughter, Sally, is going through quite a growth spurt and has terrible leg pains." *Calcarea phosphorica*
"I get excruciating cramps in my legs and my feet." *Cuprum*

Ask

What are the symptoms of the leg cramps or growing pains?
Where do you feel them?
When do they occur?
Is there anything that makes them better or worse?

Pointers for Finding the Homeopathic Medicine

For leg cramps and pains in the bones or joints that are worse from exertion and cold damp weather, try *Calcarea carbonica*. ▮ Growing pains usually respond to *Calcarea phosphorica*. If not, consider the rarer medicines, *Manganum* and *Syphilinum* in consultation with a homeopath. ▮ Severe cramps in the legs and other parts of the body in a person who is very prone to cramping may respond to *Cuprum*, especially if they come on after overwork or sex.

Dosage

- Give three pellets of 30C every four hours until you see improvement.
- If no improvement after three doses, give a different medicine.
- After you first notice improvement, give another dose only if symptoms begin to return.
- Lower potencies (6X, 6C, 30X) may need to be given more often (every two to four hours).
- Higher potencies (200X, 200C, 1M) generally need to be given only once. Repeat only if symptoms return with intensity; give only infrequently in this case.

What to Expect from Homeopathic Self-Care

Homeopathic medicines can stop leg cramps or growing pains immediately or within a few minutes. Growing pains may need to be treated constitutionally for lasting results.

Other Self-Care Suggestions

Massage the affected limb toward the heart. ▮ Apply firm rotary pressure with thumb or forefinger to any tender points in the area until the tenderness decreases by one-half. ▮ Apply a hot pack or heating pad to the area to help relax the muscles. ▮ Take a hot bath with a cup of Epsom salts dissolved in the bath water. ▮ Take Calcium (1500 mg per day) and Magnesium (750 mg per day). ▮ For severe cramps after working or exercising in the heat, drink lightly salted water or take two salt tablets while you drink fluids to restore sodium and fluid lost through excessive sweating.

	Key Symptoms	Mind	Body	Worse	Better	Food & Drink
Calcarea carbonica *(Calcium carbonate)*	**Calf, foot, and thigh cramps** **Cramps in bed** **Cramps after exertion**	Illnesses from taking on too much responsibility Worry about safety and security	**Pains in the bones and joints from cold damp weather** **Legs feel weak going uphill or up stairs** Couch potatoes Children who have large, sweaty heads and flabby bodies	**Cold damp weather** **Going uphill** **Exertion**	**Rubbing** Dry weather	**Desire for eggs, sweets, and salt**
Calcarea phosphorica *(Calcium phosphate)*	**Main medicine for growing pains** **Leg cramps while skiing** **Worse from cold, damp weather, especially going out in the snow**	Love to travel Dissatisfied, always looking for greener pastures	**Leg cramps feel better from being rubbed** **Problems with bones or teeth**	Change of weather Lifting Melting snow	Warm dry weather Lying down	**Desire for smoked meats**
Cuprum *(Copper)*	**Cramps in palms, calves, and soles** **Spasms and cramping anywhere in the body**	Avoids everyone who approaches him Great anxiety accompanying violent cramps	**Muscle twitching of lower extremities** **Jerking of hands and feet**	Motion Ascending	Lying down	

Mastitis
(Breast Inflammation)

Description
Mastitis is an inflammation of the breast, usually found in nursing mothers. It may be associated with a bacterial infection such as *Staphylococcus aureus,* but sometimes the discharge is sterile. Nursing too frequently can sometimes lead to sore breasts and cracked nipples.

Symptoms
Mastitis is acutely painful, with swelling, engorgement, and inflammation of the breast tissue. It can be extremely painful to nurse or express the milk during mastitis, but engorgement with milk without relief is also problematic.

Complications
Mastitis is usually a local problem, but systemic infection can occur in rare cases. Infection could also be transmitted to the nursing infant, requiring medical attention. If nursing is not possible, the breasts will need to be pumped when they become engorged.

Look
Is the breast red or hot?
Is it tender to touch?
What does the nipple look like?
Is there any discharge from the nipple? What does it look or smell like?
Is fever present?

Listen
"All of a sudden my breast got really red and swollen and I got a fever!" *Belladonna*
"Any time I move it hurts a lot." *Bryonia*
"My nipples are so cracked and sore." *Castor equi*
"My breasts hurt in between nursing, all the way through to my back." *Phellandrium*
"My lymph nodes are swollen and the pain in my breast goes all through my body." *Phytolacca*
"I'm so tired and I can't sleep because of the burning in my breast." *Silica*

Ask

How does your breast feel?
What makes it feel better or worse?
How does nursing affect the symptoms?
Have there been any mental or emotional changes before or during your mastitis?
Are you hungry or thirsty?
Do you want anything in particular to eat or drink?
Do you feel warm or chilly?

Pointers for Finding the Homeopathic Medicine

Mastitis that comes on suddenly with a high fever, a red face and breast, and is worse on the right side indicates *Belladonna.* ▮ When the breast pain is much worse from any motion and the woman is very irritable, think of *Bryonia.* ▮ If pain occurs just from going down stairs and the nipples are sore and cracked, the medicine is *Castor equi.* ▮ *Hepar sulphuris* is used for chilly, sensitive, and irritable women who have splinter-like pains and a foul, cheesy discharge from the breast. ▮ If the nipples are very cracked and sore to the touch, consider *Castor equi* first, then *Phytolacca.* ▮ If the breast pain radiates to the back and is unbearable between nursing times give *Phellandrium.* ▮ For swollen lymph nodes in the armpit, use *Phytolacca* if the pain radiates to the whole body, and *Silica* if there are burning pains in the breast at night.

Dosage

- Give three pellets of 30C every four hours until you see improvement.
- If there is no improvement after three doses, give a different medicine.
- After you first notice improvement, give another dose only if symptoms begin to return.
- Lower potencies (6X, 6C, 30X) may need to be given more often (every two to four hours).
- Higher potencies (200X, 200C, 1M) generally need to be given only once. Repeat only if symptoms return with intensity; give only infrequently in this case.

What to Expect from Homeopathic Self-Care

Mastitis improves with homeopathic medicines within twenty-four to forty-eight hours. If successful, homeopathic treatment allows nursing mothers to avoid antibiotics, which can complicate the problem by causing secondary yeast infections of the nipple and the infant's mouth.

Other Self-Care Suggestions

Alternating hot (five minutes)and cold (one minute) wet compresses stimulates circulation and healing. ▮ Massage techniques that specifically promote drainage of the lymph system can help. ▮ Take an echinacea and goldenseal combination; two dropperfuls of tincture in water three times a day or six capsules a day are useful to stimulate the immune system to fight infection. ▮ Take beta-carotene (50,000 IU once a day). ▮ Take Zinc (30 mg once a day). ▮ Take Vitamin C (1000 mg three times a day). ▮ If you need advice about nursing, your local La Leche League can provide excellent information, and can sometimes help you to prevent premature weaning.

	Key Symptoms	Mind	Body	Worse	Better	Food & Drink
Belladonna *(Deadly nightshade)*	**Mastitis comes on suddenly and violently** **Mastitis is often right-sided** **Breast is heavy, hard, inflamed, and red**	Irritable	**Bright red flushed face, high fever, throbbing headache**	**Jarring** **Lying down** **3:00 P.M.**	Sitting up in a quiet, dark room	**Not usually thirsty** **Desire for lemons or lemonade, sour food, and cold water**
Bryonia *(Wild hops)*	**Breast pain worse from any motion** **Has to hold the breasts when going up or down stairs** **Breasts are heavy, painful, and stony hard, but not very red**	**Wants to go home** **Extremely irritable**	**Inflamed breasts with suppressed flow of milk** **Swollen left breast, hurts when lifting arm** **Nipples very hard** Pain from motion of chest	**Touch** **Deep breathing** Coughing	**Pressure** **Lying on the painful side**	
Castor equi *(Rudimentary thumbnail of the horse)*	**Sore, deeply cracked nipples in nursing mothers** **Clothing touching the nipples is unbearable** **Dry painful nipples with red around the areola** **Ulcerated nipples**	Laughing at serious things or for no reason	**Breast abscess** **Violent itching of the breast** **Pain in the breast after the birth** Breasts are swollen and tender, feeling as if they would fall off when going down stairs Breasts feel better from firm pressure	Light touch		

Hepar sulphuris *(Calcium sulfide)*	**Breast is very painful, especially to touch** **Splinter-like pains in the breast** **Extreme sensitivity to cold air and applications**	**Extremely irritable and touchy** **Very sensitive to pain**	**Breast abscess with thick pus** **Discharge from the breast smells sour or like rotten cheese** Swollen lymph glands under the armpit	**Touch** **Lying on the painful part** **Drafts** **Uncovering**	Warmth Covering up	
Phellandrium *(Water dropwort)*	**Unbearable pain between nursing** **Pain in the nipples while nursing the child** **Pain in the right breast extending to the back between the shoulder blades**	Anxious about her health Fear that someone is behind her	**Pain in the breasts during the menstrual period** **Pain in the breasts which goes to the abdomen**	Breathing	Motion Open air	
Phytolacca *(Pokeroot)*	**Breasts heavy, stony hard, swollen, and tender** **Extreme pain in the breasts while nursing, worse in the left breast** **Breast pain radiates to the whole body**	Very afraid that she will die Doesn't care if she exposes her body to others	**Sore all over** **Swollen lymph nodes in the arm pit** **Nipples are cracked, sensitive, and can be inverted**	Motion Lifting the breast	Lying on abdomen or left side Rest	
Silica *(Flint)*	**Breast swollen, dark red, sensitive** **Burning pains prevent sleep** **Inflamed breast with a high fever**	Refined Delicate features	**Inflammation of nipples** **Darting, burning pain in left nipple** **Breast abscess** Swollen lymph nodes in the armpit Low stamina and energy	Warmth and heat	Cold, dampness Touch	Desire for eggs and sweets Aversion to fat and milk

Measles

Description

Measles is a viral disease that affects children and adults who do not have active immunity. It is highly contagious, and is spread by airborne droplets from an infected person before the rash appears and during the first few days of the disease.

Symptoms

Fever (up to 104°F), runny nose, sore throat, cough, sensitivity to light, and an extensive pink to brownish-pink, irregular, itchy rash starting around the ears, face, and neck which then lightens up as it spreads to the trunk and limbs as the fever decreases. Koplik spots, which appear only in measles, look like tiny grains of sand with a red ring and are usually seen opposite the first and second upper molars on the inside of the cheek.

Complications

Secondary infections with streptococci and other bacteria may occur causing pneumonia, ear infections, and other infections. In one out of a thousand children, measles can cause encephalitis with fever, convulsions, and coma.

Look

What does the rash look like?
Where on the body is the rash?
Are the eyes or nose running?
Is the child coughing? When does the cough come and what does it sound like?
Do you see Koplik spots inside the cheek opposite the upper molars?

Listen

"All of a sudden I feel really bad." *Aconite*
"My eyes hurt from the light and I can't stop them from watering." *Euphrasia*

"I feel dizzy and sleepy." *Gelsemium*
"Please hold me and wipe my nose for me." *Pulsatilla*
"The rash really itches a lot!" *Sulphur*

Ask

When did the symptoms start?
When did the rash appear?
Does anything make you feel better or worse?
Have there been any mental or emotional symptoms before or since you got the measles?
Do you want anything in particular to eat or drink?
Do you feel warm or chilly?

Pointers for Finding the Homeopathic Medicine

Give *Aconite* if the symptoms come on suddenly and violently with a high fever, especially after a fright or exposure to cold dry wind. ▮ *Euphrasia* is used for measles when there is a lot of sensitivity to light and a discharge from the eyes. ▮ *Gelsemium* is the medicine when measles comes on more slowly and the child is dizzy, drowsy, droopy, and dull with a fever and headache in the back of the head. ▮ *Pulsatilla* is used in the later stages of measles when thick yellow-green discharge and a low fever are present and the rash is beginning to fade. ▮ *Sulphur* is used when the rash is late to develop, and is purplish or dusky, and the itching is made worse by heat and bathing.

Dosage

- Give three pellets of 30C every four hours until you see improvement.
- If there is no improvement after three doses, give a different medicine.
- After you first notice improvement, give another dose only if symptoms begin to return.
- Lower potencies (6X, 6C, 30X) may need to be given more often (every two to four hours).
- Higher potencies (200X, 200C, 1M) generally need to be given only once. Repeat only if symptoms return with intensity; give only infrequently in this case.

What to Expect from Homeopathic Treatment

Homeopathic medicines can ease the symptoms and shorten the course of a measles infection, as well as help prevent complications. Effects of the medicine should be seen within twelve to twenty-four hours.

Other Self-Care Suggestions

Bed rest in a darkened room. ■ Drink plenty of fluids. ■ Eat a light diet, depending on appetite. ■ Vitamin C: 250 mg twice a day for young children, four times a day for older children; 1000 mg four times a day for adults. ■ Keep sores clean and avoid scratching them. ■ Apply cold compresses to the sores. ■ Oatmeal baths: use Aveno (avoid the type that contains camphor) or place one cup of dry oatmeal in the bathtub to soothe the itching. ■ To treat infected sores, apply a few drops of one part *Calendula* tincture diluted with three parts water, and cover with bandages or gauze.

	Key Symptoms	Mind	Body	Worse	Better	Food & Drink
Aconite *(Monkshood)*	**First stage of measles** **Sudden high fever** **Symptoms come on suddenly** **Measles after exposure to cold dry air or wind** **Measles after fright or shock**	**Tremendous restlessness** **Fear of death** Desire for company	**Bright red rough rash** **Redness of the eyes** **Dry, barking, croupy cough, especially during first twenty-four hours** **Itching and burning of the skin** Rapid pulse	Chill	Rest	Very thirsty for cold drinks
Euphrasia *(Eyebright)*	**Eye symptoms are the most prominent complaint of the measles** **Eyes are sensitive to light and water constantly**		**Early stage of measles** **Measles rash** Hot irritating discharge from the eyes, but a bland nasal discharge Headache in the forehead	Sunlight Wind Warm room	Open air Blinking Wiping the eyes	
Gelsemium *(Yellow jasmine)*	**At the beginning of measles with fever** **Measles following fright or from stage fright** **Dizzy, drowsy, droopy, and dull** **Muscle aching throughout body**	Mind feels extremely dull Thinking is an effort	**Measles rash** **Irritating watery discharge from the nose** **Hard, barking, croupy cough and hoarseness** Headache starts in the neck or back of head and goes to the forehead Head feels heavy and hard to lift Chills up and down the spine Overall weakness Desire to lie down and go to sleep	Fright 10:00 A.M.	Bending forward Lying down with head held high Urination	**Not thirsty**

continued on next page

	Key Symptoms	Mind	Body	Worse	Better	Food & Drink
Pulsatilla *(Windflower)*	**Later stages of measles, when fever is not high** **Measles rash in later stages when it is dusky and beginning to fade** **Warm, with desire for fresh air or open window**	**Changeable emotions** **Clingy and weepy** **Wants company when sick**	**Runny nose and eyes with thick yellow-green discharge** **Earache or diarrhea as a complication of measles** Cough usually dry at night and loose in the morning Child sits up in bed to cough	Rich food	Slow walking in the open air	**Not thirsty** Desire for butter, ice cream, and creamy foods Aversion to fat, milk, and pork
Sulphur *(Sulfur)*	**Measles rash late to appear, with lots of itching** **Measles with dusky skin and a purplish color**	**Opinionated and critical** **Thinking all the time, philosophical** **Lazy** Usually messy, but sometimes very neat	**Itching worse from heat, the heat of the bed, and bathing** **Inflammation of eyelids with redness and burning** Excessive perspiration, often bad-smelling	Heat 11:00 A.M.	Cool air	Desire for sweets, spicy foods, and fatty foods Aversion to eggs and squash

Menstrual Cramps
(Dysmenorrhea)

Description
Menstrual cramping is pain of any kind associated with the menstrual cycle. It generally occurs during the menstrual period, but occasionally occurs before or after the period, or at ovulation.

Symptoms
Mild to severe pain of the ovaries, uterus, pelvic area, or pubic area occur along with back pain or general body discomfort. Pain may also radiate to the thighs. Other symptoms of menstrual discomfort include headaches, nausea, diarrhea, or constipation and a variety of mental and emotional symptoms, including mood swings, depression, anxiety, and irritability.

Complications
Recurrent menstrual pain may be an indication of a more serious problem such as endometriosis, ovarian cysts, uterine fibroids, or, rarely, cancer.

Look
Are there any visible signs of discomfort?
Is she in any particular position?

Listen
"My right ovary is throbbing terribly and I feel so angry." *Belladonna*
"It feels like there's a tight band around my abdomen. I can't stand it." *Cactus*
"Nothing makes me feel better. Just get out of my sight." *Chamomilla*
"All I want to do is lie down and curl up tightly." *Colocynthis*
"I just want a heating pad over my uterus." *Magnesia phosphorica*
"This always happens after I drink too much before my period." *Nux vomica*

Ask
What are you feeling?
What is bothering you the most?
Where are you in your cycle?

MEDICAL CONDITIONS

Have you experienced this before?
Are you in pain? If so, where is the pain?
Does the pain remain localized, or does it radiate elsewhere?
How intense is the pain?
Does anything make the pain better or worse?
Are there any other symptoms?
What makes the pain feel better or worse?
Are there any mental or emotional symptoms that came with the menstrual pain?

Pointers for Finding the Homeopathic Medicine

If there is heavy, bright red bleeding, gushing, and throbbing pain, look first at *Belladonna.* ▮ If the pain is lessened by heat and pressure, think first of *Magnesia phosphorica,* then of *Colocynthis.* ▮ For pain so violent that she must scream out, give *Cactus grandifolia.* ▮ If the pain is very intense and the woman is terribly angry and inconsolable, look at *Chamomilla.* ▮ If the woman feels better when drawing her knees up to her chest, give *Colocynthis.* ▮ If the pain began after anger, think of *Nux vomica, Colocynthis,* and *Belladonna.* ▮ If the pain came on after too much alcohol or rich food, give *Nux vomica.*

Dosage

- Give three pellets of 30C every fifteen minutes to one hour until you see improvement.
- If there is no improvement after three doses, give a different medicine.
- After you first notice improvement, give another dose only if symptoms begin to return.
- Higher potencies (200X, 200C, 1M) generally need to be given only once. Repeat only if symptoms return with intensity; give only infrequently in this case.

What to Expect from Homeopathic Self-Care

Homeopathic medicines generally help to relieve pain within fifteen minutes to several hours. If these medicines are not helpful, we recommend constitutional homeopathic care.

Other Self-Care Suggestions

Alternating hot and cold sitz baths: soak in a tub of moderately hot water for five minutes, then in a tub of cold water up to the navel with knees bent for one minute. Alternate two to three times. ▮ Walking, stretching, and other physical exercise can sometimes help. ▮ For muscle cramps, Calcium (1000 mg) and Magnesium (500 mg) can help. ▮ Take *Viburnum* (Cramp bark) tincture: one-half teaspoon every hour, up to six doses. The dosage for capsules depends on the specific product. ▮ A heating pad is often helpful. ▮ Castor oil packs to the abdomen with a heating pad can sometimes relieve discomfort. ▮ Avoid caffeine and salt premenstrually.

	Key Symptoms	Mind	Body	Worse	Better	Food & Drink
Belladonna *(Deadly nightshade)*	**Throbbing pains, worse on the right side** **Sudden onset of symptoms** **Violent pain** **Feeling of fullness in the uterus from congested blood** **Right-sided symptoms**	Irritable Maddening pain	**Profuse, bright red, gushing, clotted menstrual flow** **Bearing down sensation, as if the pelvic organs would fall out**	**Motion** Light Noise	Semi-erect position Lying in bed Leaning against some-thing	**Great thirst for cold water, or no thirst at all** Desire for lemons and lemonade
Cactus grandifolia *(Night-blooming cereus)*	**Extreme pain that feels like a band across the abdomen** **Violent menstrual pains** **Screams with menstrual pain**	Cries without knowing why Doesn't think she'll ever feel better	**Clotted menstrual flow with pain as each clot is passed** Throbbing pain in the ovary Lumpy menstrual flow	Lying on the left side Exertion Walking	Being outside	Aversion to meat
Chamomilla *(Chamomile)*	**Intense, labor-like pain with the menstrual flow** **Profuse, dark, clotted blood with occasional gushing of bright red blood** **Menstrual pain after anger** **Hypersensitivity to pain** **Inconsolable**	**Very irritable** **Says she wants something, then changes her mind when she gets it**	**Severe menstrual pain, with pains extending down the inner thighs** **Greenish diarrhea**	Lying in bed	**Being rocked** Cold applications	Thirsty for cold drinks
Colocynthis *(Bitter apple)*	**Cramping pain that is re-lieved by bending over double** **Menstrual pain made more tolerable by hard pressure**	**Irritable and indignant** **Feelings hurt easily**	**Pain so intense that she vomits** Menstrual pain relieved by heat and pressure Ovarian pain	**Anger** **Lying on the painless side**	After a bowel movement or passing gas Heat	

Magnesia phosphorica *(Magnesium phosphate)*	Pain relieved by heat and pressure Menstrual pain before the period Pain feels better when the menstrual flow begins Menstrual flow is dark and too early	Irritable Wants nurturing, feels like she was not nurtured as a child	Great weakness with the menstrual period Intense soreness and bruised feeling in the abdomen Ovarian pain Swelling of the labia	Lying on the right side Drafts	**Hot baths** **Bending double**	
Nux vomica *(Quaker's button)*	**Cramps extend to the whole body** **Menstrual pain with the urge for a bowel movement** **Menstrual cramping after anger, rich foods, or too much alcohol**	**Irritable** **Impatient** **Obsessed with business** **Wants to be the first and the best** **Competitive and hard-driving, Type A** Easily offended Frustrated easily by little things	Menstrual flow is profuse, early, and lasts too long	Pressure	Rest Lying on either side	**Desire for fats, spicy food, alcohol, and stimulants**

Morning Sickness

(Nausea and Vomiting of Pregnancy)

Description

Morning sickness occurs most commonly in the first three months of pregnancy, but may persist in some cases until the baby is born. It is commonly experienced in the morning, but may last throughout the day or come at different times.

Symptoms

Terrible nausea with aversion to the sight and smell of food are usual symptoms. Vomiting may be pronounced, with inability to keep most food and beverages down.

Complications

Apart from the discomfort and inconvenience, the main complication of prolonged morning sickness is malnutrition and failure of the mother to gain appropriate weight, with subsequent low birth weight and congenital health problems for the child. Hyperemesis gravidarum—severe uncontrollable vomiting in pregnancy, often associated with liver disease—may cause dehydration and acidosis, requiring hospitalization and intravenous fluids.

Look

Is the woman vomiting?
Does she want to be in a particular posture or position to be comfortable?
Is her face pale?
Is she sweating?

Listen

"The nausea has been worse since I was up all night with my daughter." *Cocculus*
"I can't stand to ride in the (car, boat, airplane)." *Cocculus, Sepia, Tabacum*
"I can't stand the sight or smell of food." *Cocculus, Colchicum, Ipecac, Sepia*
"I have this terrible, constant nausea, but it doesn't help to vomit." *Ipecac*

"I want to vomit, but I can't." *Kreosotum*
"I'm totally not into sex." *Sepia, Kreosotum*
"I feel green, like when I smoked my first cigarette." *Tabacum*
"I break out in a cold sweat with the morning sickness, and all I want is fruit." *Veratrum*

Ask

How long have you been pregnant?
How long have you felt nauseous and been vomiting?
What are your symptoms like? How severe are your symptoms?
What brings on the nausea and vomiting?
Is it worse at any time of the day or night?
Does anything make the nausea and vomiting feel better or worse?
Are you hungry or thirsty?
Does any food or beverage appeal to you?
Is there anything you can't stand to eat or drink?
Are you able to keep anything down?
Are you in any pain?
Are there any other symptoms along with the morning sickness?
Do you feel warm or chilly?

Pointers for Finding the Homeopathic Medicine

The most common medicines for morning sickness are *Sepia* and *Colchicum.* ▮ When aversion to the smell of food is strongest, consider *Colchicum* first. ▮ For the worst vomiting, use *Ipecac,* and for the most deathly nausea, use *Tabacum.* ▮ When aversion to sex is a strong symptom, consider *Sepia* or *Kreosotum.* ▮ *Sepia* is for conditions that are made much better by vigorous exercise or dancing, which separates it from the motion sickness medicines such as *Tabacum* and *Cocculus;* the latter two are appropriate for conditions that are made much worse by motion. ▮ *Veratrum* is the medicine if the woman is very cold, has vomiting and diarrhea, and desires fruit, ice, and sour foods such as pickles or lemons.

Dosage

- Give three pellets of 30C twice a day until you see improvement.
- If there is no improvement after three doses, give a different medicine.
- After you first notice improvement, give another dose only if symptoms begin to return.

- It is best not to use lower potencies (6X, 6C, 12X) during pregnancy since they need to be repeated so often, and this is not desirable.
- Higher potencies (200X, 200C, 1M) generally need to be given only once. Repeat only if symptoms return with intensity; give only infrequently in this case.

What to Expect from Homeopathic Self-Care

Homeopathic medicines are very safe to use in pregnancy. The symptoms are relieved within several days to a week or ten days. Even though homeopathy is very safe, it is best not to overdo any type of treatment in a pregnant woman. If you have tried two or three medicines without success, or if the morning sickness persists past the third month, consult a homeopath for constitutional treatment.

Other Self-Care Suggestions

Eat small amounts of food frequently. ▮ Eat before getting up in the morning. ▮ Eat Saltine crackers to help relieve the nausea. ▮ Eat bland foods such as broth, rice, and pasta. ▮ Tea and toast are usually well tolerated. ▮ Sipping ginger-root tea can help relieve nausea. Use a one-quarter-inch slice of ginger root boiled in a cup of water for fifteen minutes. ▮ Many herbs, such as pennyroyal, need to be avoided during pregnancy. Research carefully before using herbs. ▮ Stimulating Stomach 36, an acupressure point in the soft place below the knee and to the outside of the leg where the tibia and fibula bones meet, often relieves nausea. Use firm rotary pressure on the spot for a few seconds. Repeat when needed.

	Key Symptoms	Mind	Body	Worse	Better	Food & Drink
Cocculus *(Indian cockle)*	**Nausea from the sight or smell of food** **Any kind of motion sickness with vertigo** **Nausea from looking at moving objects or watching things out of the window of a moving vehicle**	**Anxiety about the welfare of loved ones** Does not like to be interrupted or disturbed	**Must lie down with the morning sickness, or gets nauseated** **Headache, nausea, and vomiting with the morning sickness**	**Loss of sleep** **Taking care of a loved one who is ill** **Emotional stress** Open air	Lying on her side	**Aversion to food**
Colchicum *(Meadow saffron)*	**Intolerance of smells, especially cooking food** **Nausea from the smell of cooked meat, fish, and eggs** **Symptoms made worse by motion and turning the head** **Severe vomiting and retching**	**Ailments in response to rudeness of others** Anger at trifles	**Hungry, but disgusted at the thought of eating or when she smells food** Vomit is stringy and clear Swallowing saliva induces vomiting	**Eggs** Change of weather Cold, dampness	Warmth Rest	
Ipecac *(Ipecac root)*	**Terrible, constant nausea, not relieved by vomiting** **Nausea and vomiting with nearly all conditions** **Nausea with a clean tongue** **Hates food and the smell of food**	Difficult to please Doesn't know what she wants	**Bleeding and nausea at the same time** Cramps in the abdomen Drooling with the nausea	**Vomiting** **Warmth** Overeating	Open air	**Not thirsty** Desire for sweets, pastries

continued on next page

	Key Symptoms	Mind	Body	Worse	Better	Food & Drink
Kreosotum *(Creosote)*	**Nausea with desire to vomit, but can't** **Continuous vomiting with lots of straining** **Vomits sweetish water, undigested food, and everything that is eaten**	Dissatisfied with everything Afraid when thinking about having sex	**Vomits lots of sour, acrid fluid or foamy, white mucus** **Drooling during pregnancy** **Very irritating, burning, corrosive vaginal discharge**	Cold Lying down	Warmth Hot food	**Desire for smoked food**
Sepia *(Cuttlefish ink)*	**Sensitive to the thought or smell of food, even her favorites** **Motion sickness from walking or riding in the car** **Stomach feels empty, but eating doesn't help** **The smell of food cooking makes her nauseated**	**Aversion to her husband and sex** Irritable Depressed and crying	Crosses her legs to keep the uterus from falling out Threatened miscarriage	**Vinegar** **Afternoon** Too much sex Fasting or missing a meal Cold	**Exercise, dancing** **Keeping busy** Warmth	**Desire for vinegar,** sour food, sweets Aversion to fat, salt
Tabacum *(Tobacco)*	**Deathly nausea** **Cold, clammy, and pale with the nausea** **Motion sickness, seasickness from the least motion** **Better from cold fresh air** **Spitting with the nausea**	Feels wretched	**Violent vomiting from the least motion** Profuse sweat and saliva Sinking feeling in the stomach	**Heat** **Opening the eyes**	Uncovering the abdomen	
Veratrum album *(White hellebore)*	**Violent vomiting and diarrhea** **Cold sweat on the forehead while vomiting** **Icy cold, with cold sweat**	**Very active and busy** **Restless**	**Projectile vomiting** **Abdominal cramping** Collapse with a bluish color Diarrhea very forceful, followed by exhaustion and cold sweat	**Cold** Cold drinks Fruit	Warmth Hot drinks Covering up	**Desire for sour food, juicy fruit, pickles, lemons, salt, and ice**

Motion Sickness

Description

Motion sickness, also known as sea-, air-, or carsickness, is a complex of symptoms caused by stimulation of the balance mechanism in the inner ear by repeated motion. Disorientation, without being able to see a fixed horizon during motion, can induce motion sickness. It can be compounded by emotional stress.

Symptoms

Nausea and vomiting are the primary symptoms. Salivation, sweating, paleness, and hyperventilation are also common. Mental confusion can also be present.

Complications

Dehydration and lack of eating can produce problems if the motion sickness is prolonged.

Look

Does the person seem to want to be in any particular body position or posture to be comfortable?
Is the person flushed or pale?
Is he sweating?
How rapid is the pulse?

Listen

"Can't you please stop it from moving?" *Cocculus*
"If I could just get some sleep, I would be all right." *Cocculus*
"I can't seem to find my way home." *Petroleum*
"Strangely enough, I'm sick from walking or going in the car, but if I dance or work out I'm all right." *Sepia*
"I feel green, like when I smoked my first cigarette." *Tabacum*

Ask

How did the motion sickness start?
How long have you felt nauseated and been vomiting?
How severe is the nausea and vomiting?

What brings on the nausea and vomiting?
Does anything make the nausea and vomiting feel better or worse?
Are you hungry or thirsty?
Does any food or beverage appeal to you?
Is there anything you can't stand to eat or drink?
Are you able to keep anything down?
Are you in any pain?
Are there any other symptoms along with the motion sickness?
Do you feel warm or chilly?

Pointers for Finding the Homeopathic Medicine

Cocculus is the most common medicine for motion sickness. ▮ *Petroleum* is good for the combination of motion sickness and skin problems. ▮ *Sepia* is useful for motion sickness that is complicated by hormonal problems or relieved by vigorous exercise. ▮ *Tabacum* should be used when motion sickness is extremely severe.

Dosage

- Give three pellets of 30C every fifteen to thirty minutes until you see improvement.
- If there is no improvement after three doses, give a different medicine.
- After you first notice improvement, give another dose only if symptoms begin to return.
- Lower potencies (6X, 6C, 30X) may need to be given more often (every two to four hours).
- Higher potencies (200X, 200C, 1M) generally need to be given only once. Repeat only if symptoms return with intensity; give only infrequently in this case.

What to Expect from Homeopathic Self-Care

Homeopathic medicines can rapidly relieve motion sickness in minutes. If motion sickness is prolonged or recurrent, see an ear, nose, and throat specialist for diagnosis and a homeopath for constitutional treatment.

Other Self-Care Suggestions

Try to sit in the place in the vehicle where there is the least motion. ▮ Stare at a fixed point for orientation, not at anything that is moving. ▮ Lying down or reclining may help. ▮ Look above the horizon at a forty-five-degree angle. ▮ Get some fresh air. ▮ Eat small amounts of food frequently. ▮ Eat Saltine crackers to help relieve the nausea. ▮ Eat bland foods such as broth, rice, and pasta. ▮ Tea and toast are usually well tolerated. ▮ Sip ginger-root tea to help relieve nausea. Use a one-quarter-inch slice of ginger root boiled in a cup of water for fifteen minutes. ▮ Stimulate Stomach 36, an acupressure point in the soft place below the knee and to the outside of the leg where the tibia and fibula bones meet. Use firm rotary pressure on the spot for a few seconds. Repeat when needed.

	Key Symptoms	Mind	Body	Worse	Better	Food & Drink
Cocculus *(Indian cockle)*	**Any kind of motion sickness** **Nausea from looking at moving objects or watching things out of the window of a moving vehicle**	Doesn't like to be interrupted or disturbed	**Must lie down** **Headache, nausea, and vomiting with morning sickness** **Nausea from the sight or smell of food**	**Loss of sleep** **Caring for a loved one who is ill** Emotional stress Open air Touch	Lying on his side	**Aversion to food**
Petroleum *(Coal oil)*	**Seasickness, airsickness, or motion sickness** **Sensation of great emptiness in the stomach relieved by constant eating**	**Disoriented** Can't make up her mind Irritable	**Nausea from hunger** **Heartburn** Motion sickness with dry, cracked eczema	Cold weather	Warm air Dry weather	**Desire for beer** **Aversion to meat, fats, and cooked or hot foods**
Sepia *(Cuttlefish ink)*	**Motion sickness from walking or riding in the car** **Sensitivity to the thought or smell of food, even her favorites** **Nausea caused by the smell of cooking food**	**Aversion to partner and to sex** Irritable Depressed and crying	**Stomach feels empty but eating doesn't help** Constipation	**Vinegar** Pregnancy Fasting or missing a meal Cold	**Vigorous exercise, dancing** Keeping busy Warmth	**Desire for vinegar,** sour food, sweets Aversion to fat, salt
Tabacum *(Tobacco)*	**Deathly nausea** **Cold, clammy, and pale with the nausea** **Motion sickness, seasickness from the least motion** **Symptoms relieved by cold fresh air** **Spitting with the nausea**	Feels wretched	**Violent vomiting induced by the least motion** Profuse sweat and saliva Sinking feeling in the stomach	**Heat** **Opening the eyes**	Uncovering the abdomen	

Mumps

Description
Mumps is a contagious viral infection of the parotid gland in the upper jaw, just below and in front of the ears and other salivary glands. Mumps usually occurs in children, but can be more serious in adults.

Symptoms
The primary symptoms are moderate to high fever with chills, and painful swelling of the parotid glands and other salivary glands with fatigue and loss of appetite.

Complications
In men past puberty, the main complication of mumps is painful inflammation of the testes which can, in rare cases, cause sterility. Meningoencephalitis, which resembles bacterial meningitis, is characterized by a headache, stiff neck, and, rarely, convulsions or a coma. Pancreatitis with nausea, vomiting, and pain in the abdomen sometimes occurs at the end of the first week of mumps, and gets completely better in about a week.

Look
Does the parotid gland appear swollen in front of the ear?
Is fever present?
Is the person drooling?

Listen
"I feel faint. Please turn on the fan." *Carbo vegetabilis*
"I'm drooling, and I have a bad (metallic) taste in my mouth and bad breath." *Mercurius*
"Please hold me and take care of me." *Pulsatilla*

Ask
When did the swelling in your parotid gland appear?
Is it painful?
Does anything make you feel better or worse?
Have there been any mental or emotional changes since you got the measles?
Do you want anything in particular to eat or drink?
Do you feel warm or chilly?
Do you have any pain or swelling anywhere else (testes or breasts)?

Pointers for Finding the Homeopathic Medicine

Mercurius is the most common medicine used for mumps. ■ *Phytolacca* is used to treat stony hard parotid glands with pain extending to the ear on swallowing. ■ *Carbo vegetabilis* is used for mumps when exhaustion and bloating are prominent symptoms. ■ *Pulsatilla* and *Carbo vegetabilis* are both used when mumps causes inflammation of the testes or breasts. ■ *Pulsatilla* is appropriate when the child or adult is weepy and clingy with a lot of swelling in the testes or breasts. ■ Less common medicines which help inflammation of the testes during or after mumps are *Abrotanum* and *Jaborandi.* ■ *Abrotanum* is used to treat a large swollen parotid gland that goes down as the testes become swollen. It is given to irritable, cruel children with a failure to thrive. ■ *Jaborandi* treats mumps with increased sweating and salivation, and parotid glands double their usual size. This medicine has been used to shorten the duration of the disease.

Dosage

- Give three pellets of 30C every four hours until you see improvement.
- If there is no improvement after three doses, give a different medicine.
- After you first notice improvement, give another dose only if symptoms begin to return.
- Lower potencies (6X, 6C, 30X) may need to be given more often (every one to two hours).
- Higher potencies (200X, 200C, 1M) generally need to be given only once. Repeat only if symptoms return with intensity; give only infrequently in this case.

What to Expect from Homeopathic Self-Care

Homeopathic medicines can reduce the swelling and fever, shorten the course of the illness, and prevent or treat complications.

Other Self-Care Suggestions

Rest. ■ Eat soft foods to reduce the need for chewing. ■ Avoid spicy and sour foods and drinks, such as citrus fruit and other juices, which may cause pain by stimulating the salivary glands. ■ Isolate the person with mumps to avoid spreading the infection to those who have not had it. ■ Take Vitamin C, 500 mg two times daily for children four years or older. ■ Use a carrot poultice to relieve swelling. Blend two to three carrots, place in a cloth or cheesecloth and apply under chin for two to eight hours.

	Key Symptoms	Mind	Body	Worse	Better	Food & Drink
Abrotanum *(Lady's love)*	**Inflammation of the testes after mumps** **Emaciation in children**	Cross and irritable Anxious	**Parotid glands go down as testes begin to swell**	Cold air Getting wet Night	Motion	
Carbo vegetabilis *(Charcoal)*	**Swollen, inflamed parotid glands** **After getting chilled, the mumps go to the testes or breasts, which become swollen and inflamed** **Exhaustion or collapse with difficulty breathing** **Very chilly, yet wants to be fanned or exposed to a draft**	Apathetic Irritable	**Very bloated and full of gas** **Loud, frequent burps or loud gas** Indigestion Appetite is usually decreased	Riding in the car Rich food	**Belching** **Being fanned**	Desire for sweets and salt Aversion to rich foods and fat
Jaborandi *(Pilocarpus pinnatifolius)*	**Mumps with increased sweating and salivation** **Parotid glands double their usual size** **Inflammation of the testes after mumps**		**Face very flushed** Throat dry and inflamed Dull left-sided headache	Cold Exhaustion	Eating	

continued on next page

	Key Symptoms	Mind	Body	Worse	Better	Food & Drink
Mercurius *(Mercury)*	**Swollen, painful parotid gland** **Increased salivation** **Bad breath and bad (metallic) taste in the mouth** **Aggravated by extremes of heat and cold like the mercury in a thermometer**	**Suspicious** Hurried Restless	**Tongue is heavily coated** **Chilly and sweaty** **Trembling of the extremities**	**Heat and cold** **Night** Sweating Damp cold Drafts	Moderate temperature Rest	**Desire for bread and butter,** cold drinks, milk, lemons, sweets Aversion to sweets, salt, butter
Phytolacca *(Pokeroot)*	**Parotid gland stony hard, swollen, and tender** **Pain extends to the ear on swallowing**	Great fear of death	**Swollen lymph nodes in the neck and behind the ear** Sore all over Throat feels hot and painful	Cold Cold damp weather Night	Lying on abdomen or left side Rest Dry weather	
Pulsatilla *(Windflower)*	**Swollen, inflamed, painful parotid glands** **Enormously swollen testes in boys from mumps** **Swelling of the breasts in girls after mumps** **Temperament and symptoms change very quickly**	**Wants others around him, especially when he is sick** Clingy and weepy Indecisive	**Dry mouth but no thirst** Diarrhea in children Gas with the menstrual period	**Heat; hot stuffy rooms** **Rich foods**	**Open air** Cold applications, food, or drink	**Desire for ice cream; rich, creamy foods; and peanut butter** Aversion to fats, milk, bread, meat, and pork Aggravation from pork, fat, and rich foods

Nausea and Vomiting

(See also Indigestion, Morning Sickness, and Motion Sickness.)

Description

Nausea and vomiting are symptoms of digestive distress that can come from many causes, including strong odors, morning sickness, motion sickness, food poisoning, indigestion, intestinal obstruction, alcohol intoxication, drug use, prescription drugs, chemotherapy, and exposure to toxic materials, as well as emotional causes such as anxiety, stage fright, and disgust.

Symptoms

Nausea is queasiness of the stomach with a feeling that retching or vomiting might follow. Vomiting is the forcible emptying of the stomach contents through the esophagus and mouth. Vomiting may occur as single or repeated spasms which the body uses to empty the stomach. Unfortunately, vomiting may continue as dry heaves even after the stomach is empty if the stimulus is strong enough. In projectile vomiting, the stomach contents are ejected in a forcible stream that may extend for several feet.

Complications

Nausea and vomiting may lead to serious dehydration and possibly malnutrition if prolonged. Dehydration may require intravenous fluids if the person is unable to keep liquids down for more than a day.

Look

Is the person vomiting? How often?
What does the vomit look like?
What does the person look like? Facial expression? Body posture?

Listen

"I vomit whenever I drink milk." *Aethusa*
"I have this terrible, constant nausea but it doesn't help to vomit." *Ipecac*
"It made me so mad I could throw up!" *Nux vomica*
"I'm vomiting blood. Could you keep me company?" *Phosphorus*
"I feel deathly nauseated like I'm seasick, or like when I had my first cigarette." *Tabacum*
"I'm so cold, and it's coming out of both ends at once!" *Veratrum*

Ask

How long have you felt nauseated?
Is there vomiting?
How severe is the nausea and/or vomiting?
What brings on the nausea and/or vomiting?
Does anything make the nausea and/or vomiting better or worse?
Are you hungry or thirsty?
Does any food or beverage appeal to you?
Is there anything you can't stand to eat or drink?
Are you able to keep anything down?
Are you in any pain?
Are there any other symptoms along with the nausea and/or vomiting?
Do you feel warm or chilly?

Pointers for Finding the Homeopathic Medicine

Ipecac is the first medicine to think of for strong nausea and vomiting. ▮ Use *Bismuth* or *Phosphorus* when the vomiting is primarily of liquids, and they are vomited after becoming warm in the stomach. ▮ *Nux vomica* should be considered when the vomiting comes on from emotional stress, especially anger and frustration, and it is difficult for the person to vomit. ▮ *Phosphorus* can be considered for vomiting blood and for vomit that looks like coffee grounds, in a friendly, open, sympathetic person who desires cold drinks but vomits them. ▮ *Tabacum* is the best for deathly nausea and vomiting from motion, like seasickness. ▮ *Veratrum album* is useful for a combination of nausea, vomiting, and diarrhea, especially if the person is very cold but desires ice and sour foods such as lemons and pickles.

Dosage

- Give three pellets of 30C every one to two hours until you see improvement.
- If there is no improvement after three doses, give a different medicine.
- After you first notice improvement, give another dose only if symptoms begin to return.
- Lower potencies (6X, 6C, 30X) may need to be given more often (every hour).
- Higher potencies (200X, 200C, 1M) may need to be given only once and repeated infrequently only if the symptoms return. If the situation is very severe, they can be given every one to two hours if needed.

What to Expect from Homeopathic Self-Care

Homeopathic medicines treat nausea and vomiting quite rapidly. Results can be expected in minutes to hours. If you have recurrent attacks of nausea and vomiting, see an internist or gastroenterologist for a diagnosis to determine the cause, and see a homeopath for constitutional homeopathic treatment.

Other Self-Care Suggestions

Get some fresh air. ▮ Eat small amounts of food frequently. ▮ Eat Saltine crackers to help relieve the nausea. ▮ Eat bland foods such as broth, rice, and pasta. ▮ Tea and toast are usually well tolerated. ▮ Drink clear fluids if you can keep them down. ▮ Sip ginger-root tea to help relieve nausea. Use a one-quarter-inch slice of ginger root boiled in a cup of water for fifteen minutes. ▮ Stimulate Stomach 36, an acupressure point in the soft place below the knee and to the outside of the leg where the tibia and fibula bones meet, to relieve nausea. Use firm rotary pressure on the spot for a few seconds. Repeat when needed.

	Key Symptoms	Mind	Body	Worse	Better	Food & Drink
Aethusa *(Fool's parsley)*	**Intolerance of milk** **Love of animals**	Awkward	**Baby vomits large curds of milk** **Vomiting and diarrhea of newborns** Colic followed by vomiting and dizziness Bubbling sensation around the belly button Child lacks the power to hold up his head	Evening 3:00 to 4:00 A.M.	Open air	Not thirsty
Bismuth	**Desire for cold water which is vomited as soon as it reaches the stomach or when it becomes warm in the stomach** **Liquids are vomited more than solid food, which is retained longer** **Wants to hold the hand of the mother or father**	Afraid of death Desires company Restless and anxious	**A lot of pain, burning, and cramping in the stomach** **Pain feels like a heavy load in one spot** Nausea and gagging that is relieved by drinking cold drinks Vomiting after surgery	Warm drinks	Cold drinks Cold applications Movement	
Ipecac *(Ipeac root)*	**Terrible, constant nausea that is not relieved by vomiting** **Nausea and vomiting with nearly all conditions** **Nausea with a clean tongue**	Difficult to please Doesn't know what she wants	**Hates food and the smell of food** **Bleeding and nausea at the same time** Cramps in the abdomen Drooling with the nausea	**Vomiting** **Warmth** Overeating	Open air	**Not thirsty** Desire for sweets, pastries
Nux vomica *(Quaker's button)*	**Nausea and vomiting from anger, irritability, and frustration** **Nausea with straining to vomit, but can't** **Very irritable and impatient**	**Obsessed with business** **Wants to be the first and the best** **Competitive and hard-driving, Type A** Easily offended Frustrated easily by little things	**Violent vomiting** Wakes up at 3:00 A.M. with indigestion Abdominal cramping Sour or bitter belching, vomiting, and taste in the mouth	Anger Tight clothes Eating Cold Rich foods Stimulants Alcohol	Warmth Warm drinks After a bowel movement	Desire for fat, spicy, rich foods, and stimulants

Phosphorus	**Vomits blood or coffee grounds** **Great thirst for cold drinks which make her feel better, but are vomited after becoming warm in the stomach**	**Outgoing** **Sympathetic** **Friendly** **Desires company** Afraid of the dark, thunderstorms, and ghosts	**Stomach pain relieved by cold drinks** Nausea from putting the hands in warm water Food comes right back up after eating Sight of water makes her vomit Vomiting after surgical anesthesia	Spicy foods Warm foods Fasting	Lying on the right side Being around other people Eating	Desire for carbonated drinks Desire for salty food, spicy food, chocolate, and chicken
Tabacum *(Tobacco)*	**Deathly nausea** **Cold, clammy, and pale with the nausea** **Motion sickness, seasickness from the least motion** **Better from cold, fresh air** **Spitting with the nausea**	Feels wretched	**Violent vomiting from the least motion** Profuse sweat and saliva Sinking feeling in the stomach	**Heat** **Opening the eyes**	Uncovering the abdomen	
Veratrum album *(White hellebore)*	**Violent vomiting and diarrhea** **Cold sweat on the forehead while vomiting** **Icy cold with cold sweat**	Very active and busy Restless	**Projectile vomiting** Abdominal cramping Collapse with a bluish color Diarrhea very forceful, followed by exhaustion and cold sweat	**Cold** Cold drinks Fruit	Warmth Hot drinks Covering up	**Desire for sour food, juicy fruit, pickles, lemons, salt, and ice**

Nosebleeds

(Epistaxis)

Description

Nosebleeds are simply spontaneous bleeding from the nose. They are caused by infections of the nose and sinuses, dryness and cracking of the nasal mucous membranes, ruptured blood vessels, and trauma. Vigorous nose-blowing or nose-picking can sometimes induce a nosebleed. More serious chronic conditions, such as high blood pressure, arteriosclerosis, and bleeding diseases like hemophilia, may be involved.

Symptoms

Blood or blood-tinged mucus either drips or is blown from the nose. Clots may form in the nose. Be careful if you remove these clots, or the nose may begin bleeding again.

Complications

Low blood volume and anemia may occur if the nosebleed will not stop and blood loss is extreme. If a nosebleed will not stop readily with direct pressure and homeopathic medicines, seek medical attention to find the source of the nosebleed.

Look

How much is the nose bleeding?
Is the person conscious?
Is there evidence of any trauma, bruising, or fracture of the nose?

Listen

"My little boy, Tommy, just fell off the kitchen table and his nose is bleeding." *Arnica*

"The nosebleed started suddenly when my right ear started to throb." *Belladonna*

"Ginny, my five-year-old, has bright red cheeks and her nosebleeds seem to clot very easily. I'm worried because she tends toward anemia." *Ferrum phosphoricum*

"My nosebleed got better when my period started." *Lachesis*

"My nose feels really full inside, and there's dark blood coming out." *Hamamelis*

Ask

How much blood have you lost?
What started the nosebleed?
What color blood is coming out?
Is it painful?
Is it stopping?

Pointers for Finding the Homeopathic Medicine

For a nosebleed following an injury or trauma, give *Arnica.* ▮ For a bloody nose with a bright red face and a high fever, give *Belladonna.* ▮ If a child with a nosebleed has very pale cheeks, look at *Ferrum phosphoricum.* ▮ If the blood is dark, consider *Hamamelis.* ▮ For left-sided nosebleeds with dark blood in a talkative person, consider *Lachesis.* ▮ If the person with the nosebleed asks for cold or carbonated drinks, look at *Phosphorus.*

Dosage

- Give three pellets of 30C every ten minutes until you see improvement.
- If there is no improvement after three doses, give a different medicine.
- After you first notice improvement, give another dose only if symptoms begin to return.
- Lower potencies (6X, 6C, 30X) may need to be given more often (every fifteen to thirty minutes)
- Higher potencies (200X, 200C, 1M) usually only need to be given once. Repeat infrequently only if the symptoms return and are still severe.

What to Expect from Homeopathic Self-Care

Homeopathic medicines will help stop a nosebleed within minutes or up to about an hour, depending on the cause. Also use first-aid measures. Chronic recurrent nosebleeds respond well to constitutional treatment.

Other Self-Care Suggestions

Apply direct pressure by squeezing the sides of the nose shut with thumb and forefinger for five to ten minutes while breathing through the mouth. ▮ Put a small piece of ice under the upper lip beneath the nose, or apply pressure to the point just under the nose on the upper lip. ▮ Apply a cold compress to the nose.

	Key Symptoms	Mind	Body	Worse	Better	Food & Drink
Arnica *(Leopard's bane)*	**Nosebleed after an accident or traumatic injury** **Bleeding anywhere in the body**	**Wants to be left alone** **Insists that nothing is wrong**	**Nosebleed after washing the face** **Nosebleed after a fit of coughing** Fainting from blood loss or shock Sore, bruised feeling anywhere in the body Feels like the bed is too hard	Touch Overexertion	Lying down with the head low	
Belladonna *(Deadly nightshade)*	**Sudden nosebleed** **Nosebleed with a red, flushed face**	**Sudden outbursts of anger**	**Extreme sensitivity to noise, light, and being jarred** **Glassy eyes** **Face fiery red, hot, and dry**	**Touch** **Being jarred** **3:00 P.M.** Exposure to the sun	Bending backward in a semi-erect position Sitting up	**Great thirst for cold water or no thirst at all** **Desire for lemons and lemonade**
Ferrum phosphoricum *(Iron phosphate)*	**Nosebleed with flushed face or with round red spots on the cheeks** **Nosebleed with a very pale face** **Lots of bright red blood that clots easily**	Talkative Excited Irritable	**Nosebleeds in children** Discharges may be blood-streaked Vomiting blood	Night 4:00 to 6:00 A.M.	Cold applications Bleeding Lying down	Desire for sour foods and cold drinks Aversion to meat and milk

Hamamelis *(Witch hazel)*	**Profuse, slow bleeding from the nose that doesn't easily clot** **Nosebleeds and hemorrhoids may occur together** **Nosebleed with dark blood**	Irritable	**Weakness of veins in the nose causing nosebleed** Hemorrhoids that bleed passively	Injuries to the nose		
Lachesis *(Bushmaster snake)*	**Nosebleed with dark blood** **Nosebleed when the menstrual period should start** **Nosebleeds that decrease when the menstrual flow begins**	Intense Talkative Jealous	**Feeling of pressure inside the nose** **Symptoms tend to be more left-sided** Trickling nosebleed when blowing the nose	**Constriction of the neck or abdomen with a tight collar or belt** During and after sleep Heat	After nosebleed	
Phosphorus	**Profuse nosebleeds with bright red blood** **Nosebleed doesn't clot easily** **Nose bleeds easily with little provocation**	**Outgoing** **Sympathetic** **Friendly** **Desires company** Afraid of the dark, thunderstorms, and ghosts	Nosebleeds in the place of the menstrual period Nosebleed with cough Swollen sensation with the nosebleed Tendency toward bruising and bleeding in general	Cold air Exertion Talking and laughing Change of temperature	**Lying on the right side** Sitting	**Desire for chocolate, ice cream, fish, and spicy foods** **Very thirsty for cold and carbonated drinks**

Pinworms

Description

Pinworms are tiny white worms that come out of the anus to lay their eggs at night. They are prevalent in young children, and easily transmitted from child to child. A child with pinworms scratches his anus, then handles toys or other objects that go into his mouth or the mouths of other children, infesting them with the eggs.

Symptoms

Pinworms cause itching around the anus, which the child irritates by scratching.

Complications

Pinworms have been associated with appendicitis, convulsions, abdominal pain, and insomnia, but no cause for these problems has been found in the worms themselves.

Look

Placing scotch tape over the anal opening during sleep may trap the worms and allow identification. Scotch tape may also be touched to the area around the anus then examined under the microscope to see the eggs.

Listen

"Don't touch me. I don't like you!" *Cina*
"It feels like sharp glass is sticking in my bottom." *Ratanhia*
"It feels like something is crawling in my bottom." *Sabadilla*
"I think I have worms, but don't give me a shot!" *Spigelia*
"My butt itches so much that I can't sleep." *Teucrium*
"My bottom burns like crazy." *Urtica urens*

Ask

Does your bottom itch?
Do you scratch it?
Does anything hurt?
Have you shared your toys with anyone?

Pointers for Finding the Homeopathic Medicine

Cina is by far the most common medicine for pinworms. If pinworms are associated with: ▮ hives, give *Urtica urens.* ▮ hay fever, give *Sabadilla.* ▮ polyps, give *Teucrium.* ▮ face pain or heart palpitations, give *Spigelia.* ▮ rectal fissures, give *Ratanhia.*

Dosage

- Give three pellets of 30C twice a day until you see improvement.
- If there is no improvement after three days, give a different medicine.
- After you first notice improvement, give a different dose only if symptoms begin to return.
- Lower potencies (6X, 6C, 30X) may need to be given more often (every four hours).
- Higher potencies (200X, 200C, 1M) generally need to be given only once. Repeat only if symptoms return with intensity; give only infrequently in this case.

What to Expect from Homeopathic Self-Care

Pinworms may resolve in days to weeks with homeopathic treatment.

Other Self-Care Suggestions

Wash the bedsheets daily. ▮ Wash the child's hands frequently. ▮ Do not let small children play with known pinworm carriers. ▮ There are many herbal and dietary treatments for worms. We prefer not to use them because the herbs are very strong, because the dietary or fasting approaches are labor-intensive and may not be practical or appropriate for children, and because homeopathy is usually effective.

	Key Symptoms	Mind	Body	Worse	Better	Food & Drink
Cina *(Wormseed)*	**Restlessness, irritability** **Intense itching around the anus** **Intense scratching and boring the finger into the nose**	**Child is very cross and defiant** **Doesn't like to be looked at or touched**	Grinds teeth during sleep Boring the finger deep into the nose or ears	Touch	Rocking. Lying on the abdomen	
Ratanhia *(Krameria)*	**Pinworms and anal fissures** **Anus burns and feels like there are splinters of glass in it** **Great itching in the rectum**	Irritable and quarrelsome	**Dry, itchy anus**	Night	Hot or cool baths Walking outdoors	
Sabadilla *(Mexican grass)*	**Pinworms and hay fever with spasmodic sneezing and runny nose** **Sensation of crawling and itching in the rectum**	Easily startled Miserable	Crawling or itching feeling in the anus, alternating with itching in the nose or ears	Every one to two weeks	Heat Open air	
Spigelia *(Pinkroot)*	**Pinworms** **Crawling and itching feeling of the anus**	**Fear of pins and needles** Restless and anxious Easily offended	Twitching from worms	Cold air	Open air Heat	
Teucrium *(Cat thyme)*	**Pinworms** **Itching anus prevents sleep**	Excited Talkative Lazy		Cold, damp Change of weather	Open air	
Urtica urens *(Stinging nettle)*	**Intense burning, stinging, and itching around the anus** **Pinworms and hives**			Cold baths	Warmth	

Poison Ivy, Oak, and Sumac
(Contact Dermatitis)

Description
Poison ivy, oak, and sumac cause a contact dermatitis. Some people are highly sensitive to these plants, and some show no sensitivity. Poison ivy *(Rhus toxicodendron)* and sumac *(Rhus aromatica)* are more common in the eastern part of the United States, and poison oak *(Rhus diversiloba)* in the west. The oil of these plants can be spread around the body by touch. It can also cause a severe reaction if the plants are burned and the smoke inhaled.

Symptoms
An extremely itchy, red, blistering rash that causes great discomfort and annoyance, and often takes more than a week to heal. The blisters ooze and crust over before drying up.

Complications
These skin rashes are usually self-limiting and cause no long-term effects. The homeopathic proving of poison ivy *(Rhus toxicodendron)* suggests that arthritis could be a long-term complication if the skin rash is suppressed by external applications such as hydrocortisone cream.

Look
What does the skin rash look like?
Is the rash red?
Are there blisters (vesicles)?
Is it oozing or crusting over?
Is it spreading?

Listen
"My poison ivy feels better if I put hot water on it." *Anacardium*
"My skin feels like stiff leather." *Croton tiglium*
"I feel stiff, and better if I move around." *Rhus toxicodendron*

Ask
When did you come into contact with poison ivy, oak, or sumac?
How does your skin feel?

Does anything make it feel better or worse?
How does it feel if you scratch it?

Pointers for Finding the Homeopathic Medicine

Anacardium is often the most effective medicine for poison ivy, oak, and sumac. ▮ *Croton tiglium* can be used if the skin feels incredibly itchy and hidebound (thick and hard), and there is gushing diarrhea. ▮ *Rhus toxicodendron* is the most available medicine, and will often work.

Dosage

- Give three pellets of 30C every four hours until you see improvement.
- If there is no improvement after three doses, give a different medicine.
- After you first notice improvement, give another dose only if symptoms begin to return.
- Lower potencies (6X, 6C, 30X) may need to be given more often (every two to four hours).
- Higher potencies (200X, 200C, 1M) generally need to be given only once. Repeat only if symptoms return with intensity; give only infrequently in this case.

What to Expect from Homeopathic Self-Care

Homeopathic medicines can relieve the itching and discomfort and speed the healing process.

Other Self-Care Suggestions

Be careful not to spread the rash by scratching it, then scratching an unaffected area. ▮ Wash the area with mild soap and water and cover with sterile gauze, if needed, to keep it clean. ▮ *Calendula* lotion is soothing to the rash and irritated skin. ▮ Cold wet applications can help the rash feel better, especially cold comfrey root tea. ▮ Oatmeal bath: Use Aveno (without camphor) or place one cup of finely blended dry Oatmeal in the bath to sooth itching. ▮ If secondary infection from scratching occurs, cleanse with *Calendula* soap and water and apply *Calendula* gel or lotion. ▮ Spray on *Grindelia* tincture one part to three parts water to relieve itching.

	Key Symptoms	Mind	Body	Worse	Better	Food & Drink
Anacardium *(Marking nut)*	**Very itchy rash which feels better from very hot water** **Blistering eruption, especially on the face, hands, and fingers** **Yellow discharge oozes from the blisters and crusts over**	Two sides of the personality	**Scratches to the point of bleeding** **Itching is much worse from scratching**	Rubbing	Heat, hot bath	
Croton tiglium *(Croton oil)*	**Incredible itching of the skin, which is dry and hard** **Scratching the skin is painful** **Skin rash such as poison ivy combined with diarrhea gushing like a fire hydrant**	Anxious Dissatisfied	**Rash is most prominent on the face and genitals** **Skin feels extremely tight**	Washing As eruptions go away	Gentle rubbing	
Rhus toxicodendron *(Poison ivy)*	**Skin erruptions like poison ivy** **Water-filled blisters** **Terrible itching**	Restless Jovial	**Extreme restlessness, can't get comfortable** **Allergic skin eruptions along with joint stiffness**	**Cold baths or showers** **Scratching** Night Rest	**Hot baths or showers**	**Desire for cold milk**

Sciatica

(See also Back Pain, Acute.)

Description

Sciatica is pain along the distribution of the sciatic nerve in the back of the leg, resulting from inflammation and compression of the nerve at its root near the spine, in the buttocks, or in the pelvis. The nerve compression in the spine often comes from a herniated intervertebral disk.

Symptoms

Pain begins in the back or pelvis and radiates down the leg partially or all the way to the foot. The pain may be quite severe and accompanied by numbness and tingling. It is usually worse when sneezing, coughing, or holding the breath and bearing down.

Complications

The disk problem can get worse if lifting and straining are not done properly, increasing the sciatic pain sometimes to the point of incapacitation.

Look

Are there any visible indications of the sciatica?

Is the person moving in any way different from normal?

Listen

"My leg is twitching, and I have pain down the back of my leg." *Agaricus*

"I got so mad when he insulted me that my back and leg started hurting." *Colocynthis*

"My right leg hurts, but it's also numb." *Gnaphthalium*

"It started after I fell on my tailbone." *Hypericum*

"It wakes me up in the wee hours of the morning." *Kali iodatum*

"All my symptoms are on the left side except the pain in my leg." *Lachesis*

"It hurts when I first get up, but I've got to move around and stretch." *Rhus toxicodendron*

"It hurts when I cough or sneeze. Can you treat ringworm too?" *Tellurium*

Ask

What caused the pain?

Where do you feel it?

Describe the pain.
Does it remain localized or does it travel anywhere else?
What makes the pain better or worse?
Are there any other symptoms?
Is there numbness? Tingling? Weakness of the limbs?
Did any other physical symptoms begin along with the sciatica?
Have there been any changes in your mental and emotional state since the sciatica began?

Pointers to Finding the Homeopathic Medicine

If there are lots of twitching and spasms in a person who seems intoxicated, think of *Agaricus.* ▮ If the sciatica comes on after anger or being offended, give *Colocynthis.* ▮ If the sciatica is on the right side and has pain along with numbness, give *Gnaphthalium.* ▮ If the sciatica is from an injury to the spine, *Hypericum* is probably the right medicine. ▮ If the person wakes in the early morning (2:00 to 5:00 A.M.) with the sciatica, give *Kali iodatum.* ▮ If other symptoms are left-sided, but the sciatica is right-sided, think of *Lachesis.* ▮ If the symptoms are worse from sitting and better from moving around, consider *Rhus toxicodendron.* ▮ If a herniated disk is definitely involved, consider *Tellurium,* especially if the person also has ringworm.

Dosage

- Give three pellets of 30C every four hours until you see improvement.
- If there is no improvement after three doses, give a different medicine.
- After you first notice improvement, give another dose only if symptoms begin to return.
- Lower potencies (6X, 6C, 30X) may need to be given more often (every two to four hours).
- Higher potencies (200X, 200C, 1M) generally need to be given only once. Repeat only if symptoms return with intensity; give only infrequently in this case.

What to Expect from Homeopathic Treatment

Homeopathic medicines can substantially reduce or eliminate the pain and inflammation of acute sciatica in a day or two, or sooner. If pain persists, consult a qualified homeopath for constitutional treatment.

Other Self-Care Suggestions

Apply moist heat to the low back and buttocks. ▮ Take a hot bath with one cup of Epsom salts added. Whirlpool baths or hot tubs are also good. ▮ Rest in bed in a comfortable position. ▮ The Bowen Therapeutic Technique, an Australian bodywork practice, is very useful for treating sciatica. ▮ Acupuncture, chiropractic, osteopathy, physical therapy, or massage may be helpful if homeopathy is not producing immediate results. ▮ Take Calcium (1500 mg) and Magnesium (750 mg) daily to reduce muscle spasms. ▮ *Arnica* gel or oil or *Traumeel* ointment is very helpful when applied locally to the area. (If you are under constitutional treatment, consult your homeopath before using *Traumeel,* as it is a combination homeopathic medicine.) ▮ Back strengthening exercises and proper lifting techniques are useful to prevent future episodes of sciatica. ▮ Being overweight contributes to sciatica. Consider losing some weight.

	Key Symptoms	Mind	Body	Worse	Better	Food & Drink
Agaricus *(Fly agaric)*	**Very bad sciatica and low back pain** **Muscle spasms, twitching, tension, and tremor** **Shooting and burning pain along the spine**	**Very anxious about his health**	Legs feel heavy and limbs feel like they don't belong to him Awkward clumsiness as if drunk	**Sitting** **Cold air**	**Lying** **Slow, gentle motion**	
Colocynthis *(Bitter cucumber)*	**Sciatica after anger, being insulted, or feeling offended** **Sciatica more often right-sided**	Feelings hurt easily Indignant	**Cramps in the hips and thighs**	**The slightest motion** Rotating the leg Becoming hot in bed	**Lying on the side that hurts** **Bending double** **Hard pressure**	
Gnaphthalium *(Old balsam)*	**Numbing pain in the leg** **Alternating numbness and pain** **Right-sided sciatica with intense pain**	Irritable		**Lying down** **Motion** **Walking** **Stepping**	Flexing limbs onto abdomen Sitting in a chair	
Hypericum *(St. John's wort)*	**Injury to sciatic nerve resulting in sharp, cutting pains along the nerve** **Shooting pain in the sciatic nerve after an injury to the spine**	Sad	Aching in the left sciatic nerve after prolonged sitting Twisting or wrenching sensation in the foot	Injury Jarring	Rubbing the injured area	

continued on next page

	Key Symptoms	Mind	Body	Worse	Better	Food & Drink
Kali iodatum *(Potassium iodide)*	**Very bad sciatica that wakes him at night**	Irritable	Small of the back feels like it's in a vise	**Lying on the side that hurts** **Sitting** **Standing** **2:00 to 5:00 A.M.** **Heat**	**Walking** **Flexing the legs**	
Lachesis *(Bushmaster snake)*	**Other symptoms tend to be more left-sided, but sciatica is often right-sided** **Skin of the legs is very sensitive during the sciatica, even to the touch of the sheets**	**Feeling of pressure inside** **Very intense and talkative**	Sciatica during pregnancy	**After sleeping or on waking** Heat	Open air	Desire for oysters
Rhus toxicodendron *(Poison ivy)*	**Sciatica from overexertion or sitting too long** **The main symptom is stiffness** **Pain is worse when starts to move**	Restless Jovial	**Extreme pain when rising from sitting position** **Has to move around or stretch to find a comfortable position**	**Cold bath**	**Hot bath or shower** **Continued motion** Hard pressure or massage	
Tellurium	**Severe back pain and right-sided sciatica** **Sciatica in a person with ringworm**	Fear of being touched in sensitive places	Painful sensitivity of the spine	**Touch** **Coughing or sneezing** **Bearing down or straining to have a bowel movement**		

Shock

Description

Shock is inadequate circulation of blood and oxygen to organs or tissues because of blood loss or dehydration, weak action of the heart, or dilation of the peripheral blood vessels.

Septic shock comes from bacterial infection. Anaphylactic shock comes from allergic reactions. Electric shock comes from exposure to live electric current or lightning.

Symptoms

The person is lethargic, sleepy, and confused. Hands and feet are clammy and pale or blue. The pulse and breathing are rapid and weak. In septic shock, fever and chills are usually present. Symptoms of anaphylactic shock include agitation, flushing, heart palpitations, numbness, itching, difficulty breathing, hives, swelling, coughing, and sneezing followed by the general symptoms of shock. Electric shock may cause severe muscle contractions, loss of consciousness, heart palpitations or heart failure, and cessation of breathing; burns may also occur.

Complications

Shock is a medical emergency and can lead rapidly to death. Apply first-aid measures immediately and call 911 for emergency medical aid. Keep the person warm, raise his or her legs slightly, stop any blood loss with direct pressure if possible, check the person's airway and breathing, and give CPR (cardio-pulmonary resuscitation) if necessary. Do not give anything by mouth that must be swallowed. (Homeopathic medicines may be dissolved in a small amount of water; a few drops on the tongue are sufficient for a dose.) Turn the head to allow the person to vomit if needed. Hospitalization is strongly recommended as intravenous fluids, drugs, or surgery may be needed depending on the cause of the shock.

Look

Is the person breathing? Is the chest rising and falling?
Is the breathing rapid and weak?
What color is the person's face? Lips? Nails? Is there any paleness or blueness?
Is the person sweating? Are hands and feet clammy?

Is the pulse rapid and weak?
Look around to observe the circumstances.

Listen

"A robber came in with a gun. I was so scared." *Aconite*
"I fell off my motorcycle and took a really hard fall. I somehow just got up and walked away, thinking nothing was wrong, then I started to go into shock." *Arnica*
"I feel so cold. Don't cover me up." *Camphora*
"I was losing blood and I just keeled over." *China*
"I got a cramp while swimming. I started to drown. When they pulled me out I was blue and shivering. It felt so good when they were trying to fan me to give me air. (burp)" *Carbo vegetabilis*
"I'm icy cold, shivering, and sweating like crazy." *Veratrum album*

Ask

Is there a friend or relative present? Can he explain the situation?
What happened just before the person went into shock?
Was there a trauma or injury?
Is there blood loss, vomiting, or diarrhea?
Is the person conscious?
Did she say anything before she went into shock?

Pointers for Finding the Homeopathic Medicine

Give *Aconite* for shock from fright, panic, or emotional causes. ▮ *Arnica* is very useful for shock from traumatic injuries and blood loss. ▮ *Camphora* is used for people who are extremely cold and worse from cold, but who paradoxically want cold drinks and to be uncovered. ▮ *Carbo vegetabilis* is the best medicine for acute shock when the person feels short of breath and wants to be fanned and cooled off. ▮ *Carbolic acid* is used in anaphylactic shock, especially from a bee sting. ▮ *China* is very good for shock from loss of bodily fluids, as in dehydration and blood loss. ▮ *Veratrum album* is good for shock after excessive vomiting, diarrhea, or blood loss.

Dosage

- Use higher potencies (200X, 200C, 1M) if available; these generally need to be given only once, but may be repeated whenever symptoms return with intensity in an emergency.

- If high potencies are unavailable, give three pellets of 30C every five minutes until you see improvement.
- If there is no improvement after two to three doses, give a different medicine.
- After you first notice improvement, give another dose only if symptoms begin to return.
- Lower potencies (6X, 6C, 30X) may need to be given every few minutes until the crisis has passed.

What to Expect from Homeopathic Self-Care

Homeopathic medicines can reverse shock in minutes if blood loss can be stopped and the heart still beats. Do not hesitate to give the correct medicine if you know what it is. If you cannot tell which is the correct medicine, give *Arnica* or *Carbo vegetabilis*.

	Key Symptoms	Mind	Body	Worse	Better	Food & Drink
Aconite *(Monkshood)*	**Ailments from fright or shock** **Violent heart palpitations** **Profuse perspiration with anxiety** **Rapid pulse** **Symptoms come on suddenly**	**Extreme anxiety** **Tremendous restlessness** **Fear of impending death** Panic attacks Desire for company	Fainting from fear, fright, or anxiety Hot, heavy, burning sensation in the head	Chill	Rest Fresh air	Desire for cold drinks
Arnica *(Leopard's bane)*	**Shock after an accident or traumatic injury** **Excellent for shocks of any kind** **Shock from blood loss, bleeding anywhere in the body** **Fainting from blood loss or shock** **Any trauma with bruising**	Wants to be left alone Insists that nothing is wrong	Sore, bruised feeling anywhere in the body Feels like the bed is too hard	Touch Overexertion	**Lying down with the head low**	
Camphora *(Camphor)*	**Icy coldness but wants to be uncovered** **Everything feels cold** **Sudden loss of strength with a barely perceptible pulse** **Collapse into shock** **Shock after exposure to the elements, infection, or injury**	Forsaken, isolated feeling Fear in the night	Feels the cold in spots The cold feels painful Coma after shock	Cold drafts	Perspiring Cold drinks	

Carbolic acid	**Anaphylactic reaction and shock following a bee or wasp sting** **Pale, collapsed, bathed in cold sweat**	Worse from mental exertion Does not feel like working	Swelling of face and tongue from bee stings Vesicles that burn and itch Hives all over the body Sense of smell increased	Jarring Reading	Smoking Strong tea	
Carbo vegetabilis *(Charcoal)*	**Acute shock** **Collapsed, weak or exhausted with difficulty breathing** **Wants to be fanned**	Apathetic Irritable Harsh	Fainting from indigestion or passing gas Indigestion Excessive gas and belching Pale with bluish skin Great coldness in general and in parts of the body Cold breath	**Loss of body fluids** Warmth Rich food	**Being fanned** Cool air Belching	Desire for sweets and salty food
China *(Peruvian bark)*	**Shock from loss of bodily fluids, especially blood loss** **Septic shock from infections that resemble malaria**	**Irritable, sensitive, and moody** **Fantasies about great things he'd like to do** **Feelings of persecution**	Intermittent fever, chills, weakness, drenching sweats, and exhaustion Oversensitivity to light, noise, odors, and pain Periodic complaints	Touch Drafts Noise Fruit	Hard pressure	Desire for sips of cold water Desire for cherries, sweets, salty food, and spicy food Aversion to hot food, fats and rich food, fruit, and meat
Veratrum album *(White hellebore)*	**Collapse with bluish color, cold sweat, vomiting, and diarrhea** **Feels icy cold**	Restless Constantly busy	Shock after excessive bleeding, diarrhea, or vomiting	Cold Cold drinks Menstrual period	Warmth Hot drinks Covering up	**Desire for fruit, sour foods, salty foods, pickles, lemons, ice, and ice cold drinks**

Sinusitis

(See also Common Cold.)

Description

Sinusitis is an inflammation of the sinuses associated with viral, bacterial, or fungal infections or allergies.

Symptoms

The most common symptom is mild to severe pain in the maxillary (cheekbone) or frontal (forehead) sinuses. There may also be pain in the face or teeth. There is generally nasal discharge or stuffiness and often a sinus headache. It is the deep sinus pain that usually differentiates sinusitis from the common cold.

Complications

A severe bacterial sinusitis left untreated could potentially cause a more serious systemic infection.

Look

What color is the nasal discharge?
Are there any other visible indications of sinusitis?

Listen

"I feel so much pressure in my sinuses that I can barely breathe." *Kali bichromicum*
"My sinuses really hurt and my nose smells like rotten cheese." *Hepar sulphuris*
"My sweat and my breath smell really bad. I must be toxic." *Mercurius*
"I worked all weekend to meet a deadline; I went out in the cold air, and now I have an awful cold with lots of sneezing. I can barely breathe." *Nux vomica*
"My daughter, Sarah, complains that her nose is stuffed up and she won't leave my lap." *Pulsatilla*

Ask

When did the infection start?
Is there pain? If so, describe it.

Is the pain localized, or does it radiate?
Are there any unusual symptoms or sensations?
What makes the pain and other symptoms better or worse?
Are there any mental or emotional symptoms?

Pointers for Finding the Homeopathic Medicine

The first medicine to think of for sinusitis with pressing pain in the cheekbones and a thick, ropey nasal discharge is *Kali bichromicum.* ▮ If the sinusitis came after exposure to a draft, look first at *Hepar sulphuris* then at *Nux vomica.* ▮ If there are bad-smelling odors in the nose and sinuses, think of *Mercurius* and *Hepar sulphuris.* ▮ If the sinusitis is much worse from going outdoors, think of *Nux vomica* and *Hepar sulphuris.* ▮ In a child with a sinus infection who is clingy, weepy, and moody, give *Pulsatilla.* ▮ If the sinusitis is much better from going outside, he probably needs *Pulsatilla.*

Dosage

- Give three pellets of 30C every four hours until you see improvement.
- If there is no improvement after three doses, give a different medicine.
- After you first notice improvement, give another dose only if symptoms begin to return.
- Lower potencies (6X, 6C, 30X) may need to be given more often (every two to four hours).
- Higher potencies (200X, 200C, 1M) generally need to be given only once. Repeat only if symptoms return with intensity; administer only infrequently in this case.

What to Expect from Homeopathic Self-Care

Homeopathic medicines can relieve the symptoms of sinusitis within hours to several days.

Other Self-Care Suggestions

Hot, moist packs applied to the sinuses can relieve congestion. ▮ An echinacea and goldenseal combination (two dropperfuls of tincture in water three times a day or six capsules a day) is useful to stimulate the immune system to fight infection. ▮ Give Vitamin A (25,000 IU per day) or beta-carotene (50,000 IU per day). ▮ Give Vitamin C (1000 mg three times per day). ▮ Give Zinc (30 mg per day). ▮ Nasal irrigation with one-quarter teaspoon of salt in one cup of warm water can be very helpful. Plastic or porcelain neti pots are a particularly effective way to accomplish this. ▮ Hot, spicy food such as cayenne, black pepper, and horseradish can help clear the sinuses. ▮ Avoid dairy products, sweets, and cold and carbonated drinks. ▮ Boil four slices of fresh ginger root in a quart of water for fifteen minutes and drink three to four cups a day.

	Key Symptoms	Mind	Body	Worse	Better	Food & Drink
Hepar sulphuris *(Calcium sulfide)*	**Nose stopped up, or runs from exposure to cold air or to cold dry wind** **Sore pain at the bridge of the nose** **Painful, stuffy nose** **Nose smells like old cheese**	**Irritable** **Complaining** **Everything annoys him**	The later, fully developed stage of a cold Sneezing from every draft	**Cold air**	**Warmth** **Wrapping up**	**Desire for vinegar** Aversion to fats
Kali bichromicum *(Potassium bichromate)*	**Thick, stringy, yellow or yellowish-green nasal discharge** **Stuffiness** **Intense, pressing pain in the maxillary sinuses (cheekbones) and bridge of the nose**	Relates his symptoms in the most minute detail	**Tough, elastic mucus plugs that leave the nose raw inside when they detach** **Nasal quality to the voice** **Loss of smell** Tickling in the left nostril like a hair	Cold Morning	Heat Pressure	
Mercurius *(Mercury)*	**Yellowish-green nasal discharge** **Bad-smelling breath, perspiration, and discharges** **Coated tongue** **Sensitive to extremes of temperature, like the mercury in a thermometer** **Metallic taste in the mouth**	Suspicious Restless Hurried Reserved	**Nostrils raw and ulcerated** **Nasal discharge runny or too thick to run** **Cheeks swollen and red** Nasal discharge acrid Frequent sneezing with runny nose	**Night** **Heat** **Drafts**	**Moderate temperatures**	**Desires bread and butter**

continued on next page

	Key Symptoms	Mind	Body	Worse	Better	Food & Drink
Nux vomica (*Quaker's button*)	**Sneezing and runny nose in morning upon awakening** **Runny nose in the morning but stopped up at night** **Sniffles** **Colds that are made worse by going outdoors**	**Irritable** **Impatient** **Obsessed with business** **Wants to be the first and the best** **Competitive and hard-driving, Type A** Easily offended Frustrated easily by little things	**Pain or ulceration in nostrils** **Terrible itching inside the nose** **Nose feels plugged but there is a watery discharge** **Oversensitivity to strong odors**	**Anger** Business worries Open air or drafts Rich foods	Rest Allowing the nose to run	**Desire for hot foods, spicy foods, and meat** **Desire for stimulants and alcohol**
Pulsatilla (*Windflower*)	**A "ripe" cold with thick, bland, yellow-green mucus** **Loss of smell with nasal stuffiness** **Obstruction of the nose made worse by lying down or being indoors** **Feels better when outdoors** **Lack of thirst**	**Changeable emotions** **Weepy and clingy** **Wants company when sick**	**Nose is stuffed up** **Can't smell** Bad-smelling nasal discharge Ears feel plugged	**Warm stuffy room** **Rich food**	Slow walking in the open air	**Desire for butter, ice cream, and peanut butter** Aversion to fat, milk, pork Aggravation from fats and rich foods

Skin Infections: Boils, Folliculitis, and Carbuncles

(See also Abscesses.)

Description

Boils, folliculitis, and carbuncles are skin infections, usually associated with *Staphylococcus aureus* bacteria.

Symptoms

Folliculitis is an infection of the hair follicles with redness, tenderness, and swelling. Boils, also called furuncles, are more advanced skin infections which form a large eruption that discharges bloody pus. Boils are most common on the neck, face, breasts, and buttocks. Boils can be quite painful and especially tender to pressure. A collection of boils that forms one large infected area penetrating deeper into the tissue is called a carbuncle. Carbuncles are common at the base of the neck. They may be accompanied by fatigue and fever. They are slow to heal, slough off tissue with blood and pus, and can cause scarring.

Complications

Skin infections can lead to a serious systemic blood infection called septicemia. The symptoms of septicemia are a high fever and organ damage. Septicemia can be fatal. Red streaks extending from the infected area toward the heart are a red flag for septicemia and indicate a need for immediate medical attention.

Look

How much inflammation and swelling is at the site of the infection?
Is there discoloration of the area? If so, what color?
Is it hard or soft?
Is it oozing pus (thick, cloudy) or serum (clear fluid)?
Are any lymph nodes swollen near the infection?
Are there any red streaks up the arms or legs?
How high is the fever, if any?

Listen

"I have terrible, burning pains in the infected area." *Anthracinum* or *Arsenicum album*

"I'm really worried that this boil will be fatal." *Arsenicum album*
"I can't stand for you to touch the boil." *Hepar sulphuris*
"This boil on my left leg came out when I discovered my wife was having an affair. It's such an odd purple color." *Lachesis*
"I've been having more saliva and sweating more than usual since I got this infection." *Mercurius*
"I got this boil on my breast at the same time that I developed a dental abscess." Unless the areas are exquisitely tender, give *Silica;* if they are tender, consider *Hepar sulphuris.*

Ask

When did the infection start?
Is there pain? If so, describe it.
Are there any unusual sensations at the site of the infection?
What makes the symptoms feel better or worse?
Are there any mental or emotional symptoms?

Pointers for Finding the Homeopathic Medicine

For crusty, oozing, black eruptions, give *Anthracinum.* ▮ For infections with small, red, ulcerated pimples and burning pains, consider *Arsenicum album,* especially if the person is nervous and restless. ▮ If the person screams when you examine the infected area, give *Hepar sulphuris.* ▮ If the infected area is bluish-purple and left-sided, consider *Lachesis.* ▮ For infections with bad-smelling discharges and perspiration and bad breath, *Mercurius* is the first thought. ▮ For infections due to an ingrown nail, think first of *Silica.*

Dosage

- Give three pellets of 30C every four hours until you see improvement.
- If there is no improvement after three doses, give a different medicine.
- After you first notice improvement, give another dose only if symptoms begin to return.
- Lower potencies (6X, 6C, 30X) may need to be given more often (every two to four hours).
- Higher potencies (200X, 200C, 1M) generally need to be given only once. Repeat only if symptoms return with intensity; administer only infrequently in this case.

What to Expect from Homeopathic Self-Care

Homeopathic medicines stimulate the body's defenses against infection, promoting rapid healing and resorption of the boil or carbuncle. Boils and carbuncles should improve within one to three days. If *Silica* is the indicated medicine, healing may take longer—up to seven to fourteen days. If the boil or carbuncle is not healing well or is very inflamed and painful after homeopathic treatment, it may need to be lanced with a sterile instrument. Seek medical attention if this procedure is needed.

Other Self-Care Suggestions

Hot, moist packs can be helpful for folliculitis and boils to bring the infection to a head. ▮ An echinacea and goldenseal combination (two dropperfuls of tincture in water three times a day or six capsules a day) is useful to stimulate the immune system to fight infection. ▮ Give Vitamin A (25,000 IU a day) or beta-carotene (50,000 IU a day). ▮ Give Vitamin C (1000 mg three times a day). ▮ Give Zinc (30 mg a day).

	Key Symptoms	Mind	Body	Worse	Better	Food & Drink
Anthracinum *(Anthrax)*	**Black or bluish, blistering eruptions** **Clusters of boils or carbuncles in successive crops**	Unassertive Afraid of being alone	**Crusty, oozing eruptions** **Intolerable burning pains and bad-smelling pus** Blood poisoning or gangrene Hemorrhages of black blood from any body opening Swollen glands	Cold applications	Hot applications	
Arsenicum album *(Arsenic)*	**Painful black pustules, or pustules filled with blood** **Small red pimples that become ulcerated, with bad-smelling, bloody discharge**	**Restless and anxious** Needy and demanding Afraid of being alone Complains that he'll never get well	**Burning pains** Skin is dry, rough, and scaly, with burning and itching Tendency to gangrene	**Worse from midnight to 2:00 A.M.** **Cold air, drinks, and food**	**Heat, hot applications, warm food and drinks** Company	**Desire for frequent sips of warm, or sometimes cold, drinks** Desire for the fat on meat
Hepar sulphuris *(Calcium sulfide)*	**Boils are very painful, especially to touch** **Helps to expel foreign bodies from the boils** **Hypersensitive to pain and to cold**	**Extremely irritable and touchy**	**Thick pus** **Discharges are offensive, smelling sour or like rotten cheese** **Splinter-like pains**	**Drafts** Uncovering	**Warmth** Covering up	

Lachesis *(Bushmaster snake)*	**Boil is bluish-purple or black, filled with pus** **Symptoms tend to be more left-sided**	**Intense** **Talkative** Jealous	Boils may bleed	During and after sleep Heat	Discharges of blood or pus	
Mercurius *(Mercury)*	**Boils are inflamed, with burning and stinging pains and the rapid formation of pus** **Boils tend to open up to form ulcers and discharge bad-smelling pus**	**Suspicious** Hurried Hesitant	**Bad-smelling breath, perspiration, and discharges** **Trembling, sweating, and drooling** Moist tongue, imprinted along the edges with the teeth Metallic sweetish taste in the mouth	**Extremes of heat and cold** **Night** Damp cold Perspiring	Rest	**Desire for bread and butter** Aversion to sweets
Silica *(Flint)*	**Boil or carbuncle is filled with bad-smelling pus** **Infections from a foreign body in the tissues** **Swollen lymph nodes**	Refined Delicate features Precise	**Carbuncles may burrow deep into the tissue** **Foreign bodies like a splinter or an ingrown nail** **Infections slow to heal** Irritating, thin, foul-smelling discharge Low stamina and energy	Cold, damp Touch	Warmth and heat	

Sore Throats *(Pharyngitis)*

Description

Pharyngitis is an inflammation of the pharynx or throat which is usually associated with a virus or, as in the case of a strep throat, a bacteria.

Symptoms

The most distressing symptom is usually a mild to severe pain in the throat, which may extend to the ears. There may be a simultaneous upper-respiratory infection, bronchitis, or flu.

Complications

An untreated Group A Beta-hemolytic strep infection may lead to rheumatic fever or joint problems.

Look

Look at the throat. Is there discoloration?
Is there any discoloration or swelling of the tonsils?
Are there any pus-filled blisters on the throat or tonsils?
Are there any other visible symptoms of throat pain?

Listen

"The pain came on suddenly after I played outside in the cold." *Aconite*

"My throat feels very swollen, especially on the right side. The only thing that helps is drinking cold water." *Apis*

"My throat is extremely sore on the right side and feels hot and dry." *Belladonna*

"I have blisters with pus on my tonsils. I've never felt so much pain in my whole life." *Hepar sulphuris*

"The pain is on the left side of my throat and it's so bad that I can hardly stand to swallow my saliva." *Lachesis*

"My sore throat started on the right and went to the left. The only thing I want is hot tea." *Lycopodium*

"My breath is bad, my tongue is coated, and I have a metallic taste in my mouth." *Mercurius*

"My neck glands are swollen. I have a sore throat on the right side that makes my right ear hurt when I swallow." *Phytolacca*

Ask

When did the throat pain begin?
What seemed to bring it on?
What does it feel like?
Where does your throat hurt?
Describe the pain in detail.
What makes the pain better or worse?
Is it affected by swallowing? Warm or cold drinks?
Are there any other symptoms?
If so, what makes the symptom feel better or worse?
Are there any mental or emotional changes with the sore throat?
Are you craving anything to eat or drink?

Pointers for Finding the Homeopathic Medicine

For throat pain of very rapid onset with a high fever, give *Aconite* or *Belladonna.* ▮ If it feels better from cold drinks, first look at *Apis.* ▮ If the main symptom is swelling, give *Apis* or *Phytolacca.* ▮ For very red sore throats, the best medicines are *Belladonna* and *Apis.* ▮ For a burning, right-sided sore throat in a person with a bright red face and ear pain, give *Belladonna.* ▮ For right-sided sore throats, think of *Belladonna, Apis, Lycopodium, Phytolacca,* and *Mercurius iodatus flavus.* ▮ The medicines to give for sore throats that have the most pain on swallowing are *Lachesis, Hepar sulphuris, Belladonna,* and *Mercurius.* ▮ For left-sided sore throats, consider *Lachesis* first, then, more rarely, *Mercurius iodatus ruber.* ▮ The first medicine to consider for sore throats that start on the left then move to the right is *Lachesis.* ▮ For sore throats that begin on the right then go to the left, look at *Lycopodium.* ▮ If the sore throat feels better from warm drinks, think first of *Lycopodium.*

Dosage

- Give three pellets of 30C every two to four hours until you see improvement.
- If there is no improvement after three doses, give a different medicine.
- After you first notice improvement, give another dose only if symptoms begin to return.
- Lower potencies (6X, 6C, 30X) may need to be given more often (every two to four hours).
- Higher potencies (200X, 200C, 1M) generally need to be given only once. Repeat only if symptoms return with intensity; administer only infrequently in this case.

What to Expect from Homeopathic Self-Care

The pain and discomfort of a sore throat are usually relieved within one to twenty-four hours.

Other Self-Care Suggestions

Gargle with warm salt water three times a day. ▮ Gargle with one teaspoon of *Calendula* tincture in one cup of warm water. ▮ Suck on zinc lozenges. (Avoid any lozenges with menthol, camphor, or eucalyptus, since they interfere with homeopathic treatment.) ▮ Take Vitamin C (3000 mg a day) in divided doses of 500 mg. Cut the dose in half for a child and give a maximum of 250 mg to a baby. ▮ Take echinacea and goldenseal tincture in water (one-half teaspoon every two hours, up to six doses a day). ▮ Avoid dairy products and sweets. ▮ Drink one to two glasses of fresh carrot juice per day.

	Key Symptoms	Mind	Body	Worse	Better	Food & Drink
Aconite *(Monkshood)*	**Very sore, hot, dry, red throat after exposure to a cold, dry wind** **Sore throats of sudden onset with a high fever** **Within the first twenty-four hours of an illness**	**Tremendous anxiety and restlessness** **Fear of impending death**	Tonsils dry and swollen Chokes on swallowing	**Fright or shock** Pressure Touch	Rest	**Intense, burning thirst**
Apis *(Honeybee)*	**Swelling is the main symptom** **Right-sided, swollen, sore throats that sting and burn** **Throat pain is lessened by cold drinks**	**Busy** Doesn't like to be crossed Jealous	**Tonsils swollen and fiery red** **Throat soreness is worse from swallowing solid, sour, or hot foods**	Heat	Cool air Cold baths or showers Uncovering	**Not thirsty**
Belladonna *(Deadly nightshade)*	**Red, hot, burning sore throat, worse on the right side** **High fever (102°F to 105°F) with a sore throat** **Bright red, hot, dry face** **Sudden onset of symptoms**	**Irritable** **Hallucinations during high fevers**	**Tonsillitis worse on the right side** **Right-sided strep throat** Tonsils are swollen Throat feels tight Swallowing is painful Wants to swallow but chokes Bends head forward and lifts knees when swallowing	Drafts If perspiration is suppressed	Light covering Semi-erect position	**Great thirst for cold water, or no thirst at all** **Desire for lemons and lemonade**
Hepar sulphuris *(Calcium sulfide)*	**Exquisitely sensitive and painful sore throat** **Pus-filled blisters and abscesses on the tonsils** **Splinter-like pain in the throat** **Sensation of a fish bone stuck in the throat** **Sore throats that come on from the least exposure to a draft**	**Irritable** **Peevish** **Complaining**	**Throat with abscess that smells like old cheese** Swelling on tonsils and cervical glands Sensation of a plug in the throat Stitching pain in the throat that radiates to the ear upon swallowing	**Cold air or drafts of any kind**	**Warmth** **Bundling up**	**Desire for vinegar**

continued on next page

	Key Symptoms	Mind	Body	Worse	Better	Food & Drink
Lachesis *(Bushmaster snake)*	**Left-sided throat pain, or worse pain on the left** **Sore throats that go from left to right** **Throat pain is made much worse by swallowing saliva**	**Talkative** **Intense** **Feels tense and pressured**	**Sensation of a lump in the throat** **Throat extremely tender to any pressure; must loosen collar** Throat pain extending to the ear Tonsillitis	**After sleep** **Even slight touch or pressure**	Cold drinks	Desire for oysters and alcohol
Lycopodium *(Club moss)*	**Right-sided throat pain** **Throat feels better from warm or hot drinks** **Throat pain that goes from right to left**	**Fearful but doesn't let it show**	Swelling of tonsils, with pus formation Throat feels tight, causing constant swallowing	**Cold drinks**	Cold applications	**Desire for sweets** **Desire for warm drinks**
Mercurius *(Mercury)*	**Throat pain with bad breath and excessive salivation** **Metallic taste in the mouth** **Ulcerated tonsils and throat** **Bad-smelling perspiration and body odor** **Mercurius symptoms with pain only on the left side: *Mercurius iodatus ruber*** **Mercurius symptoms with pain on the right side: *Mercurius iodatus flavus***	Suspicious Hurried Restless Reserved	**Sore, burning throat** **Constant desire to swallow** **Brings up large lumps of mucus from the throat**	Lying on the right side Heat	**Moderate temperatures** Rest	**Desire for bread and butter**
Phytolacca *(Pokeroot)*	**Dark red or bluish, sore, puffy throat** **Throat pain extends to the ear on swallowing** **Swelling of the neck glands** **Sensation of a hot ball or lump in the throat**	Indifferent Refuses food	**Can't swallow anything hot** Throbbing of the right tonsil	Cold, damp Changes of weather	Lying on the abdomen or the left side Rest	

Sprains and Strains

Description

A sprain is an injury to the muscles, tendons, and ligaments—the connective tissues that surround joints. Strains, less severe, involve an injury only to the muscles. Sprains and strains result from twisting, turning, moving, or falling in such a way as to cause an injury. They can also result from overuse.

Symptoms

Pain (mild to severe) and stiffness are the main symptoms of sprains and strains.

Complications

In cases of severe pain, it is helpful to seek immediate attention and, if appropriate, obtain an X ray to make sure there are no fractures or dislocations.

Look

Is there visible swelling or discoloration of the injured area?
Do you notice the person favoring any particular position?

Listen

"I turned my ankle yesterday playing soccer. It's all black and blue." *Arnica*
"My ankle feels fine as long as I don't move it." *Bryonia*
"This wrist feels really cold when I touch it. The pain feels better if I ice it." *Ledum*
"My ankle feels really stiff. I just want to walk around and stretch." *Rhus toxicodendron*
"I have a bad flare-up of my tennis elbow since I played an extra set several days ago. There's no bruising. It just feels sore." *Ruta*

Ask

How did you injure yourself?
When did it happen?
What are the main symptoms that are bothering you?

Are you in pain? If so, where?
Describe the pain.
What makes the pain better or worse?
What makes your other symptoms better or worse?
Are there any mental or emotional changes since the injury?

Pointers for Finding the Homeopathic Medicine

The best medicine to give first for sprains and strains is *Arnica.* ▮ If the pain is worse from any motion, give *Bryonia.* ▮ If the injured area is cold to the touch and the pain is better from cold applications, *Ledum* is the best medicine. ▮ If the main symptom is stiffness that is better from moving around and stretching, *Rhus toxicodendron* will be of benefit. ▮ If there is injury to ligaments or tendons without any clear picture that points to one of the other medicines, give *Ruta.*

Dosage

- Give three pellets of 30C every two to four hours, depending on the severity of the symptoms, until you see improvement.
- If there is no improvement after three doses, give a different medicine.
- After you first notice improvement, give another dose only if symptoms begin to return.
- Lower potencies (6X, 6C, 30X) may need to be given more often (every two to four hours).
- Higher potencies (200X, 200C, 1M) generally need to be given only once. Repeat only if symptoms return with intensity; administer only infrequently in this case.

What to Expect from Homeopathic Self-Care

The symptoms should be considerably lessened within twenty-four to forty-eight hours.

Other Self-Care Suggestions

Ice the injured area. Sports medicine doctors used to recommend icing for the first twenty-four to forty-eight hours, then applying heat, but now many suggest continuing to apply ice to the injury. Icing reduces swelling and inflammation. ▮ Rest the injured area. If necessary immobilize it, including using crutches. ▮ Wrap the injured part with an elastic bandage. ▮ Apply an ointment, cream, or gel of topical *Arnica.* ▮ Soak in an Epsom salt tub or foot bath to help reduce swelling.

	Key Symptoms	Mind	Body	Worse	Better	Food & Drink
Arnica *(Leopard's bane)*	**The first medicine to give for any sprain or strain** **Muscles feel very sore, painful, and bruised** **Injuries from overexertion** **Shock after injuries**	**Refuses help** **Says he's fine**	Tendency to have broken blood vessels Even the bed feels too hard	Touch	Lying down with the head low	
Bryonia *(Wild hops)*	**Injuries that are painful from even the slightest motion** **Joint injuries in which *Arnica* doesn't help** **Symptoms anywhere in the body that are made worse by the least movement**	**Irritable** Wants to go home	**Stiffness and shooting pains in the joints when touched or moved**	Light touch 9:00 P.M.	**Pressure** **Lying on the affected part** **Bandaging the injured area**	**Thirst for large quantities of very cold drinks**
Ledum *(Marsh tea)*	**Injured area is cold to the touch and feels better with ice or cold applications** **He has a tremendous urge to soak his feet in cold or icy water**	Angry Dissatisfied	Body is cold, but head and face are hot	Heat	Cold air Rest	
Rhus toxicodendron *(Poison ivy)*	**Sprains and strains with stiffness and pain, made better by moving, stretching, and flexing** **Injuries to tendons and muscles after overexertion** **Restless because he can't find a comfortable position**	Active Jovial	**Restless legs in bed** **Cracking of the joints**	**Cold applications** **Getting wet and chilled**	**Warm applications** **Hot bath or shower**	**Desire for cold milk**
Ruta *(Rue)*	**Injuries to flexor tendons, joints, cartilage, and periosteum (outermost layer of the bone)** **Injuries to ankles and wrists** **Bruised, sore, aching feeling with restlessness** **Intense pain, weariness, and heaviness in the tendons**	Dissatisfied Quarrelsome	**Stiffness throughout the body** **Restlessness** **Tennis elbow**	Cold air Lying down, except on the back	Lying on the back Rubbing	

Stage Fright *(Performance Anxiety)*

Description

Stage fright is nervousness or anxiety prior to a performance or presentation.

Symptoms

Symptoms can include weakness, paleness, butterflies in the stomach, shakiness, trembling, diarrhea, rapid heartbeat and pulse, and perspiration.

Complications

There are no severe complications; however, fainting can occur.

Look

Are there any visible symptoms of stage fright?
Does the person have a pale face? Trembling? Perspiration?

Listen

"What if I forget all of my lines? What if I go blank? What if I faint?" *Argentum nitricum*
"I just feel so shaky and dizzy. I'm really, really afraid." *Gelsemium*
"I just know I'm going to get up there and make a fool of myself." *Lycopodium*

Ask

What are you feeling?
What are your physical symptoms?
Are there any mental and emotional symptoms?
When did the symptoms begin?
What's bothering you the most?
Have you experienced this before?
What seems to make the symptoms better or worse?

Pointers for Finding the Homeopathic Medicine

For extreme anxiety with rapid heartbeat and an irrational fear about what is about to occur, give *Argentum nitricum*. ■ If there is weakness, trembling, dizziness, and diarrhea, give *Gelsemium.* ▮ If the person fears he will make a fool of himself but tries to cover it up, the medicine is *Lycopodium.*

Dosage

- Give three pellets of 30C one to two hours prior to the event or performance. Repeat every thirty minutes until there is improvement.
- If there is no improvement after three doses, give a different medicine.
- After you first notice improvement, give another dose only if symptoms begin to return.
- Lower potencies (6X, 6C, 30X) may need to be given more often (every two to four hours).
- Higher potencies (200X, 200C, 1M) generally need to be given only once. Repeat only if symptoms return with intensity; administer only infrequently in this case.

What to Expect from Homeopathic Self-Care

Improvement in the symptoms should occur within five to thirty minutes.

Other Self-Care Suggestions

Count slowly from one to one hundred, taking long, deep breaths. ▮ Visualize or imagine your last successful performance or presentation. ▮ Think of sending love to all the people in the audience. ▮ Sip a glass of room-temperature water. ▮ Splash cold water on your face. ▮ Tense and relax your muscles to release your nervous feelings. ▮ If homeopathic medicines are not available, take five drops of Rescue Remedy (a Bach Flower Essence) every fifteen to thirty minutes beginning one to two hours prior to the event.

	Key Symptoms	Mind	Body	Worse	Better	Food & Drink
Argentum nitricum *(Silver nitrate)*	Anxiety in anticipation of an event Keeps asking himself, "What if this or that happens?" Fear of being late Wakes in the morning feeling that he can't face the day	Anxiety in crowds, closed rooms, elevators, theaters, airplanes Hurried Impulsive Talks a lot	Violent palpitations that make him feel that his heart will jump out of his body	Tight spaces	Cool air	Strong desire for sweets and salt
Gelsemium *(Yellow jasmine)*	Stage fright with trembling, chills, weakness, and dizziness Anxiety from anticipation Hoarseness or laryngitis from stage fright	Very frightened Confused and dazed	Tremendous fatigue Wiped out expression on her face Sticky perspiration all over the body Chills with trembling	Ordeals	Urination Alcoholic drinks	Lack of thirst
Lycopodium *(Club moss)*	Dreads the presence of new people Fear of failure or of looking like a fool Loss of self-confidence from anticipation	Hates to undertake something new, but is usually okay once he begins Can be bossy Likes appreciation and applause	Indigestion and diarrhea from fright	4:00 to 8:00 P.M. Warmth	Warm drinks	Strong desire for sweets and warm drinks

Stomach Aches and Acute Abdominal Pain

(See also Diarrhea, Food Poisoning, Indigestion and Heartburn, Colic, Nausea and Vomiting, Morning Sickness, and Motion Sickness.)

Description

Stomach and abdominal pain can range from mild discomfort to incapacitating pain. The causes are highly variable and include indigestion, gas, appendicitis, gall bladder inflammation, liver problems, menstrual cramping, acute gastroenteritis, ectopic pregnancy, miscarriage, cancer, and anxiety, as well as a number of other causes.

Symptoms

Symptoms include localized or referred pain or cramping, nausea with or without vomiting, constipation or diarrhea, gas, bloating, abnormal stools, and other symptoms of anxiety, including rapid heartbeat and pulse, and perspiration.

Complications

Many complications can occur, depending on the source of the pain. A thorough workup by a gastroenterologist should be done for persistent or significant stomach or abdominal pain. If the pain is severe or incapacitating, emergency medical care should be sought to rule out life-threatening emergencies such as appendicitis, a gall bladder attack, or an ectopic pregnancy.

Look

Are there any observable signs of distress?
Is the person in an uncharacteristic position?
Are there any abnormalities in the stool?
Is the person vomiting?

Listen

"I have terrible pain in my stomach every time I start to move" *Bryonia*
"I feel much better if I bend forward and bring up my legs." *Colocynthis*
"I've never had such terrible cramps." *Cuprum*
"I feel much worse if I bend over double. I need to stand up straight." *Dioscorea*

"Beans and cabbage don't agree with me, especially at dinner." *Lycopodium*
"The only thing that relieves the pain is to lie in bed pressing a heating pad onto my abdomen." *Magnesia phosphorica*
"The pain began after I drank too much and got into a fight with my wife." *Nux vomica*
"I love ice cream and rich foods, but they don't love me." *Pulsatilla* (or *Nux vomica*)

Ask

When did the pain or discomfort begin?
Was there something that seemed to bring it on?
Has this occurred before?
Where is the pain or discomfort? Is it severe? When does it occur?
What makes the pain or discomfort better or worse?
Are there other symptoms?
Is there anything abnormal about bowel patterns or stool?
Are these pains associated with the menstrual flow? Pregnancy?
Are there any new mental and emotional symptoms since the problem began?

Pointers for Finding the Homeopathic Medicine

If the stomach or abdominal pain is aggravated by motion, give *Bryonia*. ▮ If doubling up relieves the pain, think of *Colocynthis* or *Magnesia phosphorica*. ▮ The first medicine to think of for violent cramping is *Cuprum*. ▮ If the pain is relieved by standing up straight and made worse by bending double, the best medicine is *Dioscorea*. ▮ If the person gets bloated after eating even a small amount of food, choose *Lycopodium*. ▮ If pressure relieves the pain, consider *Magnesia phosphorica*, but if pressure aggravates the pain, look at *Lycopodium*. ▮ For stomach or abdominal pain after too much alcohol or spicy or rich foods, first think of *Nux vomica*. ▮ A plump, gentle, moody woman who doesn't do well with rich foods is likely to need *Pulsatilla*.

Dosage

- Give three pellets of 30C every fifteen minutes to four hours, depending on the severity of the pain, until you see improvement.
- If there is no improvement after three doses, give a different medicine.

- After you first notice improvement, give a different dose only if symptoms begin to return.
- Lower potencies (6X, 6C, 30X) may need to be given more often (every two to four hours).
- Higher potencies (200X, 200C, 1M) generally need to be given only once. Repeat only if symptoms return with intensity; administer only infrequently in this case.

What to Expect from Homeopathic Self-Care

Acute abdominal or stomach pain can often resolve within two to forty-eight hours.

Other Self-Care Suggestions

Charcoal absorbs gas. If there is painful gas, give two charcoal capsules every two to four hours as needed. ▮ Peppermint or fennel tea can soothe indigestion. ▮ Castor oil packs applied for one hour with a heating pad can sometimes relieve abdominal distress. ▮ Avoid overeating, especially heavy or rich foods. ▮ Avoiding fats, spicy foods, alcohol, coffee, and chocolate may be helpful. ▮ Commercial antacids may provide temporary relief. ▮ Lying on the back and bringing the knees to the chest may cause gas to pass. ▮ Applying a heating pad to the area can help relieve pain.

	Key Symptoms	Mind	Body	Worse	Better	Food & Drink
Bryonia *(Wild hops)*	**Epigastric (below stomach) tenderness and throbbing** **Abdominal wall very tender** **Appendicitis** **Severe stomach or abdominal pain caused by the least motion** **Gastritis**	**Irritable** Wants to go home	**Stomach pains worse after eating or vomiting** **Constipation with great dryness of the rectum** **Liver is heavy, sore, and swollen** Bitter vomiting of bile and water right after eating Nausea made worse by standing up	Vegetables, acidic foods	Cool air Being quiet	**Great thirst for large quantities of cold drinks**
Colocynthis *(Bitter apple)*	**Violent, gripping, clutching pain** **Pain comes in waves** **Pain is lessened by hard pressure or bending over double** **Intestines feel as if squeezed between two stones** **Pain is made worse by the least food or drink** **Vomiting from the pain**	**Symptoms come on after anger, indignation, or humiliation** **Easily offended**	**Drawing pain in the stomach** **Colicky pain with gas**	**Lying on the painless side**	Heat Rest	Potatoes and starchy foods don't agree with her
Cuprum metallicum *(Copper)*	**Violent, cramping pains and spasms anywhere in the body** **Agonizing abdominal spasms and colic** **Sudden convulsions of the stomach, accompanied by vomiting** **Abdominal cramping made worse by motion** **Violent vomiting**	Likes to be in charge	Vomiting upon first waking up in the morning Painful cramps and pressure in the epigastrium (below the stomach), made worse by touch and motion	**Motion** Vomiting	**Cold drinks**	**Desire for cold drinks**

Dioscorea *(Wild yam)*	**Unbearable sharp, cutting, twisting, gripping, grinding pains** **Gall bladder pain extending to the chest, back, and arms** **Pains that shift suddenly to different parts** **Abdominal pain made worse by bending double and better by standing erect**	Nervous Cross Depressed	Sharp pain in the liver extending to the nipples Constant ache around the navel Stomach or abdominal pain from eating too much or eating the wrong food Sharp, cramping pain in the pit of the stomach followed by belching, hiccoughs, and gas	**Lying down**	**Standing up straight**	
Lycopodium *(Club moss)*	**Sensation of a band around the waist, aggravated by tight clothing** **Excessive, noisy gas** **Bloating from even the least amount of food** **Generally weak and sensitive digestion** **Right-sided symptoms**	**Fearful and insecure, but tries to hide it** **Bossy** Wants company in the next room	Gnawing pain in the stomach Liver feels congested Sensation of something moving up and down in the abdomen upon turning to the right side Alternating diarrhea and constipation Constipation when away from home or traveling	**Pressure around the waist** **4:00 to 8:00 P.M.** Warmth	**Warm drinks** Cold applications	**Strong desire for sweets** **Aggravation from beans and the cabbage family**
Magnesia phosphorica *(Magnesium phosphate)*	**Colicky pain with lots of gas** **Pain is lessened by bending double, rubbing, warmth, and pressure** **Must loosen his clothes then walk around and pass gas** **Pain is lessened by very hot applications and drinks**	Irritable Issues about nurturing	**Trapped gas** **Pain in abdomen and around navel radiating to both sides and to back** **Colicky pain radiating from navel**	Lying on right side	Doubling up	**Thirst for very cold drinks**

continued on next page

	Key Symptoms	Mind	Body	Worse	Better	Food & Drink
Nux vomica *(Quaker's button)*	**Gallstone pain after anger** **Violent vomiting** **Pains radiate from the stomach back to the chest** **Pains lessened by vomiting and hot drinks, and made worse by eating** **Stomach or abdominal pain after eating rich foods or alcohol**	**Irritable** **Impatient** **Obsessed with business** **Wants to be the first and the best** **Competitive and hard-driving, Type A** Easily offended Frustrated easily by little things	**Sour burping** **Futile urging for a bowel movement, or no urge at all**	**Anger** **Stimulants**	**Hot drinks** Milk Rest	**Desire for and aggravation from stimulants, spicy foods, or alcohol**
Pulsatilla *(Windflower)*	**Heartburn after eating fats and rich foods** **Indigestion from eating ice cream, pork, fats, and rich foods** **Painful abdominal bloating with loud rumbling** **Rapidly changing temperament and symptoms**	**Soft, affectionate, and wants attention** **Clingy and weepy** **Highly emotional; changeable** **Wants others around, especially when sick**	**Stomach feels heavy and out of sorts** **No two stools are alike** **Wants foods that don't agree with her**	**Rich foods** **Heat; hot stuffy rooms**	Open air Cold applications, food, or drinks	**Lack of thirst** **Desire for creamy, rich foods, peanut butter** Aversion to fat, milk, bread, meat, and pork Aggravation from pork, fat, and rich foods

Styes

Description

A stye is an infection of a sweat or oil gland in the eyelid.

Symptoms

The first symptoms are usually pain, redness, swelling, and tenderness of the edge of the eyelid, followed by the appearance of a small, round, tender, hardened area. Tears, sensitivity to light, and a feeling of a foreign body in the eye may follow.

Complications

Complications are rare, but styes are often recurrent.

Look

Is there redness or swelling of the eyelid?
What does the stye look like?
Is there any discharge from the eye? If so, what is its color and consistency?

Listen

"It seems like I get a stye whenever I go out in the cold." *Hepar sulphuris*
"I only get a stye in my right eye. It's very dry and red." *Lycopodium*
"When I wake up in the morning, my eyelids are stuck together." *Pulsatilla*
"When I wake up in the morning, my eyelids are so dry that I have to pry them apart." *Staphysagria*
"My eyes itch like crazy at night." *Sulphur*

Ask

When did the stye begin?
What seemed to bring it on?
Have you had a stye before? When and under what circumstances?
What does it feel like?
What are the main symptoms?
What makes the symptoms feel better or worse?
Is there any pain? If so, describe it.
What makes the pain feel better or worse?

Are there any mental or emotional changes with the stye?
Are you craving anything special to eat or drink?

Pointers for Finding the Homeopathic Medicine

If the styes are pus-filled and sensitive to drafts, give *Hepar sulphuris.* ▮ For styes of the right eye with lots of dryness, look at *Lycopodium.* ▮ If the main symptom is profuse, thick, yellowish discharge from the eye, give *Pulsatilla.* ▮ For dry, painful eyes in a woman who never gets angry, give *Staphysagria.* ▮ If the edges of the lids are red, burning, itchy, and irritated, give *Sulphur.*

Dosage

- Give three pellets of 30C every four hours until you see improvement.
- If there is no improvement after three doses, give a different medicine.
- After you first notice improvement, give another dose only if symptoms begin to return.
- Lower potencies (6X, 6C, 30X) may need to be given more often (every two to four hours).
- Higher potencies (200X, 200C, 1M) generally need to be given only once. Repeat only if symptoms return with intensity; administer only infrequently in this case.

What to Expect from Homeopathic Self-Care

Styes can often respond within twenty-four to forty-eight hours. If the problem is recurrent or persistent, consult a qualified homeopath.

Other Self-Care Suggestions

Keep the eye clean. ▮ Place compresses soaked in hot water on the eyelid for ten minutes several times a day to bring the stye to a head and allow it to drain. ▮ Give Vitamin C (500 mg four times a day) for immune support.

	Key Symptoms	Mind	Body	Worse	Better	Food & Drink
Hepar sulphuris *(Calcium sulfide)*	**Eyelid is red, inflamed, pus-filled, and very sensitive** **Little pimples surround the inflamed eye** **Eyes tear and stick together at night due to secretion of hardened mucus** **Generally hypersensitive to pain and cold drafts**	**Irritable** **Everything annoys her**	**Eyes are very painful in bright daylight** **Inflammation and swelling of the eye with redness of the sclera (white of eye)**	**Cold air** **Uncovering**	**Warmth** **Bundling up**	**Desire for vinegar**
Lycopodium *(Club moss)*	**Styes toward the inner corner of the eyelid** **Redness of eyelid and sclera (white of eye)** **Distressing pain with dryness of the eye** **Eye goopy at night because of secretion of mucus** **Symptoms worse on the right side**	**Lack of self-confidence, but tries not to show it** **Can be bossy**	Sticking pain in the eye, worse in late afternoon	Wind Warmth Pressure	Cold applications	**Strong desire for sweets** **Prefers warm or room-temperature drinks**
Pulsatilla *(Windflower)*	**Lots of thick, yellow, bland discharge from the eye** **Sensation of something covering the eyes that needs to be rubbed away** **Watering, pain, and itching in the eye, made better by cold applications**	**Changeable moods** **Weepy and clingy** **Wants company**	Dryness of the eye as if a foreign body were in it	**Warm room**	**Outside in the fresh air**	**Lack of thirst** **Desire for creamy, rich foods, peanut butter** Aversion to pork, milk, bread, meat, and pork Aggravation from meat, fat, and rich foods

continued on next page

	Key Symptoms	Mind	Body	Worse	Better	Food & Drink
Staphysagria *(Stavesacre)*	**Painful inflammation of the sclera (white of eye)** **Eyes so dry in morning on waking that she can barely open them** **Recurrent styes** **Eyes are dry and teary**	**Suppressed anger** **Mild-mannered** **Blames herself**	Itching of the edge of the upper eyelids in open air, made better by rubbing Stinging pain of the inner corner of the eyelid	Touch	Warmth	Desire for milk and sweets Aversion to fat
Sulphur	**Eyes are red during the day, and itch violently at night** **Sensation of sand in the eye** **Redness and irritation of the edge of the eyelid**	**Critical** **Opinionated** **Lazy** **Messy**	Oily tears	Looking down	Open air	**Desire for sweets, alcohol, fatty food, and spicy food**

Sunstroke, Heatstroke, and Heat Exhaustion

Description

These are conditions resulting from oversensitivity or prolonged exposure to the heat or the sun.

Symptoms

Heatstroke, also called sunstroke, is a reaction to exposure to the sun which often begins with a headache, dizziness, and fatigue leading to heat, flushing, and dryness of the skin. Perspiration is usually, but not always, decreased. The pulse rate increases quickly, sometimes up to 180 beats per minute, and breathing rate often increases also. The person can become disoriented and unconscious, as well as having seizures. Body temperature can shoot up very quickly to 104°F or even 106°F.

Heat exhaustion, which is less severe, is characterized by gradual weakness, nausea, profuse perspiration, anxiety, and fainting. The skin is generally pale and clammy. The pulse is weak and the blood pressure is low. Notice that the primary differences between the two are the perspiration and the pulse.

Complications

In heatstroke, collapse of the heart can lead to permanent brain damage or death. Heat exhaustion is usually temporary and rarely has complications. If the body temperature is rising rapidly and the person has the symptoms of heatstroke/sunstroke, seek emergency medical attention.

Look

Are there any visible symptoms?
What color is the person's face?
Is there perspiration?
What is the person's position?

Listen

"I have a terrible throbbing headache, especially on the right side." *Belladonna*
"All I want is something cold, like lemonade." *Belladonna*
"I feel so hot and dry." *Belladonna*

"My head feels like it's about to explode." *Glonoine*
"It feels like all of my blood's gone into my head." First consider *Glonoine*, then *Belladonna*

Ask

How are you feeling?
What are your symptoms?
What makes your symptoms feel better or worse?
Are there any mental or emotional symptoms?
What would make you more comfortable?

Pointers for Finding the Homeopathic Medicine

Belladonna and *Glonoine* have very similar indications for this condition. Unless the main complaint is a bursting or exploding sensation in the head, give *Belladonna* first. ■ If there is no improvement within fifteen minutes, or if there are other clear symptoms that point to *Glonoine*, give *Glonoine*.

Dosage

- Give three pellets of 30C every fifteen to thirty minutes, depending on how severe the symptoms are, until you see improvement.
- If there is no improvement after three doses, give a different medicine.
- After you first notice improvement, give another dose only if symptoms begin to return.
- Lower potencies (6X, 6C, 30X) may need to be given more often (every two to four hours).
- Higher potencies (200X, 200C, 1M) generally need to be given only once. Repeat only if symptoms return with intensity; administer only infrequently in this case.

What to Expect from Homeopathic Self-Care

An improvement should be noticed within five to thirty minutes.

Other Self-Care Suggestions

For heatstroke: Take immediate measures to cool yourself by taking a cold shower or bath, or wrapping yourself in cold towels or ice. ■ For heat exhaustion: lie with the head down. Replace fluids and salt.

	Key Symptoms	Mind	Body	Worse	Better	Food & Drink
Belladonna *(Deadly nightshade)*	**Sudden and violent onset of symptoms** **Face is bright red, hot, and dry** **Intense body heat** **Throbbing or pounding headache, especially on the right side**	**Irritable or angry** **Hallucinations with high fever**	**Fullness and congestion of blood to the head** High blood pressure	**Heat of the sun** **Light, noise, touch, and being jarred** **Afternoon, especially 3:00 P.M.**	Bed rest	**Desire for lemons or lemonade**
Glonoine *(Nitroglycerin)*	**Quick and violent onset** **Bursting, expanding feeling in the eyes, head, and organs** **Violent throbbing and rushes of blood to the head** **Symptoms come and go with exposure to the sun**	Confused Doesn't want to talk	Bad effects from the sun, bright snow, and the heat of a fire	**Heat on the head** **Becoming overheated**	Open air Cold drinks or cold applications	

Surgery

Description

A surgical operation to remove or repair some part of the body that is causing a problem.

Symptoms

There can be mild to severe pain after surgery, depending on the type and extent of tissue or organs removed or repaired.

Complications

One of the main complications following surgery is the development of scar tissue. Some scar tissue formation is a natural part of the post-surgical healing process, but the formation of adhesions can cause considerable pain and discomfort, sometimes lifelong.

Look

What does the scar look like? Size? Color?
Are there any other visible symptoms?

Listen

"The surgery went fine. I don't need any help, thank you." *Arnica*
"I tried *Arnica* after surgery to my knee, but it didn't help." *Calendula*
"I have shooting pains up my leg since surgery for an ingrown toenail." *Hypericum*
"My pelvic area is extremely sensitive since my hysterectomy." *Staphysagria*
"My husband feels like he's in shock ever since his surgery." *Strontium carbonicum* or *Arnica*

Ask

What type of surgery did you have? When?
What are the symptoms?
Is there pain? If so, describe the pain.
What makes the pain and the other symptoms better or worse?
How is your energy level?

Have there been any mental and emotional changes since the surgery?
What makes you feel better or worse overall?

Pointers for Finding the Homeopathic Medicine

The first medicine to give is *Arnica*. ▮ If *Arnica* doesn't help and there are no indications for the other medicines listed in this section, give *Calendula* internally. ▮ If there is shooting pain, numbness, or tingling following surgery, use *Hypericum*. ▮ After clean surgery of abdominal organs where there is considerable sensitivity, give *Staphysagria*. ▮ If the person is in a shock-like state since surgery, especially if there was a lot of bleeding, give *Strontium carbonicum*.

Dosage

- Give three pellets of 30C *Arnica* the day before and the day of the surgery.
- Give three pellets of *Arnica* 30C once daily the day after surgery and for up to two weeks, until the pain is gone or considerably improved.
- If, after two doses of *Arnica* after surgery, one of the other three medicines is better indicated, begin giving it.
- If there is no improvement after three doses, give a different medicine.
- After you first notice improvement, give another dose only if symptoms begin to return.
- Lower potencies (6X, 6C, 30X) may need to be given more often (every two to four hours).
- Higher potencies (200X, 200C, 1M) generally need to be given only once. Repeat only if symptoms return with intensity; administer only infrequently in this case.

What to Expect from Homeopathic Self-Care

Homeopathic medicines can help to speed up the healing process after surgery. We recommend this program for nearly any surgery, from dental surgery to major surgery, with the exception of very simple surgery, such as just having a wart or mole removed. We strongly recommend that you follow the suggestions that follow for pre- and post-surgery. We have used this program with hundreds of patients who underwent simple surgery, and in every single case the surgeon has remarked on the rapidity of the healing and there have been no complications.

Other Self-Care Suggestions: Pre- and Post-Surgery Program

Take one dose of *Arnica* 30C or 200C the day before and the morning of surgery. ▮ Take one dose of *Arnica* 30C or 200C as soon as you are awake following surgery. ▮ If you begin with *Arnica* 30C, continue taking it once a day until the pain is nearly or completely gone. ▮ If you are using *Arnica* 200C, take another dose only if the pain returns. ▮ After two doses of *Arnica* 30C or one dose of *Arnica* 200C, if there are clear indications for one of the other medicines listed here, give it instead of the *Arnica.* ▮ As soon as you are allowed to eat or drink after surgery, begin taking a 250-mg capsule of bromelain three times a day. Continue taking these for three weeks. Note that bromelain capsules must be taken at least one hour before or after eating or drinking, or they will just act as an expensive digestive enzyme. ▮ Begin taking the following vitamins one week before surgery, and continue for one month after surgery:

Vitamin C (500 mg three times per day)
Zinc (50 mg per day)
Vitamin E (1200 IU per day; if you have high blood pressure take only 400 IU)
beta-carotene (50,000 IU per day)

▮ Apply *Calendula* and *Hypericum* tincture (diluted 1:3) topically to to prevent infection and to speed healing of the wound.

	Key Symptoms	Mind	Body	Worse	Better	Food & Drink
Arnica *(Leopard's bane)*	**Trauma, shock, surgery, and bleeding** **Bruising** **Post-surgery pain**	**Refuses help** **Says he is fine**	**Has cuts that bleed a lot or bruise** **Wants to lie down, but the bed feels too hard**	Touch Lying on a hard surface Motion	Lying down, especially with the head low	
Calendula *(Marigold)*	**Clean surgical cuts** **Pain, bleeding**	Fearful Nervous				
Hypericum *(St. John's wort)*	**Surgery of nerve-rich areas, such as fingertips and toes** **Shooting pains, numbness, and tingling after surgery**	Sad	Gaping wounds Wounds resulting in weakness from loss of blood	Jarring the injured area Touch	Rubbing the area Lying on the face Bending backward	
Staphysagria *(Stavesacre)*	**Wounds resulting from abdominal surgery of internal organs** **Area hypersensitive to the touch**	Fear of doctors		Touch Stretching the part	Rest	
Strontium carbonicum *(Strontium carbonate)*	**Shock after surgery** **Weakness after surgeries in which there was a lot of bleeding**	Angry Forgetful		Bleeding Uncovering	Wrapping up Hot bath or shower	

Swollen Glands
(See also Mumps.)

Description

Swollen glands, or lymphadenopathy, occurs most commonly with the lymph glands of the neck, but can occur with the axillary (armpit) glands, inguinal (groin) glands, or any other lymph glands in the body.

Symptoms

Characterized by swelling and sometimes pain, redness, and hardening of the lymph glands. There may be fever. The person may also have associated pain, such as a sore throat.

Complications

Untreated, severely swollen lymph glands due to bacterial infection can lead to systemic infection and even death. If the gland remains swollen for months, it is important to seek medical care to rule out such causes as cancer, especially leukemia or a lymphatic cancer such as Hodgkin's disease or lymphoma.

Look

Do the glands look swollen or discolored?
What is the appearance of the throat?
Are there any other visible symptoms?

Listen

"The gland on the left side of my neck feels like a rock." *Bromium*
"My baby, Josh, has swollen glands in his neck. He's roly-poly and sweats on the back of his head when he sleeps, and I think he's teething." *Calcarea carbonica*
"I got this swollen gland after I got chilled outside while gardening. It's so painful. All I want to do is sit in the hot tub!" *Hepar sulphuris*
"My neck glands are swollen. My breath is really bad, my tongue is coated, and I have an awful—kind of metallic—taste in my mouth." *Mercurius*
"I got this swollen gland in my neck—almost like the mumps—at the same time when I developed mastitis from nursing my baby." *Phytolacca*

"My glands are swollen and I have these weird little smelly plugs coming out of my tonsils." *Silica*

Ask

When did you first notice that your glands were swollen?
What seemed to cause the swelling?
Are you having any other symptoms? Please describe them in detail.
Is there any pain? Hardness of the lymph glands?
Do you have a fever?
Has this happened before?
Is there anything that makes you feel better or worse?
Are there any mental and emotional changes since your lymph glands became swollen?

Pointers for Finding the Homeopathic Medicine

For a stony, hard, left-sided swollen cervical lymph gland, give *Bromium*. ▮ For swollen glands in a chubby baby who sweats on his head, try *Calcarea carbonica*. ▮ If there is terrific sensitivity to pain of the swollen lymph glands, and the person is very chilly, the medicine is *Hepar sulphuris*. ▮ If the swollen lymph glands are accompanied by toxic symptoms such as bad breath, a bad taste in the mouth, drooling, body odor, and heavy perspiration, give *Mercurius*. ▮ If there is glandular swelling in the neck with a dark red sore throat that radiates pain to the right ear on swallowing, *Phytolacca* will help. ▮ In a refined person with delicate features who has swollen lymph glands and bad-smelling perspiration, especially on the feet, give *Silica*.

Dosage

- Give three pellets of 30C every four hours until you see improvement.
- If there is no improvement after four doses, give a different medicine.
- After you first notice improvement, give another dose only if symptoms begin to return.
- Lower potencies (6X, 6C, 30X) may need to be given more often (every two to four hours).
- Higher potencies (200X, 200C, 1M) generally need to be given only once. Repeat only if symptoms return with intensity; administer only infrequently in this case.

What to Expect from Homeopathic Self-Care

Lymph glands should go down in size in a matter of hours or days. *Silica,* one of the most common medicines used for glandular swelling, can sometimes act more slowly and take up to two weeks. The pain should diminish within one to forty-eight hours. If glandular swelling is a recurrent tendency, find a qualified homeopath for constitutional treatment.

Other Self-Care Suggestions

Take Vitamin C (500 mg six times a day) to reduce inflammation. ■ Take echinacea and goldenseal tincture (one-half teaspoon in water six times a day). The dosage for capsules will vary with the product. ■ Consult a licensed massage therapist for lymphatic drainage. ■ Take a combination of blood-purifying herbs, including such herbs as sanguinaria, yellow dock, and chaparral. Dosage depends on the product. ■ A carrot poultice promotes lymphatic drainage: grate three carrots, place in cheesecloth and wrap around your neck, then cover yourself with a blanket and go to sleep. ■ If you have a fever, drink two cups of sage or yarrow tea, take a hot bath, then wrap up in warm blankets and go to sleep. You will sweat profusely, then the fever should break. ■ Another time-tested naturopathic method to break a fever, especially in children, is the cold wet sock treatment. Put cold wet socks on the feet, then bundle up well in woolen blankets and go to sleep. The fever should be gone by the next morning. ■ Saunas and steam baths (no eucalyptus with homeopathy!) can speed up healing.

	Key Symptoms	Mind	Body	Worse	Better	Food & Drink
Bromium	**Large, stony hard, swollen lymph glands, especially of the neck** **Glandular swelling worse on the left side**	Despondent Indifferent	Tonsils are deep red, swollen, and made painful by swallowing liquids	Warmth Becoming overheated Lying on the left side	Motion	
Calcarea carbonica *(Calcium carbonate)*	**Swollen lymph glands of the neck in plump babies or children with sweaty heads** **Swollen lymph glands during teething** **Swelling of the tonsils**	Strong-willed Cheerful	Tendency toward chronic sore throats and tonsillitis	**Cold air, or a cold bath or shower** **Teething**	Dry weather Lying on the painful side or on the back	**Desire for eggs, cheese, milk, and salt**
Hepar sulphuris *(Calcium sulfide)*	**Swollen lymph glands that are extremely sensitive to the touch** **Glands, especially tonsils, that are filled with pus** **Swollen glands and infections from the least exposure to a cold draft** **Extremely chilly**	**Hypersensitive to pain** **Easily annoyed** Complaining	**Recurrent tonsillitis with pus pockets on the throat or tonsils** **Sensation of a splinter or a fish bone in the throat**	**Any exposure to cold**	**Warmth** **Bundling up**	**Desire for vinegar**
Mercurius *(Mercury)*	**Swollen lymph glands, especially of the neck, with increased salivation** **Bad breath, bad-smelling body odor, profuse perspiration** **Coated tongue** **Metallic taste in the mouth**	Hurried Suspicious	Stiff neck with swollen cervical glands	**Extremes of temperature** **Night**	Moderate temperature	**Desire for bread and butter**

continued on next page

	Key Symptoms	Mind	Body	Worse	Better	Food & Drink
Phytolacca *(Pokeroot)*	**Glandular swellings, especially of the parotid gland (mumps), tonsils, and breast** **Hard, painful swelling of the cervical glands** **Right-sided sore throat with pain extending to the right ear on swallowing**	Fearful Refuses to eat	Dark red sore throat Painful stiffness of the neck, worse on the right side	Cold damp weather Swallowing hot drinks	Dry weather Rest	
Silica *(Flint)*	**Swollen cervical glands, often hard and painful** **Recurrent tendency to sore throats and tonsillitis** **Tiny yellowish-green lumps of hard mucus expelled from tonsils**	**Refined and proper** Timid	**Delicate features** Swelling of submaxillary (under jaw), painful to the touch Bad-smelling perspiration of the armpits and feet	Cold air Draft Touch or pressure	Bundling up	**Desire for eggs** and sweets Aversion to milk and fat

Teething

Description

Some children have no problems at all when their first teeth break through. For others, it is quite an ordeal, and for their parents as well.

Symptoms

The most common symptoms of teething are pain in the teeth and gums, drooling, redness and swelling of the gums, fever, changes in the stool, restlessness, fussiness, and difficulty sleeping.

Complications

Teething can be a challenging event, even though there are no complications.

Look

What is the appearance of the gums?
Is there any drooling?
What position is the baby in?
Are there any changes in the stool?
Are there any other visible symptoms?

Listen

"José is such a delightful baby with chipmunk cheeks. He's always happy except when his teeth come in. He started to teethe much later than his brother." *Calcarea carbonica*

"Elijah is so miserable when he teethes. No matter what I give him, he doesn't want it. It's like he just wants to be in another body." *Calcarea phosphorica*

"My baby, Trish, turns into a little monster during teething. She kicks and screams and acts like she hates me." *Chamomilla*

"Jerrilyn is so delicate and neat. She's almost like a little adult." *Silica*

Ask

When did the symptoms begin?
What are the specific symptoms?

What makes the symptoms better or worse?
What is the baby's mood?

Pointers for Finding the Homeopathic Medicine

If the baby is chubby, contented, sweaty on the back of his head, and slow to teethe, give *Calcarea carbonica*. ■ For babies who are beside themselves and inconsolable when they teethe and whose tantrums are outrageous, give *Chamomilla*. ■ If she is peevish and nothing pleases her, but she's not as fussy as described for *Chamomilla*, give *Calcarea phosphorica*. ■ If *Calcarea phosphorica* doesn't work, give *Chamomilla*. ■ If the baby has delicate features, is constipated, and is slow to teethe, give *Silica*.

Dosage

- Give three pellets of 30C every fifteen minutes for two to four hours, depending on the severity of the symptoms, until you see improvement.
- If there is no improvement after three doses, give a different medicine.
- After you first notice improvement, give another dose only if symptoms begin to return.
- Lower potencies (6X, 6C, 30X) may need to be given more often (every two to four hours).
- Higher potencies (200X, 200C, 1M) generally need to be given only once. Repeat only if symptoms return with intensity; administer only infrequently in this case.

What to Expect from Homeopathic Self-Care

Homeopathy can relieve symptoms within fifteen minutes to one day.

Other Self-Care Suggestions

Giving the baby something cold to chew on often relieves discomfort. This can be a pacifier or teething ring that has been put briefly in the freezer, or ice wrapped in a clean, wet cloth. ■ If you cannot find homeopathic medicines, give the baby dilute chamomile tea. ■ If you cannot find any single homeopathic medicines and you are desperate, try the homeopathic combination teething tablets.

	Key Symptoms	Mind	Body	Worse	Better	Food & Drink
Calcarea carbonica *(Calcium carbonate)*	**Teething is painful and often delayed** **A chubby baby who sweats on the back of the head or neck during sleep** **Teeth hurt more from cold air or hot things**	**Strong-willed** **Cheerful**	**Baby has a large head** Tendency toward frequent colds and ear infections	**Cold damp weather**	**Warmth**	**Desire for eggs, cheese, and milk** (It is best to breast-feed your baby and not introduce dairy products for at least one year.)
Calcarea phosphorica *(Calcium phosphate)*	**Teeth are sensitive to chewing** **The child is fussy and discontented, and always wants to be somewhere else** **Teeth are delayed, soft, and susceptible to decay**	**Extreme dissatisfaction** **The baby loves to travel**	Problems with the teeth, bones, and musculoskeletal system	**Cold drafts** **Melting snow**	Warm dry weather Lying down	
Chamomilla *(Chamomile)*	**The most common medicine for teething pain in fussy, irritable babies** **Terrible tantrums with kicking, hitting, and screaming** **Hypersensitivity to pain** **Ear infections during teething** **Inconsolable with the pain** **Wants to be carried or rocked**	**Quarrelsome** **Contrary** **Capricious**	**Green diarrhea like chopped spinach during teething** Seizures during teething	**Teething** Night	**Being carried or rocked**	
Silica *(Flint)*	**Difficult or slow teething** **Teeth break down quickly and decay or lose their enamel** **Tendency to form dental abscesses** **Obstinate constipation in newborns**	**Delicate features** **Thin** Refined	**Gums are painful, inflamed, and swollen** **Gum pain is made worse by drinking cold water**	Cold air Touch or pressure	Bundling up	Desire for eggs Aversion to milk (It is best to breast-feed your baby and not introduce dairy products for at least one year.)

Tendinitis

Description
Inflammation of a tendon and, usually, of the tendon sheath.

Symptoms
The involved tendons are usually painful on motion or use. There may be swelling. The most annoying aspect of tendinitis is the need to rest the area and prevent further overuse.

Complications
In more severe or long-standing cases, there may be calcium deposits in the tendon.

Look
Is there any visible swelling?
Is the person holding the area in any particular position?

Listen
"I spent all day at the computer typing a paper, and my wrist is killing me." *Arnica*
"My elbow is fine unless I move it." *Bryonia*
"My Achilles tendon feels too short. I just can't seem to stretch it out." *Causticum*
"I'm fine once I move around and limber up." *Rhus toxicodendron*
"My brother's elbow feels sore and stiff whenever he plays tennis. Even loosening up doesn't seem to help." *Ruta*

Ask
How did the injury occur?
What are the symptoms?
Is there pain? If so, where? Is it localized or does it radiate?
Describe the pain.
What makes the pain and other symptoms better or worse?
What makes you most comfortable?
Are there any mental and emotional changes since the tendinitis began?

Pointers for Finding the Homeopathic Medicine

The first medicine to give immediately after the injury is *Arnica.* ▮ If the tendon pain is made worse by any motion, always give *Bryonia.* ▮ If there is a feeling that the tendons are too short, the medicine is *Causticum.* ▮ If there is stiffness and restlessness, the two medicines to consider are *Rhus toxicodendron* and *Ruta.*

Dosage

- Give three pellets of 30C every four hours until you see improvement.
- If there is no improvement after three doses, give a different medicine.
- After you first notice improvement, give another dose only if symptoms begin to return.
- Lower potencies (6X, 6C, 30X) may need to be given more often (every two to four hours).
- Higher potencies (200X, 200C, 1M) generally need to be given only once. Repeat only if symptoms return with intensity; administer only infrequently in this case.

What to Expect from Homeopathic Self-Care

Improvement should occur within twenty-four hours to one week. It is still necessary to rest the area.

Other Self-Care Suggestions

The most important advice in tendinitis is to rest the area. A specially designed elastic-and-Velcro bandage can be very helpful. ▮ Ice the injured area. Sports medicine doctors used to recommend icing for the first twenty-four to forty-eight hours, then applying heat, but now many suggest continuing to apply ice to the injury. Icing reduces swelling and inflammation. ▮ Vitamin C (500 mg four times a day) can help reduce inflammation. ▮ Bromelain (250 mg four times a day) at least one hour before or after meals can help relieve inflammation. ▮ Manganese can help relieve pain and promote healing. Dosage depends on the product.

	Key Symptoms	Mind	Body	Worse	Better	Food & Drink
Arnica *(Leopard's bane)*	**Any injury to a tendon** **Sore, painful, and bruised as if beaten** **Tendinitis from overexertion** **Shock after injuries**	**Refuses help** **Says he's fine**	Lack of strength in the hand when grasping something	Touch	Letting the affected part hang down	
Bryonia *(Wild hops)*	**Tendinitis that is painful from even the slightest motion** **Stiffness of the area is made worse by motion**	**Irritable** Wants to go home	**Stiffness and shooting pains in the joints when touched or moved**	Light touch	**Pressure** **Lying on the affected part** **Bandaging the injured area**	**Thirst for large quantities of very cold drinks**
Causticum *(Potassium hydrate)*	**Contracted tendons** **Feeling that the tendon is too short** **Cramp in the Achilles tendon** **Wants to stretch or bend the affected area**	**Cannot tolerate injustice** **Afraid that something bad will happen**	Hamstring under the knee seems too short	**Drafts** **Exertion** **Grasping anything**	Gentle motion	Desire for smoked meat and beer Aversion to sweets
Rhus toxicodendron *(Poison ivy)*	**Tendinitis with stiffness and pain that is lessened by moving, stretching, and flexing** **Injuries to tendons and muscles after overexertion**	Active Jovial	**Restless; must keep moving to try to find a comfortable position**	**Cold cloth or ice pack** **Getting wet and chilled**	**Warm applications** **Hot bath or shower**	**Cold milk**
Ruta *(Rue)*	**Injuries to flexor tendons, joints, cartilage, and periosteum (outermost layer of the bone)** **Injuries to ankles and wrists** **Bruised, sore, aching feeling with restlessness** **Intense pain, weariness, and heaviness in the tendons**	Dissatisfied Quarrelsome	**Stiffness throughout the body** **Restlessness** **Tennis elbow**	Cold air Sitting	Lying on the back Rubbing	

Thrush

Description

Thrush is a yeast infection of the mucous membranes inside the mouth. It is common in infants, people who have been treated with antibiotics, and people with compromised immune systems, as in AIDS.

Symptoms

There are creamy white patches on the tongue or the mucous membranes of the mouth that can be scraped off.

Complications

None, unless the thrush continues for a long time and turns into a systemic yeast infection.

Look

Observe the tongue and the inside of the mouth.
Is there any discoloration? To what extent?

Listen

"I have this white coating and canker sores all over my mouth. I'm a mess!" *Borax*
"Besides this thick coating on my tongue, my breath smells like a garbage disposal!" *Mercurius*
"My tongue burns, and there is a yucky thick white coating on it." *Sulphur*

Ask

When did the thrush begin?
What seemed to be the cause?
What are the symptoms?
Is there any pain or discomfort?
If your baby has thrush, are you nursing?
If so, do you notice any infection on your breasts?
What makes the symptoms better or worse?
Are there any mental or emotional changes since the thrush began?

Pointers for Finding the Homeopathic Medicine

By far the most common medicine for thrush is *Borax,* especially if there are also canker sores. ▮ If there is bad-smelling breath, perspiration, and body odor, give *Mercurius.* ▮ If the tongue burns and has a thick furry coating, consider *Sulphur.*

Dosage

- Give three pellets of 30C every four hours until you see improvement.
- If there is no improvement after three doses, give a different medicine.
- After you first notice improvement, give another dose only if symptoms begin to return.
- Lower potencies (6X, 6C, 30X) may need to be given more often (every two to four hours).
- Higher potencies (200X, 200C, 1M) generally need to be given only once. Repeat only if symptoms return with intensity; administer only infrequently in this case.

What to Expect from Homeopathic Self-Care

The symptoms should go away within one to several days.

Other Self-Care Suggestions

If the nursing baby has thrush, the mother should also be treated if she has a breast infection. ▮ Acidophilus or unsweetened yogurt can help reestablish healthy intestinal flora. ▮ Avoid eating anything sweet, since yeast thrives on sugar. ▮ The most common treatment for thrush in many parts of the world is topical gentian violet, but it stains and is generally unnecessary due to the effectiveness of homeopathy.

	Key Symptoms	Mind	Body	Worse	Better	Food & Drink
Borax	**Person is also susceptible to canker sores** **Tenacious, white patches in the mouth that are not easily scraped off** **Gums are sore and inflamed**	**Very sensitive** **Startles easily** **Afraid of downward motion**	**Child cries frequently while nursing and pulls away from the breast**	Fruit	11:00 P.M.	
Mercurius *(Mercury)*	**Tongue is heavily coated with thrush** **Drooling** **Gums are sore and tender** **Bad breath and metallic taste in the mouth**	Doesn't trust easily Hurried	**Bad-smelling body odor and profuse perspiration**	**Extremes of temperature** **Night**	Moderate temperature	**Desire for bread and butter**
Sulphur *(Sulfur)*	**Thickly furred tongue** **Burning pain of the tongue** **Swelling of the gums with throbbing pain** **White coating on the tongue, with a red tip and edges**	**Critical** **Opinionated** **Lazy**	**Bad breath and profuse bad-smelling perspiration** **Lips are dry and bright red**	Sweets Heat	Sweating	Desire for sweets and fats Aversion to eggs and fish

Toothache

Description

Pain in the teeth, sometimes involving the gums and mucous membranes.

Symptoms

The pain may range from mild to severe, and is often affected by chewing, hot and cold, and drafts. Common causes of tooth pain are tooth decay, dental abscesses, nerve sensitivity, dental work, sinus infections, trauma, and damage to the facial nerve.

Complications

Complications include abscesses, death of a nerve (necessitating a root canal), loss of a tooth, or a severe, untreated infection that can become systemic.

Look

Are there any visible indications of tooth pain?
Is there any discoloration of the mouth or gums?
Is there swelling?

Listen

"This toothache makes me so mad!" *Chamomilla*
"The only time my tooth doesn't kill me is when I drink ice water." *Coffea*
"I have this dental abscess, and I can't believe how sensitive I am to pain.
"My mouth smells kind of like old cheese." *Hepar sulphuris*
"My tooth hurts like crazy, I have a terrible taste in my mouth, and my pillow is wet every morning when I wake up." *Mercurius*
"My upper left molar is unbearably painful. Nothing helps." *Plantago*

Ask

When did the toothache begin?
Where is the pain? In which teeth? Is it localized or does it radiate?
Is this a problem you've had before?
Have you been to the dentist lately?
Describe the pain in detail.

What makes the pain better or worse?
Are there any problems with the gums?
Have there been any mental or emotional changes since the toothache began?

Pointers for Finding the Homeopathic Medicine

For very severe dental pain with great irritability, give *Chamomilla* or *Hepar sulphuris*. ▮ If drinking coffee aggravates the pain terribly, give *Chamomilla*. ▮ For toothaches relieved by sloshing cold water in the mouth, give *Coffea*. ▮ If the pain is due to a very sensitive dental abscess, give *Hepar sulphuris*. ▮ If the toothache is accompanied by bad breath, a very coated tongue, and a lot of salivation, give *Mercurius*. ▮ If the toothache is unbearable and is limited to the left side of the face, consider *Plantago*.

MEDICAL CONDITIONS

Dosage

- Give three pellets of 30C every fifteen minutes to four hours, depending on the intensity of the pain, until you see improvement.
- If there is no improvement after three doses, give a different medicine.
- After you first notice improvement, give another dose only if symptoms begin to return.
- Lower potencies (6X, 6C, 30X) may need to be given more often (every two to four hours).
- Higher potencies (200X, 200C, 1M) generally need to be given only once. Repeat only if symptoms return with intensity; administer only infrequently in this case.

What to Expect from Homeopathic Self-Care

Dental pain should be relieved within fifteen minutes to several hours.

Other Self-Care Suggestions

Ice may temporarily numb the pain. ▮ Clove oil acts as an analgesic, but may interfere with homeopathic medicines. ▮ Take Tylenol, white willow bark, or another pain reliever temporarily until the homeopathic medicines have a chance to act.

	Key Symptoms	Mind	Body	Worse	Better	Food & Drink
Chamomilla *(Chamomile)*	**Violent toothache** **Toothache is made worse by coffee, warm food or drink, pregnancy, eating, entering a warm room, or a cold with suppressed perspiration** **Toothache pain is relieved by cold drinks**	**Quarrelsome** **Nothing pleases him**	**Tremendous hypersensitivity to pain** **Inconsolable with the pain**	Night	Cold applica-tions Sweating	
Coffea *(Coffee)*	**Toothache is relieved by holding cold water in the mouth, and made worse again as it gets warm** **Extreme hypersensitivity to pain, stimuli, emotions**	**Excitable** **Extremely active body and mind**		Noise Touch Emotions	Sleep Lying down	
Hepar sulphuris *(Calcium sulfide)*	**Toothaches due to dental abscesses** **Extreme hypersensitivity to pain** **Toothache made much worse by the least draft** **Mouth smells like old cheese**	Irritable Everything irritates her Complaining	Swelling and inflammation of the gums, which are painful when touched The gums and mouth bleed easily	**Cold** **Touch**	**Warmth**	Desire for vinegar

Mercurius *(Mercury)*	**Tearing, shooting, or throbbing pains in decayed teeth or in roots of teeth** **Toothache extends to ears and cheek** **Tooth pain is worse at night, from eating, and from eating or drinking anything hot or cold** **Coated tongue**	Hurried Mistrustful of others	**Bad breath** **Metallic taste in the mouth** **Excessive salivation or drooling** **Body odor and profuse bad-smelling perspiration**	**Extremes of temperature** Night	Moderate temperature	**Desire for bread and butter**
Plantago *(Plantain)*	**Toothache worse on the left side of the face** **Unbearable, severe toothache made worse by touch and by extremes of hot and cold** **Teeth sore and sensitive** **Toothache shoots up left side of face** **Profuse salivation** **Piercing, digging, violent tooth pain**	Confused Muddled feeling in the head	Grinds teeth at night Teeth feel too long	Night Warm room	Sleep	

Vaginitis, Acute

Description
Vaginitis is an inflammation of the mucous membranes of the vagina. It may be caused by a viral, bacterial, trichomonal, or yeast infection, or by sexual intercourse, douching, or other irritants such as spermicides, chemicals, or a foreign body in the vagina. Atrophic vaginitis occurs in women past menopause, resulting from a decrease in estrogen levels.

Symptoms
Vaginal discharge is often the main complaint. It may be thick or thin, odorless or offensive. There may also be redness of the vaginal lips and itching, swelling, or pain of the vulva, labia, and vagina. The intensity varies greatly.

Complications
A culture of the vaginal discharge should be taken to find out the cause of the infection. If gonorrhea, chlamydia, or syphilis are found to be the cause, the diagnosis must be reported to the local public health department and immediate medical attention is required. These three infections are often asymptomatic in women and, if untreated, may lead to infertility.

Look
Is there any unusual appearance of the labia or vulva?
Is there discoloration? Swelling?
Are there eruptions?
What does the discharge look like?

Listen
"I've never had such incredible itching in my whole life." *Caladium*
"My vagina burns so badly from the discharge that I can hardly stand it." *Kreosotum*
"I always get this creamy discharge around my period. It makes me want to cry." *Pulsatilla*
"The discharge smells like old fish." *Sanicula*
"I got this yeast infection after my child was born. I've had absolutely no sex drive since." *Sepia*

Ask

When did the vaginitis begin?
What seemed to bring it on?
What does it feel like?
What are the main symptoms?
What makes the symptoms better or worse?
Is there any correlation between the vaginitis and sex?
Are there any mental or emotional changes with the vaginitis?
Are you craving anything to eat or drink?

Pointers for Finding the Homeopathic Medicine

For vaginitis with terrible itching during pregnancy, give *Caladium.* ▮ For vaginal discharges that are terribly abrading and acrid, give *Kreosotum.* ▮ For vaginitis with a yellowish-green creamy discharge in a gentle woman who cries as she tells you about it, *Pulsatilla* will probably work. ▮ If the discharge smells strongly like fish brine, look at *Sanicula.* ▮ If the symptoms occur during menopause and are accompanied by a lack of sex drive, constipation, and irritability, *Sepia* will be helpful.

Dosage

- Give three pellets of 30C every four hours until you see improvement.
- If there is no improvement after three doses, give a different medicine.
- After you first notice improvement, give another dose only if symptoms begin to return.
- Lower potencies (6X, 6C, 30X) may need to be given more often (every two to four hours).
- Higher potencies (200X, 200C, 1M) generally need to be given only once. Repeat only if symptoms return with intensity; administer only infrequently in this case.

What to Expect from Homeopathic Self-Care

Acute episodes of vaginitis can respond within twenty-four to forty-eight hours. Vaginitis is usually a chronic or recurrent problem, and requires qualified homeopathic care.

Other Self-Care Suggestions

The easiest and most effective suggestion: insert one capsule of boric acid into the vagina in the morning, and one capsule of acidophilus at bedtime, for five days. Stop during the menstrual period. ▮ Douche with one tablespoon of white vinegar in a pint of warm water daily for five days. Insert one tablespoon of unsweetened, live-culture yogurt after each douche. ▮ If the vaginitis is just on the labia and vulva and is caused by yeast, apply a preparation of half vinegar and half water topically. ▮ Some women insert a clove of garlic, wrapped in cheesecloth or gauze, vaginally for yeast infections. ▮ If there is rawness externally not due to yeast, *Calendula* cream topically can be helpful. ▮ Insert Vitamin E suppositories into the vagina for vaginal dryness. ▮ Occasionally, one tablespoon of baking soda in a quart of water works better as a douche than acidifying treatments such as vinegar or boric acid.

	Key Symptoms	Mind	Body	Worse	Better	Food & Drink
Caladium *(American arum)*	**Terrible itching of the vagina** **Vaginitis during pregnancy**	Nervous and excitable Restless after smoking Fearful of catching disease	**Dryness of labia and vulva** **Itching of vagina and vulva with burning** Desire to masturbate	**Too much sex** **Tobacco**	Cold air Sweating	
Kreosotum *(Creosote)*	**Yellow vaginal discharge that is terribly itchy and burning** **Extreme rawness of the mucous membranes** **Discharge smells putrid or like green corn**	Cross Obstinate Dissatisfied with everything	**Swelling of the labia** **Scratching makes the itching and inflammation worse** **Vaginitis is worse during pregnancy or before the menstrual period starts** Weakness of the legs	**Pregnancy** Menstrual period	Warmth Hot food Sitting	
Pulsatilla *(Windflower)*	**Thick, bland, yellow-green discharges** **Warm, with desire for fresh air or window open**	**Changeable emotions** **Clingy and weepy** **Wants company when sick**	**Discharge may be bland, thick and milky, creamy or irritating, or thin and burning** Discharge is usually painless Pain in the back and exhaustion with the discharge Vaginitis in little girls	**Warm stuffy room** Rich food	Slow walking in the open air	**Not thirsty** **Desire for butter, ice cream, and creamy foods** Aversion to fat, milk, and pork Aggravated by pork, fat, and rich foods

continued on next page

	Key Symptoms	Mind	Body	Worse	Better	Food & Drink
Sanicula *(Spring water)*	**Discharge smells like fish brine** **Body odor smells like old cheese**	Stubborn, irritable, and touchy Doesn't want to be touched	Bearing-down sensation in the pelvis, as if uterus would drop out	Motion	Uncovering Rest	**Desire for salt, bacon, and ice cold milk**
Sepia *(Cuttlefish ink)*	**Discharge makes the genitals feel raw, burning, and itching** **Discharge is white or yellow and can be slimy, lumpy, or bloody** **Symptoms caused by a hormonal imbalance**	**Depressed, sluggish, dull, and overwhelmed** **Irritable** **Cries easily**	**Discharge worse during the day, none at night** **Dryness of the vagina in menopausal women that feels worse while walking** **Aversion to her partner and to sex** Bearing-down sensation in the pelvis, as though the uterus would fall out Feels better after vigorous exercise or dancing	**Before the menstrual period** Cold Pregnancy and after childbirth	**Vigorous exercise** Warmth Crossing the legs	**Desire for vinegar and sweets** Aversion to fat

PART **3**

MATERIA MEDICA

CHAPTER **10**

All About the Medicines

We include here the main features of the most commonly used homeopathic medicines for treating first-aid and acute conditions. Other less commonly prescribed medicines that do not appear here are included under the various medical conditions in Chapter 9.

Aconite (Monkshood)

Key Symptoms
Ailments from fright or shock
Extreme anxiety
Tremendous restlessness
Fear of impending death
Ailments from exposure to cold, dry air, or wind
Symptoms come on suddenly

Mind
Claustrophobia
Fear of being in a crowd
Fear of flying in an airplane
Fear of earthquakes
Agoraphobia
Panic attacks
Desire for the company of others

Body

HEAD **One cheek red and the other pale, or both cheeks hot and red**
Hot, heavy, burning sensation in the head
Hot, watery nasal discharge
Dizziness when standing up or rising from a seat
Very painful ear infections with a high fever

CHEST **Violent heart palpitations**
Dry, croupy cough; comes on suddenly, especially during first twenty-four hours

SKIN Itching and burning of the skin

GENERAL **High fever that comes on suddenly**
Profuse perspiration with anxiety
Rapid pulse

Worse
Chill

Better
Rest

Food and Drink
Intense burning thirst for cold drinks

Allium cepa (Red onion)

Key Symptoms
Eyes and nose run like a faucet, as if the person were peeling an onion

Mind
Afraid that the pain will become intolerable

Body

HEAD **Profuse, bland discharge from the nose (*Euphrasia* is indicated for acrid discharge)**

Profuse, acrid, burning discharge from the eyes (*Euphrasia* is indicated for bland discharge)
Frequent, violent sneezing

THROAT Red, hot, dry, and tight
Hoarse
Raw

CHEST Tickling, irritating, hacking cough that will not quit

NECK Intense pain at nape of neck

GENERAL Secretion of mucus

Worse
Warm room
Cold wind
Getting the feet wet

Better
Cool, open air

Food and Drink
Desire for raw onions
Strong hunger and thirst
Aversion to cucumbers

Antimonium tartaricum (Tartar of antimony)

Key Symptoms
Loose, rattling cough with copious mucus that is hard to bring up
Hates to be looked at or touched

Mind
Irritable
Bad mood
Wants to be left alone

Body

MOUTH White, coated tongue
Lips may be blue

THROAT Mucus in throat with shortness of breath

CHEST Breathing is rapid, short, and difficult
Bronchitis, especially in infants and the elderly
Chest feels full, but they cannot bring up mucus
Vomiting from the cough
Person has to sit up in order to breathe or cough
Children bend backward on coughing
Overpowering sleepiness during bronchitis or cough

STOMACH AND ABDOMEN Nausea and vomiting with the cough
Feels as if full of rocks

SKIN Impetigo
Bluish eruptions or sores that crust over and leave a bluish-red mark

Worse

Warm room
Milk
Anger
Lying down

Better

Getting the mucus out
Belching
Vomiting
Cold, open air
Sitting up

Food and Drink

Desire for apples and other fruits
Desire for sour things, resulting in indigestion

Apis mellifica (Honeybee)

Key Symptoms

Bee stings or insect bites
Heat, redness, and stinging pain, with lots of swelling

Burning, stinging pain
Hives with burning, stinging, and itching after a bite or sting
Allergic reactions
Affected area is hot and made worse by heat, better by cold applications
Anaphylactic shock

Mind
Busy as a bee
Protects the hive (family or home)
Jealous

Body
HEAD Swelling and puffiness of the face and eyelids
Conjunctivitis (pinkeye) with redness of the eye and swelling around the eye
Hay fever

THROAT Stinging pain in the throat, especially right-sided, lessened by cold drinks
Sore throat with swelling of the uvula
Throat pain extending to right ear

SKIN Itching is intolerable at night

URINE Scalding urine, especially the last drops
Urination is frequent and can be involuntary
Feels as though the urine will not come out

GENERAL Swelling

Worse
Heat, hot rooms, hot drinks, a hot bath, or in bed

Better
Cool air, cold applications, cold bath or shower
Uncovering

Food and Drink
Not thirsty

Arnica (Leopard's bane)

Key Symptoms

Foremost medicine for trauma, injuries, falls, sprains, or strains
Any trauma with bruising
Excellent for shocks of any kind
Bleeding anywhere in the body
Used before and after surgery to promote healing

Mind

Want to be left alone
Insists that nothing is wrong

Body

HEAD **Black eyes**
Serious head trauma, especially with bruising
Concussion and bleeding, with bruising of the tissues and the brain
Nosebleed after an accident or traumatic injury

EXTREMITIES **Sprains or strains, especially of ankles**

BACK **Bruised, sore feeling in the back**

SKIN **Black and blue areas following injury**
Cuts that bleed a lot or bruise

GENERAL **Sore, bruised feeling anywhere in the body**
Wants to lie down, but the bed feels too hard and he looks for a softer spot
Fainting after an accident or traumatic injury, blood loss, or shock

Worse

Touch
Overexertion

Better

Lying down with the head low

Arsenicum album (Arsenic)

Key Symptoms

Tremendous anxiety
Fear of death
Restlessness
Burning pains anywhere in the body

Mind

Very anxious about health
Hypochondriacal
Afraid of germs and contagion
Irritable
Despair of never recovering

Body

HEAD **Burning in the eyes**
Thin, watery, burning discharge from nose
Nose feels plugged
Hay fever

CHEST **Asthmatic attacks, with great anxiety**

STOMACH AND ABDOMEN **Heartburn**
Diarrhea that is made worse by acidic foods or fruit
Food poisoning
Stomach flu
Nausea and vomiting after eating or drinking

SKIN Hives (can be from shellfish)

GENERAL **Insomnia**
Very chilly

Worse

Midnight to 2:00 A.M.
Cold food or drinks

Better

Heat
Warm drinks

Food and Drink
Desire to sip cold drinks frequently
Desire for milk, fat on meat, sour foods

Belladonna (Deadly nightshade)

Key Symptoms
High fever when child has a bright red face
Right-sided symptoms
Bright red bleeding
Sunstroke or heat exhaustion
Sudden onset of symptoms
Extreme sensitivity to noise, light, and being jarred

Mind
Sudden outbursts of anger
Child has high fever but plays normally, as if not sick at all

Body
HEAD Maddening, violent headaches
Right-sided headaches with severe throbbing pain
Fiery red, hot, dry face
Nosebleed with a red flushed face
Eyes glassy with fever
Right-sided ear infections with severe pain
Migraines made worse by the least movement or jarring

THROAT Throat red, dry, very painful, and worse on right side (sometimes strep throat)

CHEST Short, croupy, dry, barking cough

WOMEN Profuse, gushing, bright red menstrual flow
Breasts are heavy, hard, inflamed, and red

GENERAL Fever is often above 103°F
Throbbing pains
Hallucinations during fever
Sunstroke or heat exhaustion

Worse
Light
Noise
Jarring
3:00 P.M.
Touch
Exposure to sun
Lying down
Getting chilled or overheated

Better
Sitting up in a quiet, dark room
Bending backward in a semi-erect position

Food and Drink
Great thirst for cold water or no thirst at all
Desire for lemons or lemonade, sour food

Borax

Key Symptoms
The main medicine for canker sores in children, especially if thrush is also present
Symptoms are made worse by any downward motion

Mind
Afraid of downward motion, such as going downstairs or being put down
Startles easily from noise
Sensitive
Nervous

Body
MOUTH Thrush (white, furry patches) of mucous membranes of mouth
Mouth feels hot and dry
Mouth is sensitive to acids, salty foods, and spicy foods

GENERAL **Hand, foot, and mouth disease**
Child wakes up screaming from nightmares

Worse
Sudden noises
Being tossed up and down
Nursing
Fruit

Better
Pressure
Cold weather

Bryonia (Wild hops)

Key Symptoms
Symptoms made worse by any motion
Extremely irritable
Talks of business
Dry mouth and lips, with extreme thirst for cold drinks
Worse at 9:00 P.M.

Mind
Wants to go home

Body
HEAD Bursting, splitting headache, made worse by motion
Pain over left eye
Dizzy when getting up from a seat or bed
Holds the head to keep it from moving

MOUTH Extremely dry, chapped mouth and lips

CHEST Hard, dry cough that is made worse by any movement
Motion or cough causes pain in the chest and severe headache
Holds on to chest to keep it from moving during the cough

Cough dry at night
Pain from motion of chest

BACK **Neck very stiff and painful**
Back pain worse from any movement

STOMACH AND ABDOMEN Appendicitis
Large, hard, dry stool
Gushing diarrhea

STOOL **Large, hard, dry stool**
Constipation

ARMS AND LEGS Joints red, hot, swollen
Injuries or fractures that are made worse by any movement

Worse
Moving the eyes
Coughing

Better
Pressure
Lying on the painful side
Warm drinks

Food and Drink
Great thirst for cold drinks
Desire for meat

Calcarea carbonica (Calcium carbonate)

Key Symptoms
Large, sweaty heads and flabby bodies
Fair, fat, flabby
Worried about safety, security, and home
Practical
Illnesses from taking on too much responsibility

Mind
Independent
Obstinate
Overwhelmed
Afraid of flying, heights, mice, insanity
Anxious about health

Body
MOUTH **Sour taste in the mouth**
Tip of tongue feels scalded
Cold air makes the teeth hurt

EXTREMITIES **Calf, foot, and thigh cramps**
Cramps after exertion
Pains in the bones and joints from cold damp weather
Legs feel weak when going uphill or up stairs

GENERAL **Sour perspiration**
Low thyroid
Couch potato

Worse
Cold, damp weather
Exertion
Going uphill
Teething

Food and Drink
Desire for eggs, milk, sweets, and salt

Cantharis (Spanish fly)

Key Symptoms
Bladder infections, especially of sudden onset
Burns of any kind
Burning pains

Mind
Excessive sexual energy

Body

BLADDER AND KIDNEYS **Violently acute bladder infection**

Severe pain in the bladder or urethra at the beginning of or during urination

Bloody urine

Burning or scalding urine

Constant urge to urinate

Urine is passed one drop at a time

Sensitive kidney region

SKIN **Burns and scalds that are made better by cold water**

Skin eruptions that burn when touched

Worse

Urinating

Cold

Hearing the sound of water

Better

Warmth

Rest

Lying quietly on her back

MATERIA MEDICA

Carbo vegetabilis (Charcoal)

Key Symptoms

Most common medicine for fainting or collapse

Weakness in which the person is blue and the pulse is faint

Person is cold and yet wants to be uncovered or to be fanned

Tremendous amount of gas and bloating

Feels better after belching

Mind

Sluggish

Anxious

Irritable

Indifferent

Body

STOMACH AND ABDOMEN **Everything he eats turns to gas**

Loud, rancid-smelling belches

Even a small amount of food causes abdominal discomfort

Burning in the stomach with a cold feeling

Indigestion in nursing mothers

Can't stand tight clothing around the waist

GENERAL **Cold sweat**

Worse

Lying down

Rich food

Warmth

Better

Being fanned or exposed to a draft

Food and Drink

Desire for salty food

Causticum (Potassium hydrate)

Key Symptoms

Constant desire to clear throat of mucus

Fear that something bad will happen

Hoarseness

Aggravation from drafts

Mind

Indignation from injustice or authority

Empathetic people who can't bear to hear about the suffering of others

Body

THROAT Scraping, burning, or rawness of the throat

CHEST Coughs with burning pain or soreness in the chest

BLADDER AND KIDNEYS Loss of urine from coughing, walking, sneezing, or blowing the nose

ARMS AND LEGS Carpal tunnel syndrome
Contracted muscles and tendons

SKIN **Deep burns and the after-effects of severe burns**
Burns that are slow to heal
Warts

Worse
Wind
Dry, cold air
Evening

Better
Cold drinks
Damp weather

Food and Drink
Desire for smoked meat
Aversion to sweets

Chamomilla (Chamomile)

Key Symptoms
Cross, contrary child, especially an infant during teething
Demands to be carried or rocked
Great pain, with irritability, impatience, and restlessness
Inconsolable child

Mind
Screaming and crying
Extremely fussy

Quarrelsome, especially if a child
Asks for something, then, when he receives it, wants something else
Cannot bear to be touched or examined
Doesn't want anyone near him

Body

EAR **Ear infection, especially during teething**
Child is inconsolable with ear pain
Cannot stand to listen to music

FACE One cheek may be red and hot, the other pale

STOMACH AND ABDOMEN **Colic in infants, in which child screams and arches his back**
Green diarrhea, like chopped eggs or spinach
Abdominal pain is made worse by touch
Belching and diarrhea with an odor like rotten eggs

RECTUM AND STOOL **Greenish diarrhea, like spinach, during teething**

GENERAL **Tremendous hypersensitivity to pain**
Symptoms are often worse during teething

Worse

Anger
Teething
Cold wind
Night
9:00 P.M.

Better

Being carried

Food and Drink

Desire for cold drinks
Aversion to warm drinks

Cocculus (Indian cockle)

Key Symptoms

Motion sickness, seasickness, airsickness

Nausea and dizziness made worse by motion

Dizziness from looking at moving objects or watching things out of the window of a moving vehicle

Sickness after caring for ill family member or from loss of sleep

Mind

Weakness after excessive worrying and caring for a loved one

Nervous exhaustion

Profound sadness

Body

HEAD Significant dizziness, generally accompanied by nausea

Headache made worse by riding in a vehicle

STOMACH AND ABDOMEN Tremendous nausea, especially due to dizziness

Nausea made worse by thinking about or smelling food

ARMS AND LEGS Cracking of knee joints

WOMEN Morning sickness with headache, nausea, and vomiting

Must lie down with the morning sickness or gets nauseated

GENERAL Sensation of hollowness or emptiness, as if body parts are asleep

Worse

Traveling in boats, cars

Loss of sleep, especially from caring for a loved one

Better

Sitting

Lying on the side

Food and Drink

Aversion to food

Coffea (Unroasted coffee)

Key Symptoms

Overstimulation, hypersensitivity, and hyperexcitability
Nervous agitation and restlessness
Unusual activity of body and mind
Exquisite sensitivity to pain
Hypersensitivity to noise, light, and touch

Mind

Overactive mind
Overreaction to all emotions, even joy and surprise
Extreme nervous tension and anxiety
Abundance of ideas
Boundless energy to complete tasks
Can't tolerate noise

Body

HEAD **Severe toothache, made better by holding ice water in the mouth**

CHEST **Violent heart palpitations**
Palpitations after excessive joy or surprise

GENERAL **Insomnia; wide awake at 3:00 A.M. with mind full of thoughts**
Fainting from joy or excitement

Worse

Excessive emotions, including joy
Strong odors
Noise
Touch

Better

Lying down
Sleep
Warmth

Colocynthis (Bitter cucumber)

Key Symptoms

Abdominal cramping lessened by bending over double
Illness after indignation or humiliation
Colic in newborns

Mind

Offended at everything; Indignation
Everything annoys her
Angry when questioned

Body

STOMACH AND ABDOMEN **Violent, cramping abdominal pain**
Colicky baby lies on abdomen and screams if moved even slightly
Repeated episodes of diarrhea after the least food or drink
Gas is made worse by eating, especially fruit
Watery diarrhea with gas and pain
Intestines feel like stones are grinding inside

ARMS AND LEGS **Sciatica after anger, being insulted, or feeling offended**
Sciatica more often right-sided
Cramps in the hips and thighs

WOMEN Clutching ovarian pain, lessened by drawing legs up into abdomen

GENERAL Restlessness during pain

Worse

Becoming angry
Lying on the painless side

Better

Hard pressure
Bending over
Drawing the legs up
Lying on the side that hurts

Food and Drink

Desire for bread

Cuprum (Copper)

Key Symptoms

Spasms and cramping anywhere in the body

Mind

Wants to be in charge

Avoids everyone who approaches her

Great anxiety accompanying violent abdominal cramps

Body

CHEST Cough with violent fits

Coughs relieved by cold drinks

STOMACH AND ABDOMEN **Severely painful colic**

Violent vomiting with abdominal cramping and diarrhea

Profuse, gushing diarrhea

Vomiting prevented by drinking cold water

ARMS AND LEGS **Cramps in palms, calves, and soles of feet**

Jerking of hands and feet

Muscle twitching of lower extremities

WOMEN Violent menstrual cramps that make her scream

Worse

Mental or emotional overwork or exhaustion

Suppression of symptoms

Motion

Going uphill or up stairs

Better

Cold drinks

Lying down

Food and Drink

Desire for cold drinks

Drosera (Sundew)

Key Symptoms

Violent fits of hard coughing with choking
Can barely breathe while coughing
Dry, barking, croupy, spasmodic cough that ends in gagging or vomiting
Periodic and spasmodic fits of deep, barking cough
Whooping cough
Croup

Mind

Becomes angry easily
May feel harassed or persecuted

Body

CHEST **Episodes of dry, incessant coughing following each other rapidly**
Deep, hoarse voice
Cough from tickle in the larynx, like a crumb or feather
Harassing cough beginning as soon as the head touches the pillow at night
Cough made worse by singing, talking, or eating

STOMACH **Gagging and retching from coughing**
Vomiting from coughing

Worse

Lying down
After midnight
Talking

Better

Pressure
Open air

Euphrasia (Eyebright)

Key Symptoms

Profuse, acrid tearing with a bland discharge from the nose (opposite of *Allium cepa)*

Colds, allergies

Hay fever centers on the eyes

Mind

Irritable

Body

HEAD Eyes water all the time

Eyes are burning, irritated, sensitive to light

Frequent blinking of the eyes

Headache from nasal congestion, with profuse discharge from eyes and nose

Worse

Evening

Better

Open air

Dark

Ferrum phosphoricum (Iron phosphate)

Key Symptoms

First stage of infections with fever where no specific symptoms are present

Useful in the very first stage of the cold; she feels she is coming down with something, but there are no clear symptoms

High fever with flushed face, especially with round red spots on the cheeks or sometimes very pale

Fever is generally 102°F or higher

Mind
Irritable
Talkative

Body
HEAD **Face red and flushed or very pale**

NOSE **Nosebleed with flushed face or with round red spots on the cheeks**
Nosebleed with very pale face
Lots of bright red blood that clots easily
Nosebleeds in children

THROAT **Inflammation of throat or lungs with fever, but few definite symptoms**
Throat red, inflamed, ulcerated
Throat pain made worse by swallowing saliva
Tonsils red and swollen

CHEST Bruised, sore muscles of chest and shoulders

GENERAL Tendency to come down with a cold easily
Very weak
Bright red bleeding from any part of the body
Discharges may be blood-streaked
Anemia
Bruised soreness of the muscles

Worse
Night
4:00 to 6:00 A.M.
Motion
Right side

Better
Cold cloth or ice pack
Bleeding
Lying down

Food and Drink
Desire for sour foods and cold drinks
Aversion to meat and milk

Gelsemium (Yellow jasmine)

Key Symptoms

Most common medicine for an exhausting flu
Dizzy, drowsy, droopy, and dull
Muscle aching throughout body
Stage fright
Illness following fright

Mind

Mind feels extremely dull
Thinking is an effort

Body

HEAD **Pressing headache across forehead and back of head**
Dizziness, as if drunk, with heaviness of the eyelids
Blurred vision

STOMACH AND ABDOMEN **Diarrhea from stage fright**

BACK **Dull pain and chills up and down the spine**

GENERAL **Overall weakness**
Wants to lie down and go to sleep
Lack of thirst

Worse

Fright

Better

Bending forward
Lying down with head held high

Glonoine (Nitroglycerin)

Key Symptoms

Sunstroke
Violent throbbing with rushing of blood

Mind

Confused and bewildered
Becomes lost in familiar places

Body

HEAD **Terrible bursting, pounding headache, especially after exposure to the sun**
Face flushed and hot

CHEST **Violent palpitations and throbbing in the heart and whole body**

BACK Hot sensation down the spine

Worse

Direct sun, especially on the head

Better

Open air
Cold applications

Hepar sulphuris (Calcium sulfide)

Key Symptoms

Oversensitive and annoyed by every little thing
Hypersensitive to pain
Splinter-like pains
Abscesses
Tendency to form pus
Extreme chilliness

Mind

Irritable
Everyone gets on her nerves
Complains constantly
Dissatisfied about everything

Body

THROAT **Sensation of a splinter or fish bone stuck in the throat**

Exquisitely painful sore throat with ulceration

Swollen tonsils and neck glands

Sharp pain in the throat extending to the ear on swallowing

SKIN **Extremely painful abscesses**

Boils very painful, especially to touch

Expelling foreign bodies lessens the pain

WOMEN Breast abscess with thick pus

Discharge from the breast smells sour or like rotten cheese

GENERAL **Discharges or body parts smell sour or like old cheese**

Worse

Drafts

Uncovering the body

Touch

Lying on the painful part

Better

Heat

Covering up

Food and Drink

Desire for vinegar

Hypericum (St. John's wort)

Key Symptoms

Excellent for puncture wounds or smashed fingers or toes

Numbness, tingling, and radiating pain along nerves

Cuts with sharp, shooting pain

Pain in the coccyx tailbone) from a fall or blow

Shooting pain from injury to the spine or nerves

Mind

Confused; forgets what he wanted to say

Dull and forgetful after head injury

Body

HEAD **Head injury and concussion, especially if the spinal nerves are also involved**

BACK **Herniated disk**

Injuries to the spine or tailbone with sharp, shooting pains

SKIN Lacerations or injuries to areas with lots of nerves, such as the tips of the fingers and toes

GENERAL **Shooting pain radiating upward from the injured area**

Worse

Injury

Jarring of the affected area

Better

Rubbing the injured area

Food and Drinks

Desire for wine, pickles, and cold drinks

Ignatia (St. Ignatius bean)

Key Symptoms

Most common medicine to use immediately following grief or loss

Uncontrollable crying, loss of appetite, and extreme sadness

Great mood swings

Frequent sighing

Numbness and cramping anywhere in the body

Mind

Upset after hurt or disappointment

High-strung and emotionally reactive

Says or does the opposite of what you would expect

Body

THROAT **Throat pain that is lessened by swallowing**

Sensation of a lump in the throat, especially after grief

CHEST A feeling of pressure or tightness

GENERAL Symptoms that are just the opposite of what you would expect

Worse
Grief or disappointment

Better
Deep breathing
Changing positions

Food and Drink
Strong desire for or dislike of fruit
Desire for cheese

Ipecac (Ipecac root)

Key Symptoms
Most important medicine for nausea and vomiting
Terrible, constant nausea not relieved by vomiting
Nausea and vomiting with nearly all conditions
Bright red, gushing bleeding
Bleeding and nausea at the same time

Mind
Irritable
Full of desires but doesn't know what he wants
Difficult to please

Body
MOUTH **Tongue usually clean**
Copious saliva

CHEST **Loose, rattling cough**
Unable to bring up mucus
Cough incessant and violent with every breath

STOMACH AND ABDOMEN **Hates food and the smell of food**
Nausea and vomiting from coughing
Nausea with a clean tongue
Vomiting in infants during breast-feeding
Cramps in the abdomen

Worse
Vomiting
Overeating
Warmth

Better
Open air
Closing eyes
Cold drinks

Food and Drink
Lack of thirst

Kali bichromicum (Bichromate of potash)

Key Symptoms
Pressure in the sinuses, and pain at the root of the nose
Thick, ropey, greenish-yellow discharge from nose
Sinus infection with pressing pain in cheekbones and bridge of nose
Thick postnasal drip
A cold that develops into a sinus infection; a ripe or late-stage cold

Mind
Tends to talk in excessive detail
Avoids people

Body
HEAD **Nose dry and constantly feels stopped up**
Voice sounds very nasal

Bones of the head feel sore
Sensation of a hair on the tongue

CHEST **Cough with thick, stringy mucus in bronchitis or asthma**
Rattling breathing during sleep
Tickling sensation in the chest
Dry, metallic, hacking cough

GENERAL **Pain in small spots**
Pains that move quickly from place to place

Worse
Beer, alcohol
Cold, damp weather
Morning
2:00 to 3:00 A.M.

Better
Heat

Food and Drink
Desire for beer and sweets
Aversion to meat

Lachesis (Bushmaster snake)

Key Symptoms
Symptoms are worse on the left side of the body
Symptoms move from left to right
Symptoms are worse on waking or after sleep
Dislike of tight clothing around the neck or abdomen
Fear of snakes

Mind
Intense
Very talkative
Jealous
Suspicious
Jumps from one subject to the next

Body

HEAD Headaches worse on the left side and better when the period begins
Nosebleed, especially left-sided
Nosebleed with dark blood
Nosebleed when the menstrual period should start

THROAT **Worse on left side**
Sensation of a lump in the throat
Extremely painful sore throat, made much worse by swallowing saliva or liquids

WOMEN **Hot flashes of menopause**
Premenstrual symptoms, including headaches and irritability, which are lessened as soon as the period begins

SKIN Purplish areas
Varicose veins

GENERAL **Feels tense and pressured**

Worse

After sleep
Slightest touch
Constriction of any kind
Suppression of emotions or symptoms

Better

Discharge, such as onset of menstrual flow or expression of emotions

Ledum (Marsh tea)

Key Symptoms

Puncture wound or smashed fingers or toes
Injured area feels cold and person wants cold application
Insect bites or stings

Mind

Dissatisfied
Bad mood

Body

EXTREMITIES Sprains with significant bruising
Sore heels and soles of feet
Swelling of ankle and ball of big toe

Worse

Warmth
Moving joints

Better

Cold
Putting feet in cold water

Lycopodium (Club moss)

Key Symptoms

Symptoms that are right-sided or move from right to left
Desire for warm or room-temperature drinks
Worse from 4:00 to 8:00 P.M.
Stage fright

Mind

Insecurity or lack of courage, which the person tries to cover up
Fearful inside, but may seem bossy
Desire to have someone in the next room

Body

THROAT **Right-sided sore throat, feels better with warm drinks**

STOMACH AND ABDOMEN **Gas and bloating**
Bloating after eating even a small amount of food
Aggravation from cabbage, broccoli, or beans
Can't handle the pressure of clothing around the abdomen

GENERAL Chilly

Worse

After eating
Warmth

Better
Warm drinks

Food and Drink
Strong desire for sweets and warm or room-temperature drinks

Magnesia phosphorica (Magnesium phosphate)

Key Symptoms
Abdominal cramping lessened by warm applications and pressure
Colic in infants

Mind
Complains about symptoms

Body
STOMACH AND ABDOMEN Gassy colic relieved by bending double, drawing the legs up, rubbing, warmth, and pressure
Colic with watery diarrhea
Tendency to belch with colic, but discomfort not relieved by belching
Abdominal bloating with a desire to loosen the clothes around the abdomen
Menstrual cramps relieved by bending double, warmth, and pressure
GENERAL Exhausted

Worse
Cold
Drafts
Night
Milk

Better
Hot bath
Doubling up
Rubbing

MATERIA MEDICA

Mercurius (Mercury)
(also called *Mercurius solubilis* and *Mercurius vivus*)

Key Symptoms

Bad-smelling discharges, breath, or perspiration
Drooling
Toxic states (as though one had ingested poison)
Like the mercury in a thermometer; very sensitive to both heat and cold

Mind

Distrustful of those around her
Hurried
Restless
Emotionally reserved

Body

HEAD **Green or yellow discharge from the nose or ears**
Raw, ulcerated nostrils
Ear pain, with constant desire to swallow
Teeth marks on the tongue
Metallic taste in the mouth

THROAT Burning, raw throat with ulcers on the tonsils
Stitching throat pain radiating to the ears on swallowing

WOMEN Thick, white vaginal discharge

GENERAL **Night sweats**

Worse

Extremes of heat or cold
Night
Drafts
Becoming heated

Better

Moderate temperatures

Food and Drink

Desire for bread and butter, lemons

Natrum muriaticum (Sodium chloride)

Key Symptoms

Wants to be left alone when not feeling well
Feelings hurt very easily
Headaches from exposure to the heat or sun

Mind

Often has a history of grief or disappointment in relationships
Very sensitive to the slightest reprimand or insult
Pouty, sulky
Deeply affected by music

Body

HEAD Canker sores in the mouth
Cold sores on the lips
Extremely runny nose
Deep crack in the center of the lower lip
Hay fever
Nasal discharge with egg-white consistency
Headaches that throb or feel like hammers knocking on the brain
Headaches over the eyes

SKIN Hives

Worse

10:00 A.M.
Heat
Being in the sun

Better

Open air

Food and Drink

Desire for salty food, pasta, bread, lemons
Aversion to slimy food

Nux vomica (Quaker's button)

Key Symptoms
Highly irritable and impatient
Chilly

Mind
Obsessed with business
Wants to be the first and the best
Competitive and hard-driving, Type A
Easily offended
Frustrated easily by little things

Body
HEAD Painfully stiff neck

BACK Muscle tension, cramping, and spasms

NOSE Colds with stuffy nose and sniffles
Nose is stuffed up at night and when outside

STOMACH AND ABDOMEN Heartburn that is made worse by spicy foods
Constipation without a desire to have a bowel movement
Fussy, colicky infant who arches her back
Nausea with retching

STOOL Constipated with urge to go, but no stool comes out

GENERAL Heightened sensitivity to light, noise, sound, and other stimuli
Insomnia at 3:00 A.M.

Worse
Abuse of alcohol or drugs
Eating too much food or excessively spicy food
Early morning
Cold, dry air

Better
Discharges from the body
Rest

Food and Drink
Desire for spicy food, fat, coffee, alcohol, and tobacco

Petroleum (Coal oil)

Key Symptoms
Seasickness, airsickness, or motion sickness
Severe dryness and cracking of skin, even to the point of bleeding

Mind
Gets lost in familiar places
Can't make up his mind
Irritable

Body
STOMACH AND ABDOMEN Sensation of great emptiness in the stomach, relieved by constant eating
Heartburn
Hunger immediately after bowel movement
Must get up during the night to eat
SKIN Ragged, chapped, cracked fingertips and heels, especially in the winter

Worse
Traveling in a car, plane, train, or boat
Cold weather

Better
Warm air
Dry weather

Food and Drink
Desire for beer
Aversion to meat, fats, and cooked or hot foods

Phosphorus

Key Symptoms
Bright red bleeding
Chronic tendency to bruise and bleed easily
Desire for company
Great thirst for cold drinks

Mind

Outgoing
Sympathetic
Friendly
Desires company
Afraid of the dark, thunderstorms, and ghosts

Body

HEAD **Nosebleeds with bright red blood**

THROAT **Hoarseness**
Loss of voice

CHEST Hard, dry, exhausting cough
Cough dry at first, then loose
Dry, hot, burning sensation in chest
Pneumonia with coughing up of blood

STOMACH AND ABDOMEN **Craves cold drinks but vomits them as soon as they become warm in the stomach**

Painless, watery, exhausting diarrhea
Stomach pain relieved by cold drinks

WOMEN **Excessive, bright red menstrual bleeding**

GENERAL Tendency to dehydration

Worse

Spicy foods
Warm foods
Fasting

Better

Lying on the right side
Being around other people
Eating

Food and Drink

Desire for chocolate, ice cream, fish, and spicy foods
Very thirsty for cold and carbonated drinks

Phytolacca (Pokeroot)

Key Symptoms

Glandular swelling and inflammation, especially of breasts, tonsils, and parotid glands (mumps)

Throat pain radiating to the right ear on swallowing

Mind

Fear of death

Body

THROAT **Tonsils inflamed, swollen, painful, dark red**

Throat or tonsil pain worse on the right side

Throat pain made worse by warm drinks and better by cold drinks

Painful swelling of the cervical (neck) glands

CHEST **Breasts heavy, hard, swollen, and tender in mastitis**

Swollen lymph glands in the armpit

GENERAL **Swollen lymph nodes**

Faintness or weakness when standing up from a sitting or lying position

Worse

Exposure to cold, damp weather or a change of weather

Better

Dry weather

Lying on abdomen or left side

Rest

Podophyllum (May apple)

Key Symptoms

Traveler's diarrhea or dysentery

Explosive diarrhea with abdominal cramping, rumbling, and weakness

Diarrhea at 4:00 or 5:00 A.M.

Mind

Fear of becoming seriously ill or dying
Mental burnout from overwork

Body

STOMACH AND ABDOMEN **Early-morning urgent diarrhea, forcing the person out of bed**
Profuse, gurgling, rumbling, gushing, painless diarrhea
Sensation of hollowness and emptiness in the stomach
Liver problems; liver feels sore under right rib cage

Worse

Early morning
Hot weather

Better

Lying on abdomen
Rubbing the liver area

Pulsatilla (Windflower)

Key Symptoms

Temperament and symptoms change very quickly
Cries very easily
Easily overheated and uncomfortable in warm, stuffy rooms
Wants to be outside in the open air
Wants others around her, especially when she is sick

Mind

Child is weepy, whiny, and clingy, and wants to be carried and cuddled
Soft, affectionate, and wants attention
Indecisive
Highly emotional

Body

HEAD **Conjunctivitis with yellowish-green, goopy discharge from eyes**
Eyelids stick together on waking because of thick, gluey discharge

Abundant, thick mucus from nose in morning; nose stopped in evening
Dry mouth, but no thirst

CHEST **Dry cough in evening and at night, changing to loose cough in morning**
Needs to sit up in bed in order to get relief from the cough

STOMACH AND ABDOMEN Diarrhea in children

WOMEN **Irregular, clotted, changeable menstrual periods**
Symptoms may be worse during pregnancy or menopause, or before or during menstrual periods

Worse
Heat
Rich foods

Better
Open air
Slow walking in the open air
Cold applications, food, or drink

Food and Drink
Desire for rich and creamy foods such as peanut butter, butter, or ice cream
Aversion to fat, milk, and pork
Aggravation from pork and rich foods
Not thirsty

Rhus toxicodendron (Poison ivy)

Key Symptoms
Stiffness of the joints, relieved by moving around or hot baths
Sprains and strains with a lot of stiffness
Restlessness of the body, with a constant need to move around and find a comfortable position

MATERIA MEDICA

Mind

Busy, active, good-humored person who likes to make jokes
Tremendous apprehension at night forces him out of bed
Thinks someone wants to poison him

Body

EXTREMITIES **Injuries after overexertion**
Injuries to tendons and muscles
Bursitis, tendinitis
Cracking of the joints

SKIN **Fine, water-filled, crusty blisters**
Skin is dry, hot, burning, and very itchy
Shingles
Chicken pox

Worse

Getting cold or wet
Cloudy weather, change of weather, or before a thunderstorm

Better

Warmth

Food and Drink

Strong desire for cold milk

Rumex (Yellow dock)

Key Symptoms

Dry cough made worse by uncovering, undressing, or a change in temperature
Teasing cough that prevents sleep

Mind

Spirits are low
Serious
Indifferent to surroundings

Body

CHEST **Barking, suffocating cough**

Cough from a tickle, like a feather or dust, in the pit of the throat

Dry, tickling cough, preventing sleep

Cough made worse by cold air, talking, or breathing deeply

Continuous cough lessened by closing or covering the mouth

Large amounts of mucus in the trachea

Rawness under the clavicle

Worse

Lying in bed, as soon as the head touches the pillow

Uncovering

11:00 P.M.

Morning upon awakening

Inhaling cold air, or change of temperature

Touch or pressure on the throat

Talking

Better

Covering the mouth

Sucking on a lozenge (don't use mentholated lozenges)

Wrapping up

Ruta (Rue)

Key Symptoms

All parts of the body feel sore and bruised

Injuries to the tendons, cartilage, and periosteum (the outer layer of bones), especially the wrists and ankles

Bruises to the periosteum, such as the shin

Mind

Dissatisfied

Quarrelsome

Anxious from becoming overheated

Body

HEAD **Burning, red eyes and headache following eyestrain from close work or reading**

BACK Back pain relieved by pressure and by lying on the back

Spine and limbs feel bruised

EXTREMITIES **Sensation like a sprain and stiffness in the wrist**

Pain and stiffness in wrists and hands

Stiffness of muscles and tendons

Injured area feels bruised, sore, and achy, causing restlessness

Soreness of tendons

GENERAL **Easily fatigued, especially after overexertion**

Flu in which the whole body feels bruised

Worse

Overuse of the eyes

Cold, damp weather

Better

Lying on the back

Warmth

Motion

Sarsaparilla (Wild licorice)

Key Symptoms

Very common medicine for women with bladder infections

Bladder infection in which the main symptom is burning at the urethra (where the urine comes out) at the close of urination

Mind

Depression and anxiety from the pain

Body

BLADDER AND KIDNEY **Urine may be difficult to pass while sitting, only dribbling out**

In some cases, she can only urinate while standing
Considerable pain at the close of urination; almost unbearable
Constant desire to urinate, but little or nothing comes out
Gas released from the bladder during urination

Worse
Getting cold and wet
Night
Yawning
Motion

Better
Standing
Uncovering the neck and chest

Sepia (Cuttlefish ink)

Key Symptoms
Hormonal problems in women
Lack of sexual desire
Desire for vigorous exercise or dancing
Desire for vinegar, pickles, and other sour foods

Mind
Irritable, weepy
Indifferent or feels aversion toward her husband and family
Wants to be left alone
Depressed and crying

Body
HEAD Thick, greenish discharge from the nose
Mask of pregnancy across the nose and cheeks
STOMACH AND ABDOMEN **Morning sickness**
Constipation
BLADDER AND KIDNEYS Loss of urine from coughing or sneezing

WOMEN Yellowish-green or white, foul-smelling vaginal discharge
Lots of vaginal itching
Sensation that the pelvic organs are pulling or bearing downward
Falling out of the uterus or rectum

SKIN Ringworm in isolated spots, worse every spring

Worse
Vinegar
Pregnancy
Fasting or missing a meal
Cold
4:00 to 6:00 P.M.

Better
Vigorous exercise
Keeping busy
Warmth

Food and drink
Desire for vinegar
Desire for sour and sweet foods
Aversion to fat, salt

Silica (Flint)

Key Symptoms
Abscesses, cysts, or boils anywhere in the body
Bad-smelling or sour perspiration, especially from the feet
Problems of the nails or teeth
Swollen lymph glands, often filled with pus
Low stamina and energy
Refined temperament
Delicate features, like a porcelain doll

Mind
Shy
Proper, fastidious, timid

Body

HEAD **Dental abscesses**

Ear infections, especially chronic

Parotid gland swelling (mumps)

Blocked tear ducts in newborns

THROAT **Sore throat with splinter-like pain**

Tonsils swollen with pus

Hard, swollen glands

STOMACH AND ABDOMEN **Constipation with bashful stool** (starts to come out, then goes back in) and rabbit-pellet stools

EXTREMITIES Ingrown toenails

WOMEN **Abscess or cyst of the vulva or labia**

Acrid vaginal discharge, with itching of the vulva and vagina

Mastitis in nursing mothers

SKIN **Useful to expel splinters and other foreign bodies**

GENERAL **Low stamina**

Worse

Suppressed perspiration

After vaccinations

Cold weather and drafts

Better

Warmth

Food and Drink

Desire for eggs and sweets

Aversion to fat and milk

Spongia (Toasted sponge)

Key Symptoms

Dry, croupy, barking cough

Hollow cough, like a saw cutting through wood or a barking seal

Cough relieved by eating or drinking

Croupy cough wakes him

Dry cough made worse by talking or singing

Mind
Fear of suffocation

Body
THROAT **Hoarseness**
Constant clearing of throat
Larynx is dry, tight, and burning; all made worse by touching larynx, singing, talking, or swallowing
Feeling of a plug in the larynx, with anxious, gasping breathing

CHEST **Cough is made worse by inhaling and before midnight**
Cough is relieved by eating or drinking, especially warm drinks
Irrepressible cough comes from deep in the chest
Chest feels so weak that she can barely talk
Suffocating feeling
Breathing is short and difficult
Cough is quite dry
Air passages feel dry
Heart palpitations with bronchitis

Worse
Cold air
Hot room
Lying down
After midnight
Exertion

Better
Warm things
Lying with the head low
Going downward

Staphysagria (Stavesacre)

Key Symptoms
"Honeymoon cystitis," bladder infections after sex
Symptoms that come on after holding in anger or after being insulted or humiliated

Mind
Ailments
Mild personality
Wants to please
Blames herself
Trembling from anger

Body
HEAD Styes
Inflammation of eyelids
BLADDER AND KIDNEYS **Desire to urinate, but can't do so after sex with a new partner or during pregnancy**
Sensation as if a drop of urine were rolling along the urethra
Frequent need to urinate
Urge to urinate, but nothing comes out
Bladder does not feel empty, even right after urinating
Burning in urethra during urination or, especially, when not urinating

Worse
Too much sex
Masturbation

Better
Expressing emotions, especially anger
Warmth
Rest

Food and Drink
Desire for sweets and milk
Aversion to fat

Sulphur

Key Symptoms
Red, burning skin eruptions with lots of itching
Heartburn after overeating or eating wrong foods
Hungry at 11:00 A.M.
Sudden, explosive diarrhea makes him get out of bed in the morning (5:00 A.M.)

Mind

Critical
Opinionated
Thinking all the time; philosophical
Messy
Lazy

Body

HEAD Inflammation of eyelids with redness and burning

STOMACH AND ABDOMEN Sudden urge to go to the bathroom for diarrhea
Bad-smelling bowel movements
Stool is loose and burning
Rectal itching
Burning pain in the stomach and esophagus
Belching with a bad taste in the mouth

SKIN Itching made worse by heat, the heat of the bed, wool, and bathing

GENERAL Very smelly (like rotten eggs) diarrhea, gas, perspiration, and discharges
Excessive sweat, often bad-smelling

Worse

Heat
11:00 A.M.
Bathing

Better

Cool air

Food and Drink

Desire for sweets, spicy foods, fatty foods, and alcohol
Aversion to eggs, squash

Symphytum (Comfrey or knitbone)

Key Symptoms

Acute fractures and non-union of previous fractures
Injuries to cartilage or periosteum (covering of bones)

Specific medicine for blunt injuries to the eyes ("*Arnica* of the eye")
Black eye

Worse
Injuries

Tabacum (Tobacco)

Key Symptoms
Deathly nausea with violent vomiting, made worse by the least motion
Motion sickness, seasickness from the least motion
Cold, clammy, and pale with the nausea
Better in cold, fresh air
Spitting with the nausea

Mind
Wretched feeling

Body
STOMACH AND ABDOMEN Severe vomiting with lots of spitting
Incapacitating nausea
Nausea of pregnancy (morning sickness)
Nausea relieved by uncovering the abdomen
Nausea made worse by opening the eyes

Worse
Traveling in a car or on a boat
Heat
Opening the eyes

Better
Fresh air
Uncovering the abdomen

Urtica urens (Stinging nettle)

Key Symptoms

Stinging pain after burns or insect bites
Nettle rash
First- and second-degree burns or scalds, with intense burning and itching

Mind

Restless, nervous

Body

EXTREMITIES Joint pains alternating with nettle rash

MEN Herpes of the scrotum with heat and itching

WOMEN Herpes of the labia with heat and itching
Itching, stinging, and swelling of the vulva

SKIN **Hives or allergic reaction from shellfish**
Itchy, raised blotches
Hives after overheating or overexertion
Chicken pox

Worse

Cool, moist, or snowy air
Cool bathing

Veratrum album (White hellebore)

Key Symptoms

Severe abdominal cramping with diarrhea and profuse sweating
Violent vomiting and diarrhea

Mind

Extremely restless and busy

Body

STOMACH AND ABDOMEN **Abdominal cramping with chills, vomiting, diarrhea, and cold sweats**

Stomach flu with diarrhea and vomiting at the same time

Diarrhea profuse and rapidly exhausting

Diarrhea from drinking cold water on hot days

Vomit shoots out violently from the mouth

Wants ice water, then vomits as soon as it is swallowed

WOMEN **Violent menstrual cramps with diarrhea, chills, vomiting, and fainting**

GENERAL **Icy cold with cold sweat**

Collapse with a bluish color

Worse

Cold

Cold drinks

Fruit

Exertion

Better

Warmth

Hot drinks

Covering up

Food and Drink

Desire for very cold drinks, ice, juicy fruits, lemons, pickles, sour foods, and salty foods

Answers to the Practice Cases

1. *Ledum*
2. *Urtica urens* (second choice is *Cantharis*)
3. *Bryonia*
4. *Hepar sulphuris*
5. *Staphysagria*
6. *Chamomilla*
7. *Belladonna*
8. *Podophyllum*
9. *Lycopodium*
10. *Causticum*
11. *Kali bichromicum*
12. *Arnica*
13. *Glonoine, Belladonna*
14. *China*
15. *Allium cepa*

Glossary

acute illness condition that is self-limiting and short-lived, generally only lasting a few days to a couple of months.

aggravation temporary worsening of already existing symptoms after taking a homeopathic medicine.

allopathic medicine treatment of disease through the use of drugs that produce opposite effects; conventional medicine.

antidote a substance or influence that interferes with homeopathic treatment.

casetaking the process of the in-depth homeopathic interview.

centesimal a type of preparation of homeopathic medicines that is based on serial dilutions of 1 to 99, designated by the letter "C".

chief complaint the main problem that causes a patient to visit a healthcare practitioner.

classical homeopathy a method of homeopathic prescribing in which only one medicine, based on the totality of the patient's symptoms, is given at a time, followed by a period of waiting to evaluate the action of the medicine.

combination medicine a mixture containing more than one homeopathic medicine.

common symptoms those signs and symptoms that are common to any person carrying a particular diagnosis.

constitutional treatment homeopathic treatment based on the whole person, involving an extensive interview and careful follow-up.

decimal a type of preparation of homeopathic medicines that is based on serial dilutions of 1 to 9, designated by the letter "X".

defense mechanism that aspect of the vital force whose purpose is to maintain health and defend the body against disease.

general symptoms those symptoms pertaining to the body as a whole.

high-potency remedies remedies of a 200C potency or higher.

homeopathic medicine a medicine that acts according to the principles of homeopathy.

homeopathy the treatment of an illness by giving minute quantities of a substance as a medicine that in a healthy person would cause the same symptoms.

indication a symptom that leads one to prescribe a certain homeopathic medicine.

law of similars the concept that like cures like.

low-potency remedies remedies of a 30C potency or lower.

materia medica a book that includes individual homeopathic remedies and their indications.

medicine another name for a homeopathic medicine.

minimal dose the smallest quantity of a medicine that produces a change in the patient.

modality those factors that make a particular symptom better or worse.

mother tincture the initial, standardized alcohol preparation from which homeopathic dilutions are subsequently made.

particular symptoms those symptoms pertaining to an individual part of the body.

polychrests the fifty or so most commonly used homeopathic medicines.

potency the specific strength of a homeopathic medicine, determined by the number of serial dilutions and succussions.

potentization the preparation of a homeopathic medicine through the process of serial dilution and succussion.

prover a participant in a systematic experiment of taking a particular medicine for the purpose of eliciting symptoms.

proving an experiment in which a substance or medicine is taken repeatedly and the effects carefully documented.

relapse the return of symptoms when a homeopathic medicine is no longer acting.

repertory a book that lists symptoms and the medicines known to have produced such symptoms in healthy provers.

simillimum the one medicine that most nearly responds to the totality of the symptoms of the patient and that will produce the greatest relief.

single medicine one single homeopathic medicine given at a time.

succussion the systematic and repeated shaking of a homeopathic medicine after each serial dilution.

suppression the elimination of a particular symptom without the strengthening of the vital force; sometimes even weakens the vital force.

symptom picture all of the symptoms that describe the person's illness, or the symptoms that are characteristic of a homeopathic medicine.

totality of symptoms a comprehensive picture of the whole person: physical, mental, and emotional.

underlining a method of emphasizing symptoms in the case record.

vital force the invisible energy present in all living things that creates harmony, balance, and health.

vitalism the philosophy that views each living organism as being imbued with an all-pervading life energy.

Bibliography

Allen, T.F. *Allen's Encyclopedia*. New Delhi: B. Jain, 1986.

Berkow, Robert, ed. *The Merck Manual*. Rahway, NJ: Merck and Co., Inc, 1995.

Boericke, William. *Pocket Manual of Materia Medica with Repertory*. New Delhi: B. Jain, 1982.

Bruning, Nancy and Corey Weinstein. *Healing Homeopathic Remedies*. New York: Dell, 1996.

Castro, Miranda. *The Complete Homeopathy Handbook*. New York: St. Martin's, 1990.

Clarke, John Henry. *Dictionary of Practical Materia Medica*. New Delhi: B. Jain, 1985.

Cummings, Stephen and Dana Ullman. *Everybody's Guide to Homeopathic Medicines*. New York: J.P. Tarcher/Putnam, 1991.

Hammond, Christopher. *How to Use Homeopathy*. Rockport, ME: Element, 1991.

Hayfield, Robin. *The Family Homeopath*. Rochester, NY: Healing Arts Press, 1994.

Hering, Constantine. *Guiding Symptoms*. New Delhi: B. Jain, 1989.

Idarius, Betty. *The Homeopathic Childbirth Manual*. Ukiah, CA: Idarius Press, 1996.

Jonas, Wayne and Jennifer Jacobs. *Healing with Homeopathy*. New York: Warner, 1996.

Kent, James Tyler. *Lectures of Homeopathic Materia Medica with New Remedies*. New Delhi, Jain, 1982.

Kruzel, Thomas. *The Homeopathic Emergency Guide*. Berkeley: North Atlantic, 1992.

Lockie, Andrew and Nicola Geddes. *Homeopathy: The Principles and Practice of Treatment.* New York: Dorling Kindersley, 1995.

Morrison, Roger. *Desktop Guide to Keynotes and Confirmatory Symptoms.* Albany: Hahnemann Clinic Publishing, 1993.

Murphy, Robin. *Lotus Materia Medica.* Pagosa Springs: Lotus Star Academy, 1995.

Phatak, S.R. *Materia Medica of Homeopathic Medicines.* New Delhi: Indian Books and Periodicals Syndicate, 1977.

Reichenberg-Ullman, Judyth and Robert Ullman. *Ritalin-Free Kids.* Rocklin, CA: Prima, 1996.

Rose, Barry. *The Family Health Guide to Homeopathy.* Berkeley: Celestial Arts, 1992.

Ullman, Dana. *The Consumer's Guide to Homeopathy.* New York: J.P. Tarcher/Putnam, 1995.

Vermeulen, Frans. *Synoptic Materia Medica I.* Haarlem: Merlijn Publishers, 1992.

Ullman, Robert and Judyth Reichenberg-Ullman. *The Patient's Guide to Homeopathic Medicine.* Edmonds, WA: Picnic Point Press, 1995.

Index

B

W

Y

Z